TEXTBOOK OF
MEDICINAL CHEMISTRY

Volume II

TEXTBOOK OF MEDICINAL CHEMISTRY

Volume II

V. Alagarsamy
M Pharm, PhD, FIC, DOMH
Professor and Principal
MNR College of Pharmacy, Sangareddy
Gr. Hyderabad

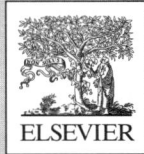

ELSEVIER
A division of
Reed Elsevier India Private Limited

Textbook of Medicinal Chemistry, Volume II
Alagarsamy

ELSEVIER
A division of
Reed Elsevier India Private Limited

Mosby, Saunders, Churchill Livingstone, Butterworth Heinemann and Hanley & Belfus are the Health Science imprints of Elsevier.

© 2010 Elsevier
Reprinted - 2010

All rights reserved. No part of this publication may be reproduced or transmitted in any form or by any means, electronic or mechanical including photocopying, recording, or any information storage and retrieval system without the prior written permission from the publisher and the copyright holder.

ISBN: 978-81-312-2190-7

Medical knowledge is constantly changing. As new information becomes available, changes in treatment, procedures, equipment and the use of drugs become necessary. The authors, editors, contributors and the publisher have, as far as it is possible, taken care to ensure that the information given in this text is accurate and up-to-date. However, readers are strongly advised to confirm that the information, especially with regard to drug dose/usage, complies with current legislation and standards of practice. ***Please consult full prescribing information before issuing prescriptions for any product mentioned in the publication.***

Published by Elsevier, a division of Reed Elsevier India Private Limited

Registered Office: Gate No. 3, Building No. A-1, 2 Industrial Area, Kalkaji, New Delhi-110019
Corporate Office: 14th Floor, Building No. 10B, DLF Cyber City, Phase II, Gurgaon-122002, Haryana, India

Commissioning Editor: Nimisha Goswami
Development Editor: Subodh K. Chauhan
Manager Publishing Operations: Sunil Kumar
Manager Production: N.C. Pant

Typeset by Televijay Technologies (P) Ltd., Chennai.

Printed and bound at Rajkamal Electric Press, Kundli, Haryana.

Preface

Medicinal chemistry emerged as a specialized area due to the development in chemistry and biology, hence it is considered as a highly interdisciplinary science combining a wide variety of subjects such as organic chemistry, pharmacology, biochemistry, toxicology, pharmacognosy, molecular biology, genomics, proteomics, computational chemistry, physical chemistry and statistics. Now, the growth of medicinal chemistry has reached a stage where the activity-guided synthesis of compounds is possible rather than screening of synthesized compounds for different biological activities. This field also penetrates into the areas of gene therapy and biochemistry-based virtual drug receptors with the help of computer-aided molecular modelling techniques.

This book is an upshot of my vision to discover the best book on medicinal chemistry, which deals about the concise description of diseases, clear classification of drugs with their chemical structures, synthesis of each drug with different routes, mode of action, metabolism, physical and pharmacological properties along with their therapeutic uses, assay technique, dose, official dosage forms and summary of structure–activity relationship (SAR) studies. Swathing the entire features of medicinal chemistry, first of its kind, is the unique feature of this book. It facilitates the students to understand the subject more easily and interestingly.

While writing this book, I felt that the book will bring about a re-orientation in the teaching and learning process of medicinal chemistry. Academic community in India is faced with scarcity of books to cater to their needs. Numerous foreign writers' books deal well about basics and pharmacological aspects related to medicinal chemistry, but lack two major requirements, i.e. synthesis and clear classification of drugs used. Some Indian authors filled this lacuna to a certain extent by including the synthesis, but failed to give a clear classification of drugs with their chemical structure. For this, the content of this book has been carefully tailored to cater the needs of the academicians belonging to all Indian universities, pharmacologists, clinical and industrial pharmacists by incorporating the missing links between general synthetic organic chemistry and medicinal chemistry.

This *Textbook of Medicinal Chemistry* is presented in two volumes. Volume II consists of six sections. The first section is devoted to drugs acting on inflammation and allergy. Sections II to V deal about the drugs acting on different systems of human body such as respiratory system, digestive system, blood and endocrines. Section VI is dedicated to chemotherapy, where detailed discussion from the history of development of antibiotics to the recent drugs approved for HIV infection is provided. In all these sections, chemical, pharmacological, biochemical and toxicological aspects of organic medicinal compounds are described elaborately.

We hope that this special volume will be a good source of information and reference for not only graduate and postgraduate students but also basic and applied researchers in this field. Moreover, it will also be of interest to a wide range of scientists, including organic chemists, biochemists, pharmacologists and clinicians, who are interested in drug research. I welcome suggestions and constructive criticism from all corners of scientific community.

V. Alagarsamy

Acknowledgements

I wish to place on record my heartfelt thanks to everyone who have made this book possible, especially my beloved teachers from first standard to doctoral programme guides, Dr Rajani Giridhar and Dr M.R. Yadav.

I am immensely grateful to Dr B. Suresh and Dr R.K. Goyal for inspiring and initiating me to write the book.

I am grateful to Shri M.N. Raju, Chairman, and Mr Ravi Varma, Director, MNR Educational Trust, Hyderabad, for providing constant encouragement and moral support to achieve this goal.

I express my sincere appreciation to my students, Dr V. Raja Solomon (postdoctoral researcher, Laurentian University, Canada), Mr J.C. Hanish Singh, Mr P. Parthiban, Mr S. Thiru Senthil Murugan and Ms J. Rajeshwari, for helping me author this book. I also thank my colleagues, especially, Mr S. Satheesh Kumar, Mr B. Subba Rao, Mr R. Chandrasekar and Mr M. Shahul Hameedh, for their untiring support in making this book.

The friendly interaction I had experienced with the Elsevier team, Ms Ritu Sharma, Ms Nimisha Goswami, Mr Subodh K. Chauhan, and Televijay Technologies Project Manager Ms Usha K. Nair, offered a plenty of energy to eliminate the fatigue during the preparation of this book. If the author gets such a cooperative and energetic publication team, publishing any number of books will not be a difficult task. I thank them wholeheartedly for helping me reach this target and am requesting them to continue their service to the author community in the same intensity.

The stimulation I got from my father, mother, sister, brothers and wife to reach this target is more than analeptics, and the patience and cooperation extended by my children, Aish and Abhi, made me think of the goal without any diversion. To express my thankfulness, I pray The Almighty to bless my children with teachers like those I got in my life so that they too are inspired by their teachers and dedicate to the field of medicinal chemistry and, in turn, serve for the suffering humanity.

V. Alagarsamy

Contents

Preface			v
Acknowledgements			vii
SECTION I		**Drugs Acting on Inflammation/Allergy**	**1**
Chapter 1		**Antihistamines**	**3**

• Structure–Activity Relationship—H_1 Receptor Antagonists • Classification • Synthesis and Drug Profile

Chapter 2   **Prostaglandins**   **46**

• Functions of PGs • Biosynthesis • Synthesis and Drug Profile

Chapter 3   **Analgesics, Antipyretics, and NSAIDs**   **56**

• Classification • SAR of Salicylates; Synthesis and Drug Profile; SAR of p-Amino Phenol Derivatives; SAR of 3,5-Pyrazolidine Diones; SAR of Anthranilic Acid Derivatives; SAR of Aryl Alkanoic Acid Derivatives; SAR of Indole Acetic Acid Derivatives; SAR of Oxicams

SECTION II		**Drugs Acting on Respiratory System**	**107**
Chapter 1		**Expectorants and Antitussives**	**109**

• Introduction to Respiratory System • Expectorants and Antitussives • Classification • Synthesis and Drug Profile

Section III		**Drugs Acting on Digestive System**	**119**
Chapter 1		**Antiulcer Agents**	**121**

• Classification • Synthesis and Drug Profile • SAR of H_2-Receptor Antagonists

Chapter 2		**Antidiarrhoeals**	**137**

- Synthesis and Drug Profile

SECTION IV — Drugs Acting on Blood and Blood-Forming Organs — 143

Chapter 1 Coagulants 145

- Classification • Anticoagulants; Classification; Synthesis and Drug Profile

Chapter 2 Plasma Expanders 160

SECTION V — Drugs Acting on Endocrine System — 163

Chapter 1 Oral Hypogylcaemic Drugs 165

- Classification • Synthesis and Drug Profile • SAR of Sulphonyl Ureas

Chapter 2 Steroids 192

- Steroid Nomenclature and Structure • Progestogens • Oestrogens • Androgens and Anabolic Agents

Chapter 3 Antithyroid Drugs 215

- Classification • Synthesis and Drug Profile

SECTION VI — Chemotherapy — 221

Chapter 1 History and Development of Chemotherapy 223

- Historical Background • Spectrum of Activity of Chemotherapeutic Agents

Chapter 2 Antibacterial Sulphonamides 229

- SAR of Sulphonamides • Classification • Synthesis and Drug Profile

Chapter 3 Quinolone Antibacterials 254

- Effective Antibacterial Quinolone Derivatives • Synthesis and Drug Profile • SAR of Quinolones

| Chapter 4 | **Antibiotics** | **265** |

• Classification • Penicillins; Cephalosporins; Amino Glycoside Antibiotics; Tetracyclins; Polypeptide Antibiotics; Macrolide Antibiotics; Lincomycins; Other Antibiotics

| Chapter 5 | **Antitubercular Agents** | **331** |

• Synthesis and Drug Profile

| Chapter 6 | **Antifungal Agents** | **344** |

• Classification • Synthesis and Drug Profile

| Chapter 7 | **Antiviral Agents** | **364** |

• Introduction • Classification • Synthesis and Drug Profile • SAR of Amantadine Analogues

| Chapter 8 | **Antiamoebic Agents** | **401** |

• Classification of Amoebicides • Synthesis and Drug Profile

| Chapter 9 | **Antimalarials** | **409** |

• Life Cycle of Plasmodium • Classification • Synthesis and Drug Profile • Structure–Activity Relationship

| Chapter 10 | **Anthelmintics** | **435** |

• Classification • Synthesis and Drug Profile

| Chapter 11 | **Antineoplastic Agents** | **455** |

• Classification • Synthesis and Drug Profile

| Chapter 12 | **Antileprotic Drugs** | **511** |

• Classification • Synthesis and Drug Profile

Contents of Medicinal Chemistry, Volume I

SECTION I	Physicochemical Factors in Relation to Biological Activity of Drugs	9
Chapter 1	**Physicochemical Properties**	11
Chapter 2	**Ferguson Principle**	13
Chapter 3	**Hydrogen Bonding**	15
Chapter 4	**Ionization and pKa Value**	19
Chapter 5	**Redox Potential**	22
Chapter 6	**Surface Tension**	25
Chapter 7	**Complexation**	27
Chapter 8	**Steric Features of Drugs**	30
Chapter 9	**Bioisosterism**	36
SECTION II	Drug Design	41
Chapter 1	**Concepts of Drug Design**	43
	• Design of Analogues and Pro-drugs • Design of Lead and Lead Discovery • Rational Approach to Drug Design	
Chapter 2	**Receptors**	49
	• Types of Receptors • Theories of Receptors • Forces Involved in Drug Receptors Interaction • Factors Affecting the Drug-Receptors Interaction	
Chapter 3	**Computer-Aided Drug Design**	54
	• Bioinformatics Hub	

Chapter 4	**Structure–Activity Relationship and Quantitative Structure–Activity Relationship**	56
	• Historical Development of QSAR • Basic Requirements for QSAR Analysis • Model Development Procedures	
Chapter 5	**Combinatorial Chemistry**	66
	• Combinatorial Compound Libraries	
Chapter 6	**Pro-Drugs**	71
	• Classification of Pro-drugs • Application of Pro-drugs	

SECTION III	Drugs Acting on Central Nervous System	83
Chapter 1	**Central Nervous System**	85
Chapter 2	**Sedatives and Hypnotics**	88
	• Molecular Basis of Inhibitory Neurotransmitters • Classification • Synthesis and Drug Profile • SAR of Barbiturates; SAR of Benzodiazepines	
Chapter 3	**General Anaesthetics**	130
	• Stages of Anaesthesia • Classification • Synthesis and Drug Profile	
Chapter 4	**Local Anaesthetics**	150
	• Classification • Synthesis and Drug Profile • SAR of Benzoic Acid Derivatives • SAR of Anilides	
Chapter 5	**Tranquillizers**	178
	• General Mode of Action • Classification • Synthesis and Drug Profile • SAR of Phenothiazines; SAR of Butyrophenones	
Chapter 6	**Antidepressants**	204
	• Classification • Synthesis and Drug Profile • SAR of Dibenzazepines; SAR of Dibenzocylcoheptane Derivatives	
Chapter 7	**CNS Stimulants**	229
	• Classification • Synthesis and Drug Profile	

Chapter 8	**Narcotic Analgesics**		**247**

• Synthesis and Drug Profile
• SAR of Morphine Derivatives; SAR of Meperidine Analogues; SAR of Methadone Derivatives; SAR of Benzomorphan Derivatives • Narcotic Antagonists • Classification
• Synthesis and Drug Profile

Chapter 9	**Anticonvulsants**		**286**

• Classification • Synthesis and Drug Profile
• SAR of Hydantoins; SAR of Oxazolidine Diones; SAR of Phenacemide Analogues

Chapter 10	**Anti Prakinsonism Agents**		**317**

• Classification • Synthesis and Drug Profile

Chapter 11	**Skeletal Muscle Relaxants**		**329**

• Classification • Synthesis and Drug Profile

Chapter 12	**Alzheimer's Disease**		**344**

• Pathogenesis; Treatment

SECTION IV	**Drugs Acting on Autonomic Nervous System**		**349**
Chapter 1	**Autonomic Nervous System**		**351**
Chapter 2	**Adrenergic Drugs**		**356**

• Physiological Basis of Adrenergic Receptors Function • General Classification of Adrenergic Agonists
• Synthesis and Drug Profile • Structural–Activity Relationship

Chapter 3	**Cholinergic Drugs**		**378**

• Spectrum of Cholinomimetic Drugs
• Classification • Synthesis and Drug Profile • Structure–Activity Relationship

Chapter 4	**Andrenergic Blockers**		**398**

• Physiological Basis of Adrenergic Receptor Antagonists • Classification • Synthesis and Drug Profile
• Structure–Activity Relationship

| Chapter 5 | **Anticholinergic Drugs** | **419** |

• Difference Between the Quaternary and the Tertiary Antimuscarinics • Classification • Synthesis and Drug Profile • SAR of Atropine Analogues; SAR of Muscarinic Antagonists

| SECTION V | Drugs Acting on Cardiovascular System | 445 |

| Chapter 1 | **Cardiovascular System** | **447** |
| Chapter 2 | **Antihypertensive Drugs** | **449** |

• Classification • Synthesis and Drug Profile

| Chapter 3 | **Antiarrhythmic Drugs** | **476** |

• Classification • Synthesis and Drug Profile

| Chapter 4 | **Antihyperlipidaemic Agents** | **499** |

• Classification • Synthesis and Drug Profile

| Chapter 5 | **Antianginals** | **520** |

• Principles of Therapy for Angina
• Classification • Synthesis and Drug Profile • SAR of Dihydropyridine Derivatives

| SECTION VI | Drugs Acting on Urinary System | 547 |

| Chapter 1 | **Urinary System** | **549** |
| Chapter 2 | **Diuretics** | **551** |

• Classification • Synthesis and Drug Profile; SAR of Thiazide Derivatives; SAR Carbonic Anhydrase Inhibitors; SAR of Loop Diuretics

SECTION I

DRUGS ACTING ON INFLAMMATION/ALLERGY

1	Antihistamines	03
2	Prostaglandins	46
3	Analgesics Antipyretics and NSAIDs	56

Chapter 1

Antihistamines

INTRODUCTION

Histamine, [2-(imidazol-4-yl) ethylamine], which is biosynthesized by decarboxylation of the basic amino acid histidine, is found in all organs and tissues of the human body.

$$\text{Histidine} \xrightarrow[-CO_2]{\text{Histidine decarboxylase}} \text{Histamine}$$

The histamine is stored in the secretory granules of mast cells (pH 5.5) as positively charged and ionically complexed with negatively charged acidic group on other secretory granules, which constitutes heparin. The principal target cells of immediate hypersensitivity reactions are mast cells and basophils to generate IgE antibodies that binds to FC€ receptor on the granule surface. This leads to transmembrane activation of tyrosine protein kinase, which phosphorylates and activates the phospolipase. The phosphotidyl inositol biphosphate is converted into inositol triphosphate, which triggers the intracellular release of calcium ion. The calcium ion causes exocytic release of histamine with the transfer of Na^+ ion from extracellular space. The released histamine targets the histaminergic receptors (H_1, H_2, and H_3) to elicit the actions.

Histamine is an important chemical messenger, communicating information from one cell to another, and is involved in a variety of complex biological actions. It is mainly stored in an inactive bound form, from which it is released as a result of an antigen–antibody reaction, initiated by different stimuli, such as venoms, toxins, proteolytic enzyme, detergents, food materials, and numerous chemicals. Systemically, histamine contracts smooth muscles of the lungs and the gastrointestinal system and cause vasodialation, low blood pressure, and increases the heart rate. It also causes symptoms such as itching, sneezing, watery eye, and running nose.

4   Drugs Acting on Inflammation/Allergy

Histamine exerts its biological function by interacting with at least three distinctly specific receptors H_1, H_2, and H_3. Historically, the term antihistamine has been used to describe a drug that acts on H_1 and H_2 receptors. An antihistaminic agent should ideally prevent the production or release of these autocoids by inhibiting the response of sensitized mast cells and basophils to specific antigens.

1. Antihistamines are drugs that competitively blocks the H_1 receptors.
2. Antihistamines antagonize the stimulant action of histamine on the smooth muscles of gastro intestinal tract (GIT), uterus, and blood vessels, and inhibit histamine augmented salivary secretion.
3. H_1-receptor antagonists have been used clinically to treat various allergic disorders, such as seasonal or perennial allergic rhinitis and chronic urticaria.

Release and Function of Endogenous Histamine

Histamine is released because of the interaction of an antigen with IgE antibodies on the mast cell surface and plays a central role in immediate hypersensitive reactions (Fig. 1.1).

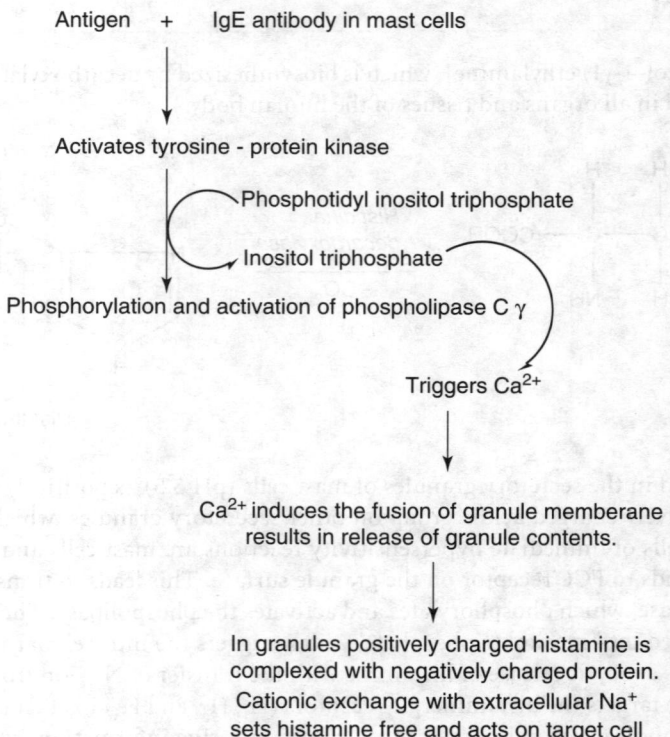

Figure 1.1 Steps involved in the release of histamine.

The release of histamine, in addition to the stimulation of IgE receptors, also activates the phospholipase A_2, leading to the production of host mediators, including platelet activating factors and metabolites of arachidonic acid. Leukotriene D_4 is also generated, which is a potent constrictor of smooth muscles. This mediates the constriction of bronchi.

Histamine and Gastric Acid Secretion

Histamine is a powerful gastric acid secretagogue and evokes a copious secretion of acid from the parietal cells by acting on the H_2 receptors. The output of pepsin and intrinsic factors are also increased. However, the secretion of acid is evoked by the stimulation of vagus nerve and by the enteric hormone gastrin. The mechanism operating at the gastric parietal cells is through $H^+ K^+$ ATPase (proton pump), which secretes H^+ ions in the apical canaliculi of parietal cells and also which can be activated by histamine (Fig. 1.2).

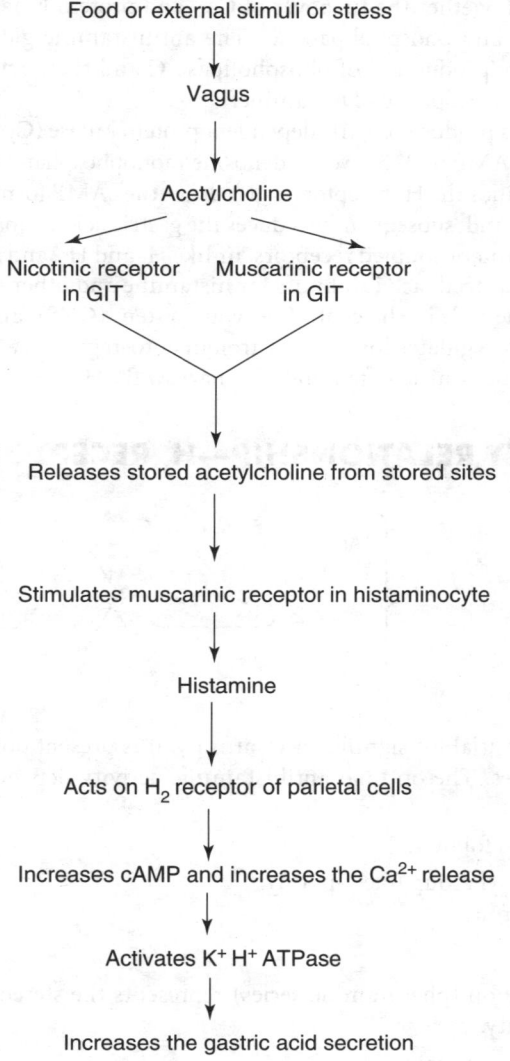

Figure 1.2 Histamine induced gastric acid secretion.

The therapeutically available antagonists of histamine receptors are used as antiallergic drugs by targeting H_1 receptors and as antiulcers by targeting H_2 receptors.

6 Drugs Acting on Inflammation/Allergy

Mode of Action of Antihistamines

After the release of histamine by the mast cells, it binds with histaminergic receptors (H_1, H_2, and H_3) to elicit a series of events that mediates the characteristic responses through second messenger systems. The histaminergic receptors are G-protein coupled type. H_1 receptors are coupled to phospholipase-C and their activation leads to the formation of inositol phosphate (Ip_3) and diacylglycerol (DAG), respectively, from phospholipids in cell membrane. Ip_3 causes rapid release of Ca^{2+} from endoplasmic reticulum. DAG activates the protein kinase C. Altogether the turnover of Ca^{2+} and protein kinase-C activates Ca^{2+}/calmodulin dependent protein kinase and phospholipase A_2. The antihistaminergic (H_1-antagonist) binds to the H_1 receptors and decreases the production of phospholipase-C and their activation to form IP_3 and DAG thereby blocks the characteristic response of histamine.

Histamine on H_2 receptors produces cAMP-dependent protein kinase (Cyclic adenosine monophosphate (cAMP), also known as cyclic AMP or 3′-5′-cyclic adenosine monophosphate) to elicit a response in the GIT. The H_2 antagonist reversibly binds the H_2 receptors and reduces the cAMP formation, which is responsible for the activation of proton pump and, subsequently, reduces the gastric acid formation in the GIT.

H_3 receptors are also G-protein coupled receptors, unlike H_1 and H_2, and they produce a decreased Ca^{2+} influx. H_3 receptors function as feedback inhibitors for histamine and other neurotransmitters by decreasing the calcium influx into the cells in the central nervous system (CNS), and in the GIT, they reduce the secretion of gastrin and down-regulates histamine through auto-regulatory effects. Blocking H_3 receptors antagonize these effects, but the clinical extendibility is narrow for H_3.

STRUCTURE ACTIVITY RELATIONSHIP—H_1 RECEPTOR ANTAGONISTS

$$1 \begin{cases} Ar^1 \\ \diagdown \\ \underset{2}{X}-\underset{\underbrace{}_{3}}{C-C}-\underset{4}{N} \\ \diagup \\ Ar \end{cases}$$

1. Aryl groups

The diaryl substitution is essential for significant H_1 affinity. It is present both in first generation and second generation antihistamines. The optimal antihistaminic activity depends on the co-planarity of two aryl substitutions.

Active aryl substitutions are as follows:

- Ar is phenyl and hetero aryl group like 2-pyridyl
- Ar^1-Aryl or aryl methyl group

2. Nature of X

Antihistamines with X = carbon (pheniramine series) represents the stereo selective receptor binding to the receptors due to its chirality.

The active substitutions of X are as follows:

- Where X = oxygen (amino alkyl ether analogue)
- X = nitrogen (ethylene-diamine derivative)
- X = carbon (mono amino propyl analogue)

2. The Alkyl Chain

Most of the antihistamines have ethylene chain, and branching of this chain results in a less active compound.

$$-C-C-N\begin{subarray}{l}R^1\\R\end{subarray}$$

All antihistamines contain this general chain.

3. Terminal nitrogen atom:
The terminal N-atom should be a 3° amine for maximum activity. The terminal nitrogen may be a part of heterocyclic ring. For example, antazoline and chlorcyclizine, retains high antihistaminic activity. The amino moiety deserves the protonation on interaction with H_1 recptor due to the basicity with pka 8.5-10.

Chlorcyclizine

CLASSIFICATION

I. H_1-Antagonists with classical structures
According to the chemical features, they are further classified as follows:

a. Ethylene diamine derivatives
b. Amino alkyl ether analogues
c. Cyclic basic chain analogues
d. Mono amino propyl analogues
e. Tricyclic ring system or Phenothiazine derivaties
f. Dibenzocyclo heptenes
g. Miscellaneous agents
h. Newer agents

a. Ethylene diamine derivatives

8 Drugs Acting on Inflammation/Allergy

Name	Ar¹	Ar²
Tripelennamine	2-pyridyl	$-H_2C-C_6H_5$
Pyrilamine	2-pyridyl	$-H_2C-C_6H_4-OCH_3$ (para)
Methapyrilene	2-pyridyl	$-H_2C-(2\text{-thienyl})$
Thonzylamine	2-pyrimidyl	$-H_2C-C_6H_4-OCH_3$ (para)
Zolamine	2-thiazolyl	$-H_2C-C_6H_4-OCH_3$ (para)

b. Amino alkyl ethers

$$Ar^1\text{-}\underset{Ar^2}{\overset{R}{C}}\text{-}O\text{-}CH_2\text{-}CH_2\text{-}N(CH_3)_2$$

Name	Ar¹	Ar²	R
Diphenhydramine	$-C_6H_5$	$-C_6H_5$	$-H$
Bromodiphenhydramine	$-C_6H_5$	$-C_6H_4-Br$ (para)	$-H$
Doxylamine	$-C_6H_5$	2-pyridyl	$-CH_3$

(Continued)

(*Continued*)

Name	Ar¹	Ar²	R
Carbinoxamine	4-Cl-phenyl	2-pyridyl	–H
Medrylamine	4-H₃CO-phenyl	phenyl	–H

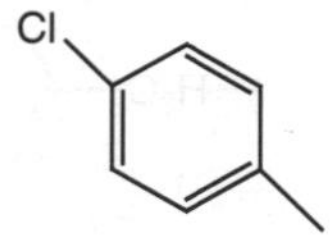

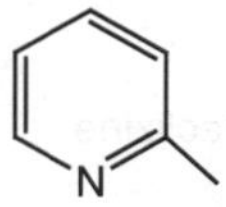

Name	Structure
Clemastine	4-Cl-C₆H₄–C(CH₃)(C₆H₅)–O–CH₂CH₂–(2-(1-methylpyrrolidinyl))
Diphenylpyraline	(C₆H₅)₂CH–O–(4-(1-methylpiperidinyl))

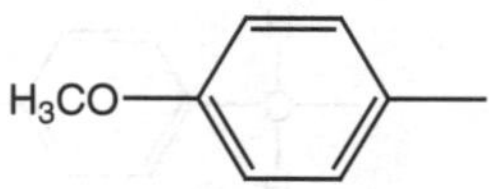

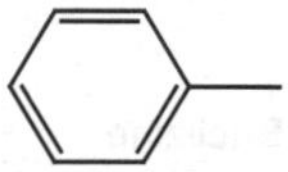

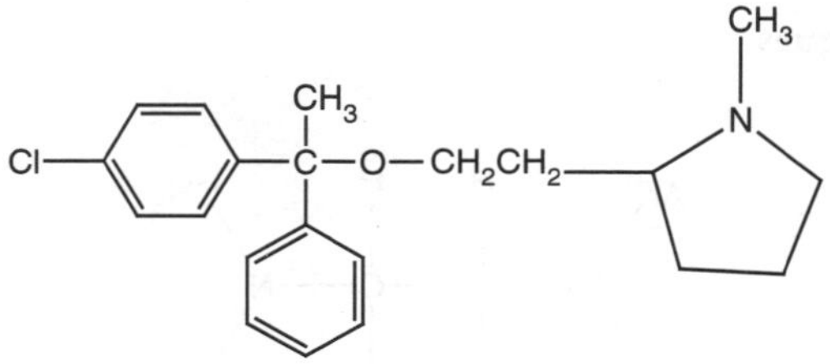

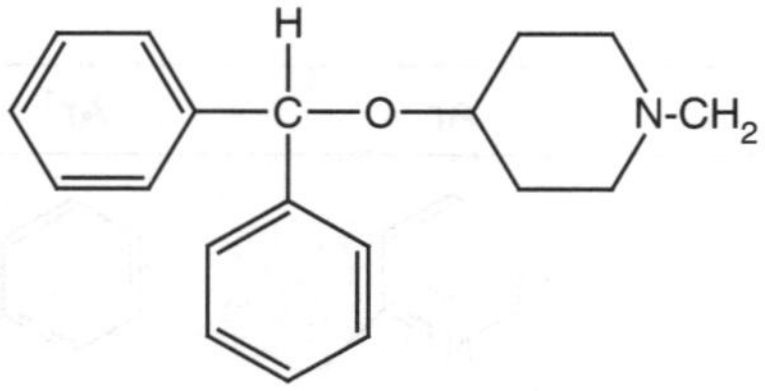

c. Cyclic basic chain analogues or piperazine derivatives

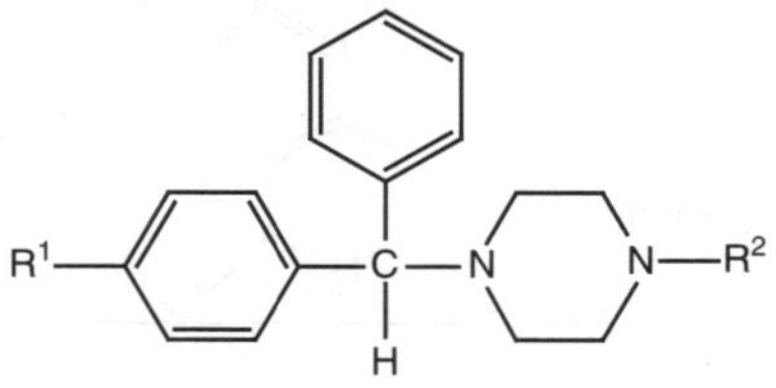

R¹–C₆H₄–CH(C₆H₅)–N(piperazine)–R²

Name	R¹	R²
Cyclizine	–H	–CH₃
Chlorcyclizine	–Cl	–CH₃

(*Continued*)

(Continued)

Name	R¹	R²
Meclizine	–Cl	–H₂C–(3-methylphenyl) (–CH₂–C₆H₄–CH₃, meta)
Buclizine	–Cl	–CH₂–(4-tert-butylphenyl)

d. Mono amino propyl analogues
i. Saturated analogues

General structure: Ar(Ar¹)CH–CH₂–CH₂–N(CH₃)₂

Name	Ar	Ar¹
Pheniramine	2-pyridyl	phenyl
Chlorpheniramine	2-pyridyl	4-chlorophenyl
Bromopheniramine	2-pyridyl	4-bromophenyl

ii. Unsaturated analogues

General structure: Ar(Ar¹)C=CH–CH₂–N(pyrrolidine)

Name	Ar	Ar¹
Pyrrobutamine	4-chlorobenzyl (4-Cl-C₆H₄–CH₂–)	phenyl
Triprolidine	4-methylphenyl (H₃C–C₆H₄–)	2-pyridyl

e. Tricyclic ring systems or phenothiazine derivatives

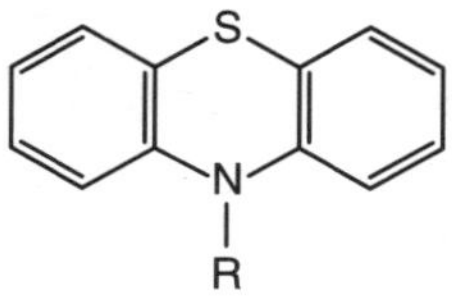

Name	R
Promethazine hydrochloride	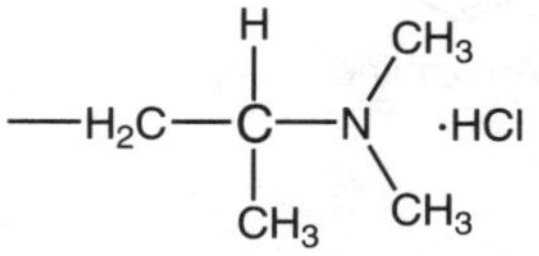 —H₂C—CH(CH₃)—N(CH₃)₂ · HCl
Trimeprazine	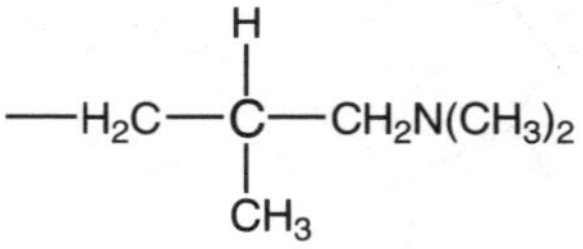 —H₂C—CH(CH₃)—CH₂N(CH₃)₂
Methdilazine	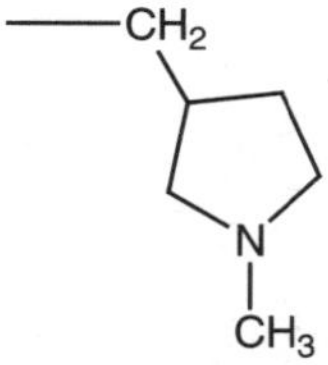 —CH₂—(1-methylpyrrolidin-3-yl)

f. Dibenzocyclo heptenes

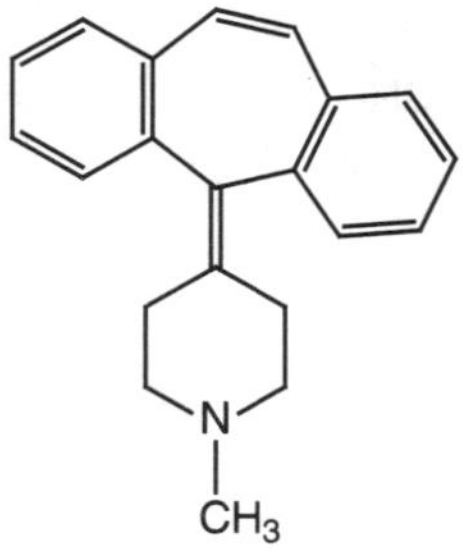

Cyproheptadine (periactin)

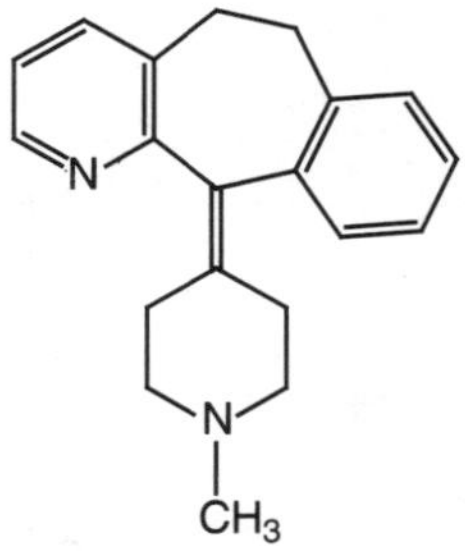

Azatadine

12 Drugs Acting on Inflammation/Allergy

g. Miscellaneous

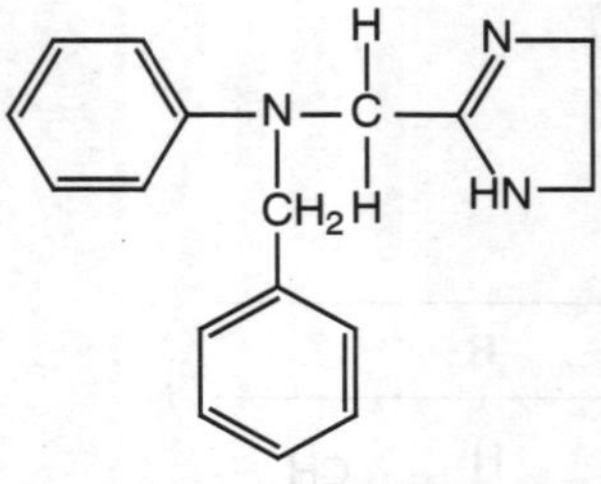

Antazoline

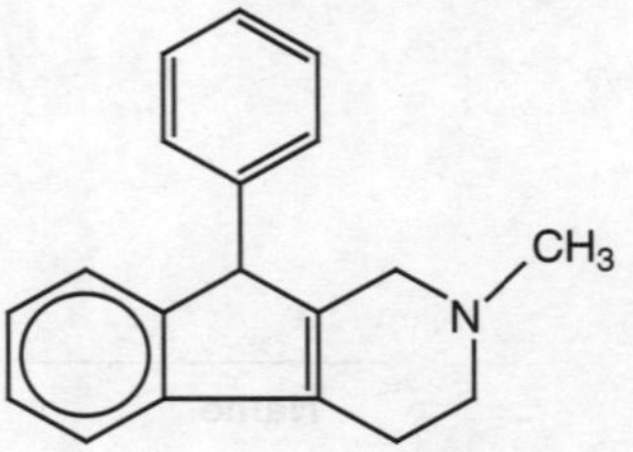

Phenindamine

h. Newer agents

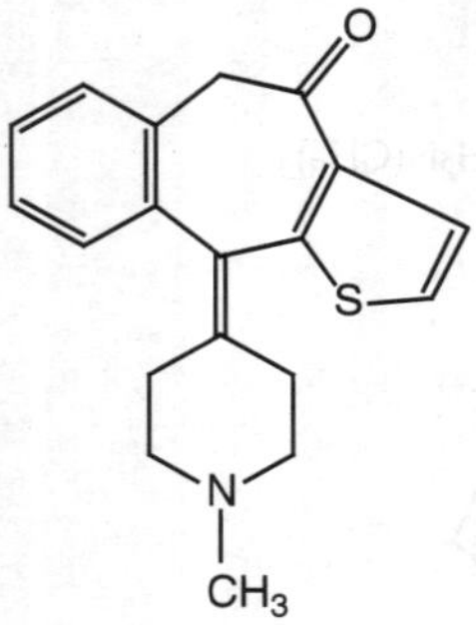

Ketotifene

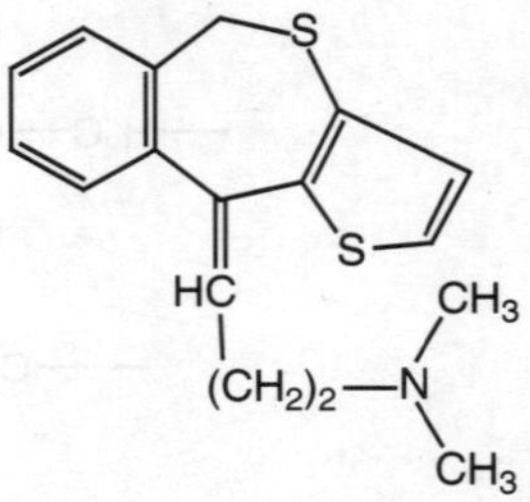

Dithiadene

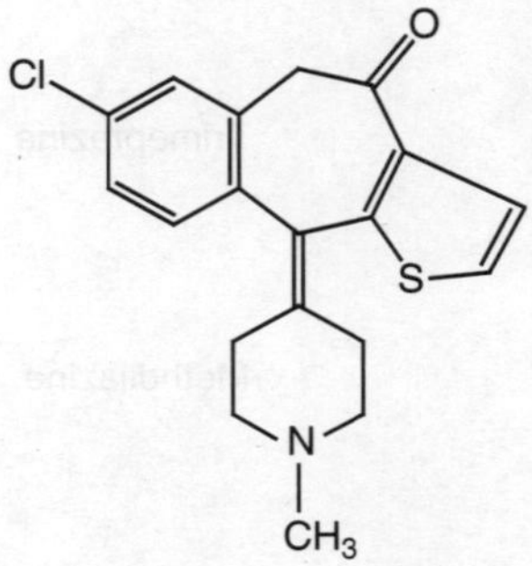

7-Chloro ketotifene

II. H_1-Antagonists with nonclassical structures
i. Azelastine

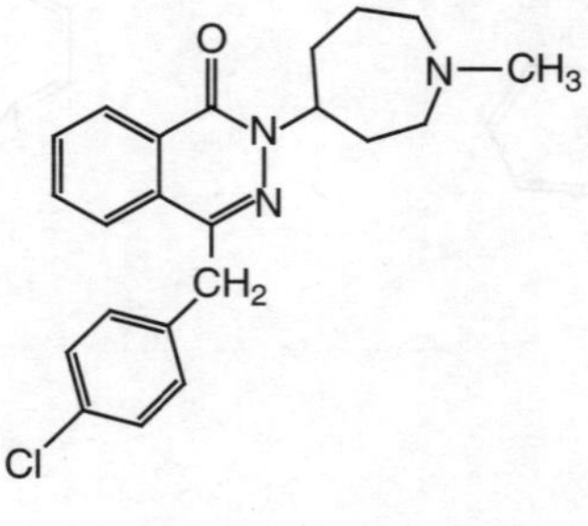

ii. Tazifylline

iii. Astemizole

III. Nonsedative H$_1$-antihistamines

Nonsedative antihistamines bind only to peripheral H$_1$-receptors and produce with little or no sedation because of poor CNS penetration and lower affinity for central histaminic activity.

These are divided into two main classes:

1. Piperazine derivatives—Cetirizine
2. Pyridine and piperidine derivatives—Loratadine, Fexofenadine, Terfenadine, Astemizole, Acrivastine

i. Loratadine

ii. Epinastine

iii. Rocastine

iv. Cetirizine

v. Fexofenadine

vi. Acrivastine

IV. Inhibition of histamine release (mast cells stabilizers)
i. Cromolyn sodium

ii. Nedocromil sodium

SYNTHESIS AND DRUG PROFILE

I. H$_1$-antagonists with classical structure
a. Ethylene diamine derivatives

Metabolism of ethylene diamine derivatives: These antihistaminic drugs undergo N-demethylation and subsequent deamination. In addition, some compounds produce quaternary N-glucuronide as urinary metabolites, a process that occurs to some extend in many relatively unhindered tertiary aliphatic amines among the antihistamines and also in other liphophilic tertiary aliphatic amine drugs.

i. Tripelennamine (Pyribenzamine HCl)

2-(Benzyl[2-(dimethylamino)ethyl]amino)pyridine

Synthesis

Pyridine $\xrightarrow{\text{NaNH}_2, \text{ Chichibabin reaction}}$ 2-Aminopyridine + 2-Chloro-N,N-dimethylethanamine $\xrightarrow{-\text{HCl}}$ intermediate + Benzyl chloride $\xrightarrow{-\text{HCl}}$ Tripelennamine

Properties and uses: It is a white, crystalline powder, soluble in water, freely soluble in alcohol and ether, but insoluble in chloroform or benzene. Tripelennamine is the first ethylenediamine developed in the American laboratories; it appears to be effective as diphenhydramine and may have the advantage of fewer and less severe side reactions. Drowsiness may occur and may impair the ability to perform tasks requiring alertness. The concurrent use of alcoholic beverage should be avoided. It is used in the treatment of allergic rhinitis, allergic conjunctivitis, angioedema, dermagraphism, and anaphylactic reactions.

Dose: Usual dose is 25–50 mg for adults consumed orally four to six times a day.

ii. Pyrilamine (Mepyramine, Anthisan)

N-(4-Methoxybenzyl)-N-(2-(dimethylamino)ethyl)pyridin-2-amine

Synthesis

Pyridine → (NaNH₂, Chichibabin reaction) → 2-Aminopyridine + 2-Chloro-N,N-dimethylethanamine → (−HCl) → intermediate + p-Methoxy benzyl chloride → (−HCl) → Mepyramine

Properties and uses: Mepyramine maleate is a white or slightly yellowish crystalline powder, soluble in water and in ethanol. Pyrilamine differs structurally from tripelennamine having a methoxy group in the para position of the benzyl radical. It differs from its more toxic and less potent precursor phenbenzamine (antergan) having a 2-pyridyl group on the nitrogen atom in the place of a phenyl group. Clinically, pyrilamine and tripelennamine are considered to be among the less potent antihistamines. It is used as an antihistaminic agent with a low incidence of sedative effects; it is also used as an antiemetic.

Assay: Dissolve the sample in anhydrous acetic acid and titrate against 0.1 M perchloric acid. Determine the end point potentiometrically.

Dose: Usual dose is 25–50 mg for adults taken orally three to four times per day.

Dosage forms: Mepyramine tablets B.P.

iii. Thonzylamine (Resistab)

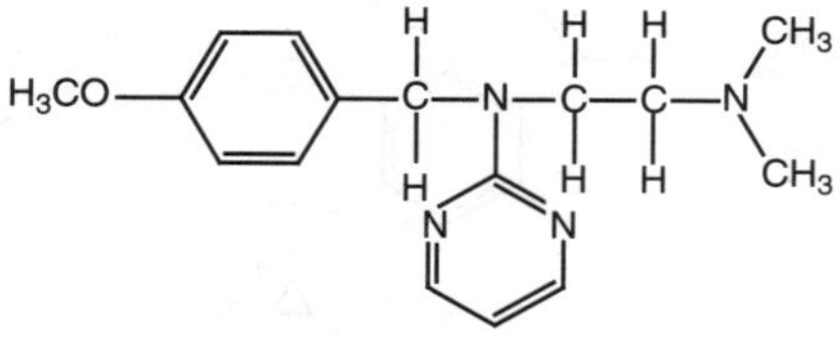

N-(4-Methoxybenzyl)-N-(2-(dimethylamino)ethyl)pyrimidin-2-amine

Synthesis

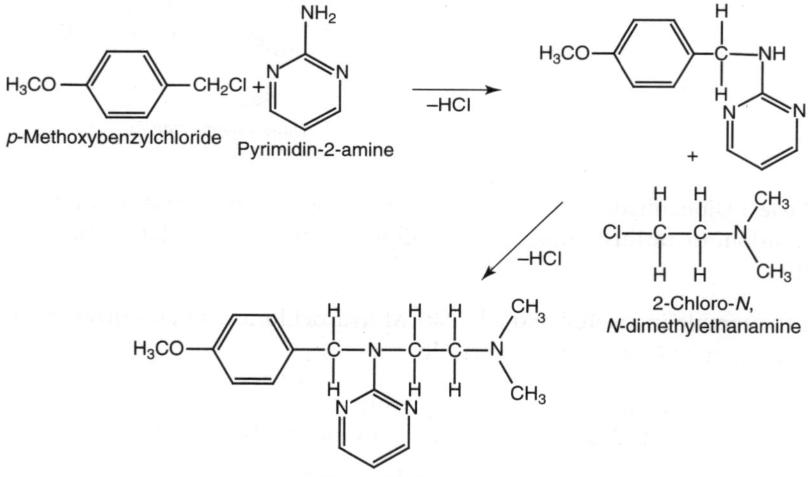

p-Methoxybenzylchloride + Pyrimidin-2-amine

2-Chloro-N,N-dimethylethanamine

Thonzylamine

Properties and uses: It is recommended for use with streptomycin in exudative human tuberculosis. It is used in treating the symptoms of diseases, such as hay fever, utricaria, and other mild allergic conditions.

Dose: Usual dose is 50 mg for adults consumed orally up to four times a day.

I. b. Amino alkyl ether analogues

i. Diphenhydramine (Benadryl, Bendylate)

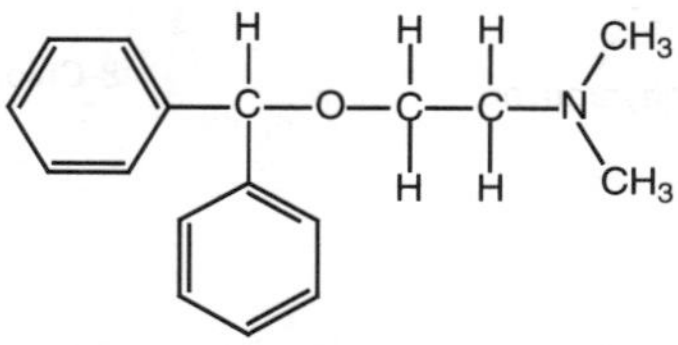

2-(Benzhydryloxy)-N,N-dimethylethanamine

Synthesis

Diphenylmethane →(Br₂/Light)→ bromodiphenylmethane + HO–CH₂–CH₂–N(CH₃)₂

→ (Δ, K_2CO_3) → Diphenydramine

Properties and uses: Diphenhydramine hydrochloride is a white crystalline powder, soluble in water and in alcohol. In addition, to antihistaminic activity, diphenhydramine exhibits antiemetic, antitussive, and sedative properties.

Assay: Dissolve the sample in alcohol and add 0.01 M hydrochloric acid and titrate against 0.1 M sodium hydroxide. Determine end point potentiometrically.

Dose: Usual dose is 25–50 mg for adult taken orally three to four times per day with maximum of 400 mg per day; for skin: used topically 2% of the cream three or four times per day.

Dosage forms: Diphenhydramine oral solution B.P.

ii. Dimenhydrinate (Dramamine)

[Diphenhydramine]⁺ · [8-Chlorotheophylline]⁻

Synthesis

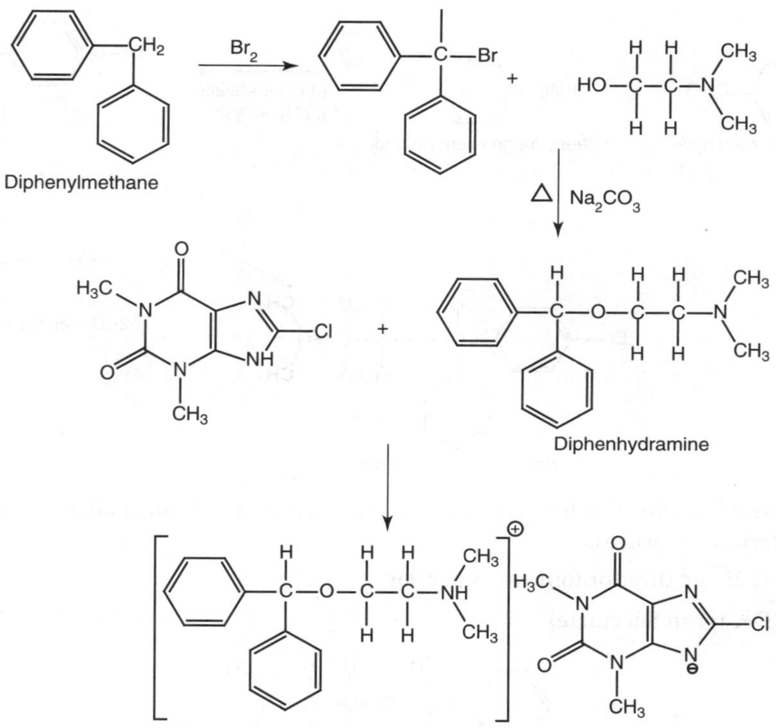

Diphenylmethane

Diphenhydramine

Dimenhydrinate (Mixture of Diphenhydramine and 8-chlorotheophylline)

Properties and uses: Dimenhydrinate is a white crystalline powder or colourless crystals, slightly soluble in water and in alcohol. Used as histamine H_1-receptor antagonist, antinauseant, in motion sickness, radiation sickness, and also in the case of nausea during pregnancy.

Assay: Dissolve the sample in anhydrous acetic acid and titrate against 0.1 M perchloric acid. Determine the end point potentiometrically.

Dose: Usual dose is taken orally as 50 mg thrice/day.

Dosage forms: Dimenhydrinate tablets B.P.

iii. Bromodiphendhydramine (Ambodryl hydrochloride)

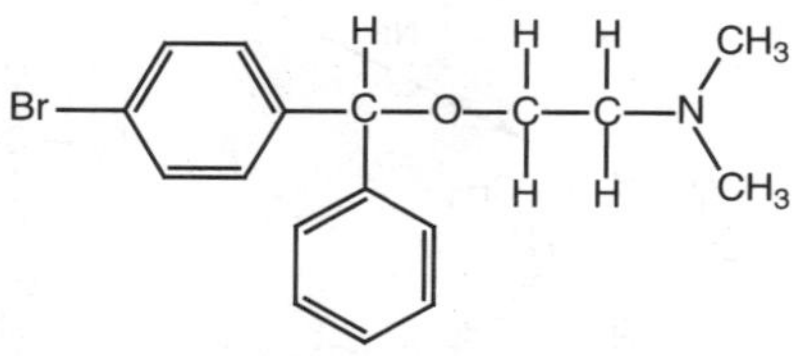

2-[(4-Bromophenyl)(phenyl)methoxy]-*N,N*-dimethylethanamine

Synthesis

[Reaction scheme: 4-Bromobenzaldehyde + Phenylmagnesium bromide → (i) Condensation (ii) Hydrolysis → 4-bromo-diphenylmethanol; then with SOCl₂, −HCl, and 2-(Dimethylamino)ethanol → Bromo diphenhydramine]

Properties and uses: It is effective for mild, local allergic reactions, physical allergy, and for minor drug reactions, characterized by pruritis.

Dose: Usual dose is 25 mg three or four times per day.

iii. **Doxylamine** (Decapryn Succinate)

[Structure: N,N-Dimethyl-2-(1-phenyl-1-(pyridin-2-yl)ethoxy)ethanamine]

Synthesis

[Reaction scheme: 2-Acetylpyridine + Phenylmagnesium bromide → 1-phenyl-1-(pyridin-2-yl)ethanol; then Na + Dimethylamino ethyl chloride → Doxylamine]

Properties and uses: Doxylamine succinate is a white powder, highly soluble in water and in alcohol. It is a relatively selective histamine H_1-receptor antagonist. In vivo studies have shown that concentrations dependent upon the inhibition of histamine stimulated vascular permeability in the conjunctiva following topical ocular administration. It appears to be devoid of effects on adrenergic, dopaminergic, and serotonin receptors. It is used with antitussives and decongestants for the relief of cough and cold.

Assay: Dissolve the sample in anhydrous acetic acid and titrate against 0.1 M perchloric acid. Determine the end point potentiometrically.

Dose: Usual dose is 12.5 to 25 mg for adult taken orally four to six times per day.

iv. Carbinoxamine

2-((4-Chlorophenyl)(pyridin-2-yl)methoxy)-N,N-dimethylethanamine

Synthesis

Piconaldehyde + p-Chloro phenylmagnesium bromide $\xrightarrow{H^+/H_2O}$

+ Dimethylamino ethyl chloride $\xrightarrow{-HCl}$ Carbinoxamine

Properties and uses: Carbinoxamine is available as white, crystalline powder with no odour, soluble in water, alcohol, chloroform, or ether. It is a potent antihistaminic and is available as the racemic mixture. It differs structurally from chlorpheniramine only in having an oxygen atom separate from the asymmetric carbon atom in the aminoethyl side chain. The levo isomer of carbinoxamine is more active than dextro isomer (s-configuration) of chlorpheniramine.

v. Clemastine

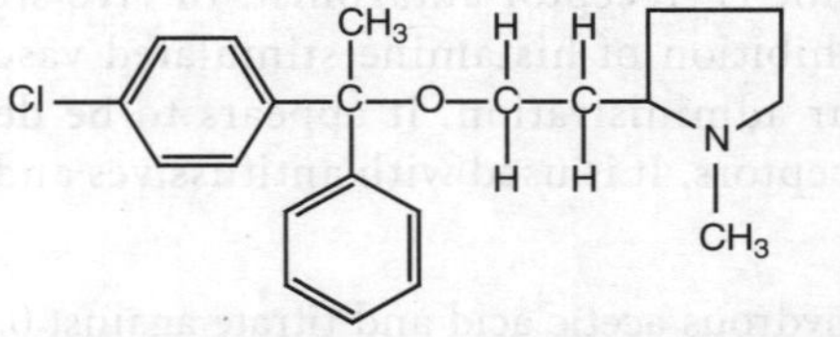

2-(2-1-(4-Chlorophenyl)-1-(phenylethoxy)ethyl)-1-methylpyrrolidine

Synthesis

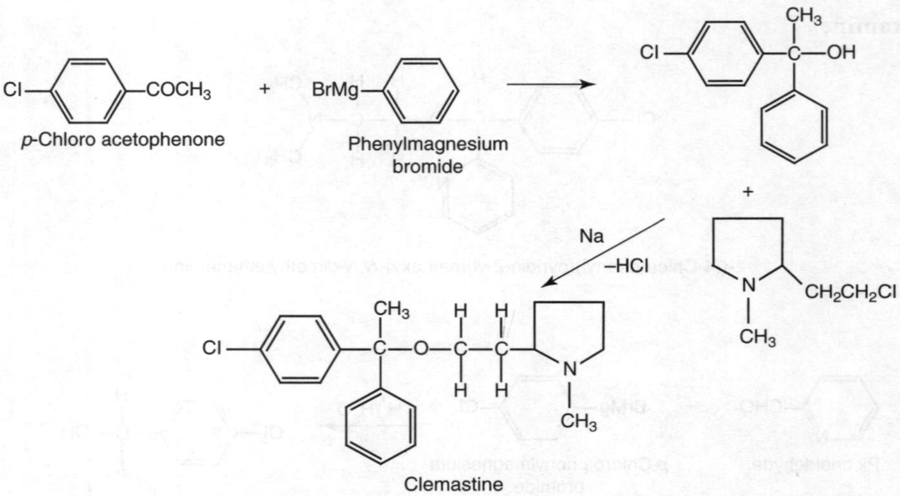

p-Chloro acetophenone + Phenylmagnesium bromide →

Na, –HCl

Clemastine

Properties and uses: Clemastine fumarate is a white crystalline powder, very slightly soluble in water, slightly soluble in alcohol and methanol. It has two chiral centres, each of which is (R) absolute configuration. A comparison of the activities of the antipodes indicates that the asymmetric centre close to the side chain of nitrogen is of lesser importance to antihistaminic activity. It is a long-acting ethanolamine antihistamine with sedative and anticholinergic side effects.

Assay: Dissolve the sample in anhydrous acetic acid and titrate against 0.1 M perchloric acid. Determine the end point potentiometrically.

Dosage forms: Clemastine oral solution B.P., Clemastine tablets B.P.

vi. Diphenylpyraline (Diaben)

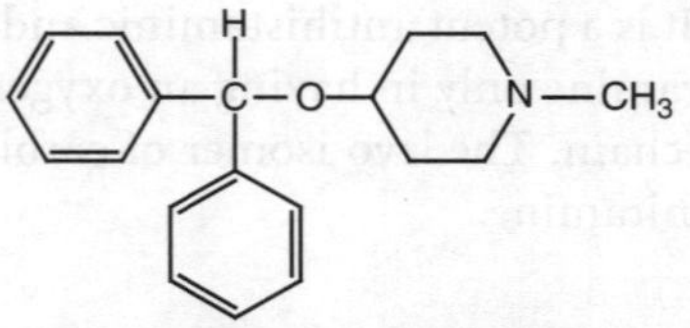

4-(Diphenylmethoxy)-1-methylpiperidine

Synthesis

Metabolism: This type of drugs undergoes *N*-demethylation (formation of corresponding secondary amine) and subsequent deamination (formation of carboxylic acid metabolites) is the major pathway for diphenylpyraline and some of its analogues. Minor metabolites that are conjugates of the ether cleavage products have been found in some animal species.

Properties and uses: Diphenylpyraline hydrochloride is a white powder, soluble in water and ethanol, practically insoluble in ether. It is structurally related to diphenhydramine with the aminoalkyl side chain incorporated in a piperidine ring. It is a potent antihistaminic agent.

Assay: Dissolve the sample in anhydrous acetic acid and add mercury (II) acetate solution and titrate against 0.1 M perchloric acid using oracet blue B solution as indicator.

Dose: Usual dose for adults taken orally is 5 mg two times per day.

I.c. Piperazines derivatives
i. Cyclizine (Marezine)

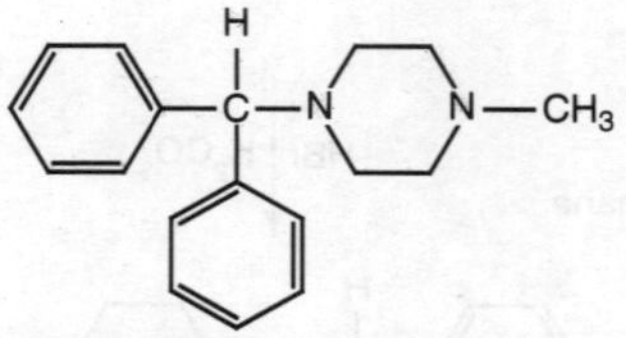

1-Benzhydryl-4-methylpiperazine

Synthesis

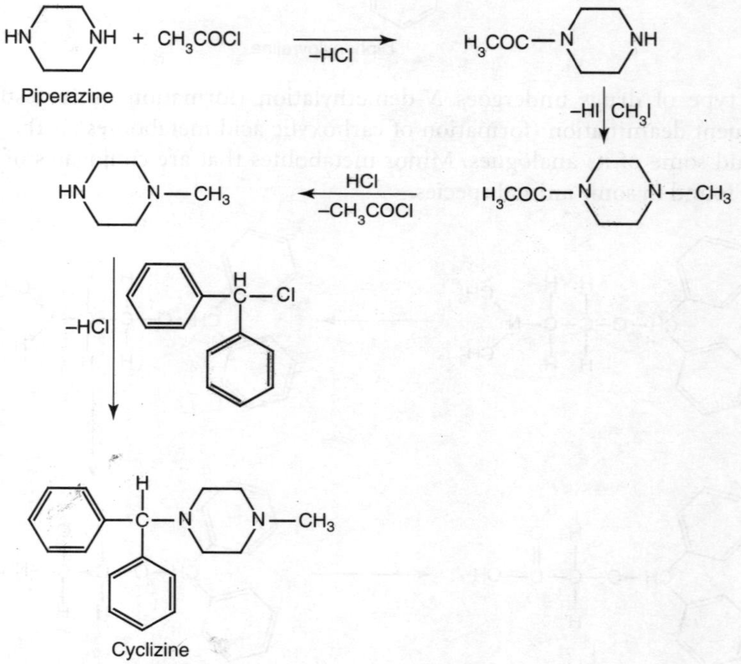

Cyclizine

Properties and uses: Cyclizine hydrochloride is a white crystalline powder, slightly soluble in water and in alcohol. It is mostly employed as a prophylaxis and for the treatment of motion sickness.

Assay: Dissolve the sample in anhydrous formic acid, add acetic anhydride and titrates against 0.1 M perchloric acid. Determine the end point potentiometrically.

Dose: Usual dose is 25–100 mg per day.

Dosage forms: Cyclizine HCl tablets I.P., Cyclizine injection B.P., Cyclizine tablets B.P., Dipipanone and cyclizine tablets B.P.

ii. Chlorcyclizine (Diparalene)

Structure: 1-((4-Chlorophenyl)(phenyl)methyl)-4-methylpiperazine

Synthesis

(4-Chlorophenyl)(phenyl)chloromethane + 1-Methylpiperazine

1-Chloro-4-((chloro phenyl)methyl)benzene → (−HCl) → **Chlorcyclizine**

Properties and uses: Chlorcyclizine hydrochloride is a white crystalline powder, soluble in water, methylene chloride and in alcohol. Substitution of halogen in the 2nd or 3rd position of either of the benzhydryl rings results in a much less potent activity. Chlorcyclizine is indicated in the symptomatic relief of utricaria, hay fever, and certain other allergic conditions.

Assay: Dissolve the sample in a mixture of 0.1 M hydrochloric acid and methanol and titrate against 0.1 M sodium hydroxide. Determine end point potentiometrically.

Dose: Usual dose is 50–200 mg per day.

iii. Meclizine (Antivert, Bonine)

1-(p-Chlorophenyl benzyl)-4-(3-methylbenzyl) piperazine

Synthesis

[Synthesis scheme: 1-Chloro-4-((chloro phenyl)methyl)benzene + 1-(Piperazin-1-yl)ethanone → (−HCl) intermediate → (−CH₃COOH, H₃O⁺) → piperazine intermediate + ClH₂C-(3-methylphenyl) → (−HCl) → **Meclizine**]

Properties and uses: It is a white or slightly yellowish, crystalline powder with no characteristic odour and taste. It is insoluble in water and in ether, but soluble in chloroform and alcohol. It is a moderately potent antihistaminic agent. It is used primarily as an antinauseant in the prevention and treatment of motion sickness; in the treatment of nausea and vomiting associated with vertigo and radiation sickness.

Assay: Dissolve the sample in alcohol and titrate against 0.1 M sodium hydroxide. Determine the end point potentiometrically.

Dose: Usual dose is 25–50 mg per day.

I. d. Monoamino propylamine derivatives

i. Saturated analogues

1. Pheniramine Maleate (Avil, Polarmine)

N,N-Dimethyl-3-phenyl-3-(pyridin-2-yl)propan-1-amine

Properties and uses: Pheniramine maleate is a white crystalline powder, freely soluble in water, alcohol, methanol, and methylene chloride. This drug is the least potent member of the series and is marketed as the racemate.

Assay: Dissolve the sample in anhydrous acetic acid and titrate against 0.1 M perchloric acid. Determine the end point potentiometrically.

Dose: Usual dose is 25–30 mg per day in divided doses.

Synthesis

Route I. From: 2-Phenylacetonitrile

Route II. From: Picolinaldehyde

Phenylmagnesium bromide + **Picolinaldehyde** → (i) Nu - addition (ii) Hydrolysis → [α-(pyridin-2-yl)benzyl alcohol]

Catalytic reduction → [2-benzylpyridine] + N,N-Dimethylamino chloroethane → NaNH$_2$, –HCl → **Pheniramine**

2. Chlorpheniramine HCl (Piriton, Alermine)

3-(4-Chlorophenyl)-N,N-dimethyl-3-(pyridin-2-yl)propan-1-amine

Synthesis
Route-I. From: 2-(4-Chlorophenyl)acetonitrile

2-(4-Chlorophenyl)acetonitrile + **2-Bromopyridine** → [α-(4-chlorophenyl)-α-(pyridin-2-yl)acetonitrile]

+ **N,N-Dimethylamino chloro ethane** → [intermediate with CN group]

→ –CO$_2$, (i) Hydrolysis (ii) –CO$_2$ (iii) HCl → **Chlorpheniramine**

Route-II. From: Picolinaldehyde

(4-Chlorophenyl)magnesium bromide + Picolinaldehyde → (i) Nu-addition (ii) H₂O → [chlorophenyl-pyridyl carbinol]

Catalytic reduction ↓

[2-(4-chlorobenzyl)pyridine] + N,N-Dimethylamino chloro ethane

↓ NaNH₂

Chlorpheniramine

Properties and uses: Chlorpheniramine HCl is a white crystalline powder, soluble in water and in ethanol. Chlorination of pheniramine in the para position of the phenyl ring increases potency by almost 10-fold, with no appreciable change in toxicity. Most of the antihistaminic activity resides with the dextro isomer.

Assay: Dissolve the sample in anhydrous acetic acid and titrate against 0.1 M perchloric acid. Determine the end point potentiometrically.

Dose: Usual oral dose is 5 mg three or four times per day.

Dosage forms: Chlorpheniramine maleate injection I.P., B.P., Chlorpheniramine maleate tablets I.P., B.P., Chlorpheniramine oral solution B.P.

I. d. Monoaminopropyl analogues
ii. Unsaturated analogues
1. Triprolidine (Actidil)

2-(3-(Pyrrolidin-1-yl)-1-*p*-tolylprop-1-enyl)pyridine

Synthesis

Scheme:

1-p-Tolylethanone + HCHO + Pyrrolidine →(Mannich reaction) p-tolyl-CO-CH₂-CH₂-N(pyrrolidine) intermediate + 2-pyridyl-MgBr →
(i) Nu-addition
(ii) Hydrolysis →
carbinol intermediate (with OH, pyridyl, tolyl, CH₂-CH₂-pyrrolidine) →
−H₂O, Dehydration → **Triprolidine**

Properties and uses: Triprolidine hydrochloride is a white crystalline powder, practically insoluble in ether, soluble in water and in ethanol. The activity is mainly confined to the geometric isomer in which the pyrrolidino-methyl group is *trans* to the 2-pyridyl group. Pharmacological studies confirm the high activity of triprolidine and the superiority of (E) over corresponding (Z) isomers as H_1-antagonists. In guinea pig ileum sites, the affinity of triprolidine (E) for H_1-receptors was more than 1000 times the affinity of its (Z) partner.

Assay: Dissolve the sample in a mixture of anhydrous acetic acid and acetic anhydride and titrate against 0.1 M perchloric acid using crystal violet solution as indicator.

Dose: Usual dose is 5–7.5 mg per day.

Dosage forms: Triprolidine HCl tablets I.P., Triprolidine tablets B.P.

I. e. Tricyclic ring system or phenothiazines
1. Promethazine HCl (Phenargen)

N,N-Dimethyl-1-(phenothiazin-10-yl)propan-2-amine hydrochloride

Synthesis

Diphenylamine + S (Sulphur) $\xrightarrow{I_2/AlCl_3}$ phenothiazine

Promethazine hydrochloride

Properties and uses: Promethazine hydrochloride is a white or faintly yellowish crystalline powder, highly soluble in water, soluble in alcohol and in methylene chloride. It may be used effectively in perennial and seasonal allergic rhinitis, vasomotor rhinitis, allergic conjunctivitis due to inhalant allergens and foods, and certain milder type of skin manifestations of urtricaria. It also possesses some anticholinergic, antiserotonergic, and marked local anaesthetic properties.

Assay: Dissolve the sample in a mixture of 0.01 M hydrochloric acid and alcohol and titrate against 0.1 M sodium hydroxide. Determine end point potentiometrically.

Dose: Usual dose is 20–50 mg per day.

Dosage forms: Promethazine hydrochloride injection I.P., Promethazine hydrochloride tablets I.P., B.P., Promethazine hydrochloride syrup I.P., Promethazine injection B.P., promethazine oral solution B.P.

2. Trimeprazine (Temaril)

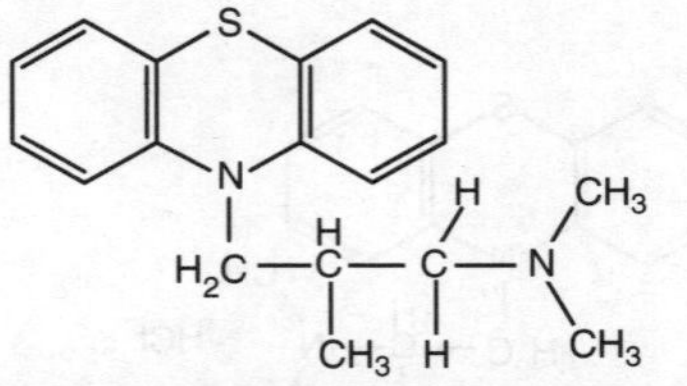

N,N,2-Trimethyl-3-(phenothiazin-10-yl)propan-1-amine

Synthesis

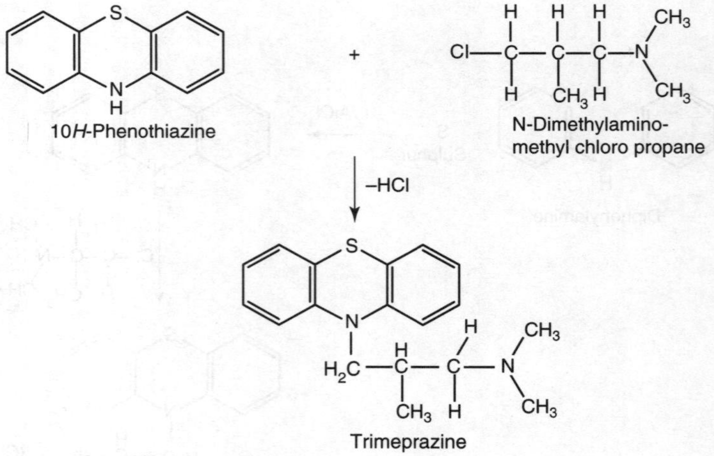

10*H*-Phenothiazine + N-Dimethylamino-methyl chloro propane

−HCl

Trimeprazine

Properties and uses: It is a white crystalline powder, soluble in water. It is used as histamine H_1-receptor antagonist.

Dose: Usual dose for adults is 10–40 mg per day orally.

3. Methdilazine (Tacaryl HCl)

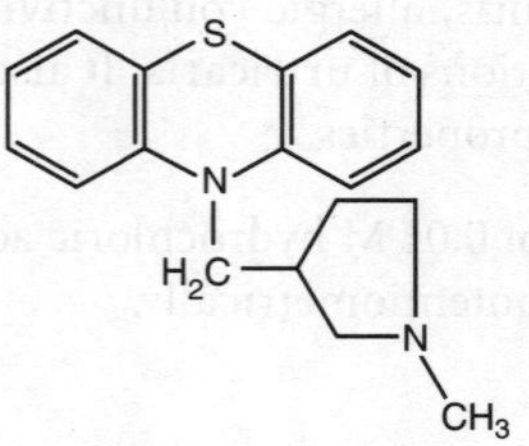

10-((1-Methylpyrrolidin-3-yl)methyl) phenothiazine

Synthesis

10H-Phenothiazine + N-Methyl-3-chloro methyl pyrrolidine

−HCl →

Methdilazine

Properties and uses: It may be used for the symptomatic relief of urtricaria. It has also been used successfully for the treatment of migraine headache.

Dose: Usual dose for adults is 8 mg taken orally two to four times a day.

I. f. Dibenzocyclo heptene derivatives
1. Cyproheptadine (Periacetin)

4-Dibanzo(a,d) cyclohepten-5-ylidene)-1-methyl piperidine

Properties and uses: Cyproheptadine hydrochloride is a white or slightly yellow crystalline powder, slightly soluble in water and methanol, sparingly soluble in alcohol. This dibenzocycloheptene may be regarded as a phenothiazine analogue in which the sulphur atom has been replaced by an isosteric vinyl group and the ring nitrogen replaced by a sp^2 carbon atom. It also possesses antiserotonin activity and is used as an antipruritic agent associated with skin disorders (utricaria, allergic dermatitis, neurodermatitis). It is used to stimulate the appetite in under-weight patients and those suffering from anorexia nervosa.

Synthesis

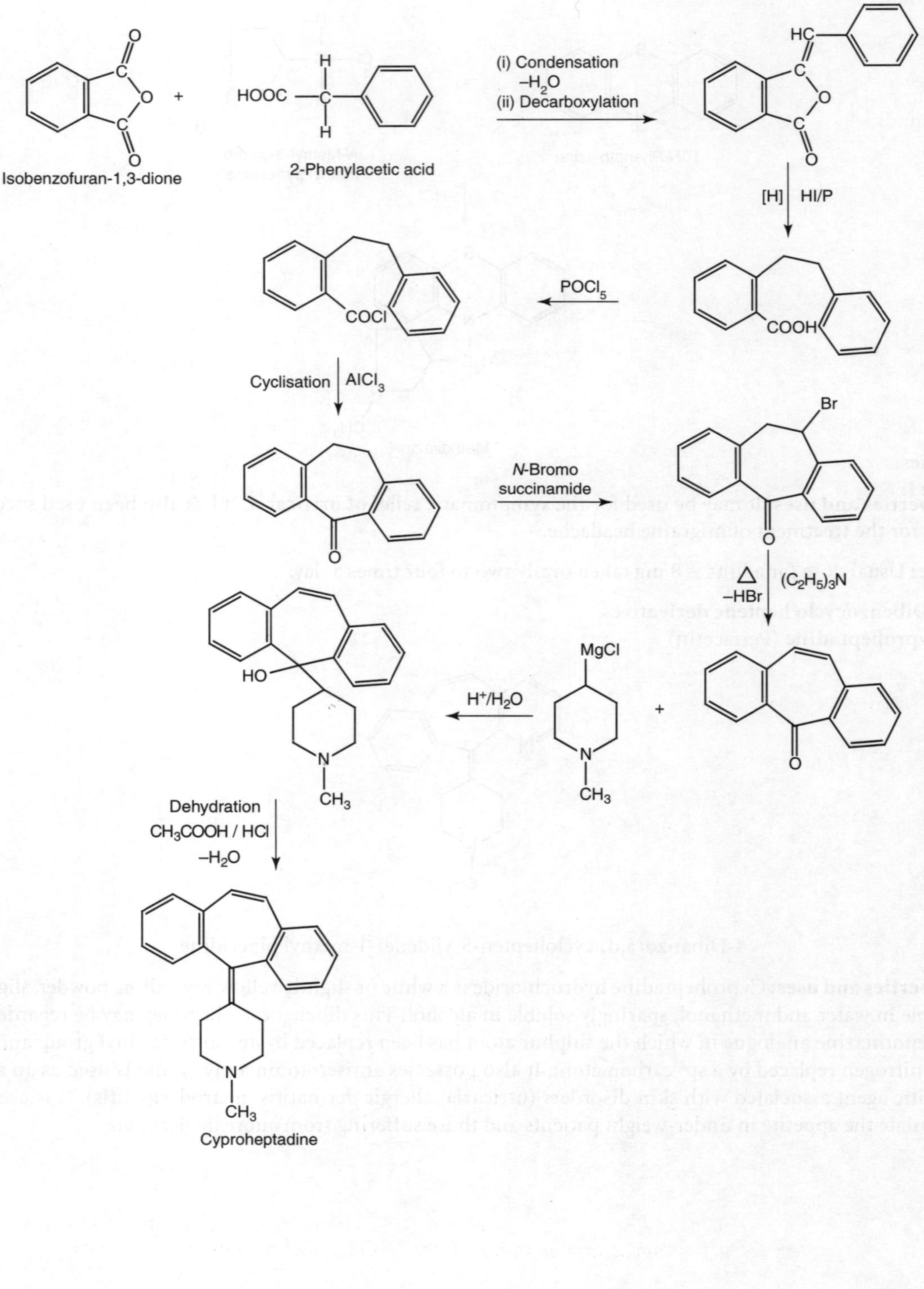

Isobenzofuran-1,3-dione + 2-Phenylacetic acid (HOOC-CH₂-Ph)

(i) Condensation, $-H_2O$
(ii) Decarboxylation

→ benzylidene phthalide

[H] HI/P → 2-(2-phenylethyl)benzoic acid

$POCl_5$ → acid chloride (COCl)

Cyclisation / $AlCl_3$ → dibenzosuberone precursor (ketone)

N-Bromosuccinamide → α-bromoketone

Δ / $(C_2H_5)_3N$, $-HBr$ → dibenzosuberenone

+ 1-methyl-4-piperidinyl MgCl →

H^+/H_2O → tertiary alcohol (HO-)

Dehydration CH_3COOH / HCl, $-H_2O$

→ **Cyproheptadine**

Assay: Dissolve the sample in a mixture of 0.01 M hydrochloric acid and alcohol and titrate against 0.1 M sodium hydroxide. Determine end point potentiometrically.

Dose: Usually, the dose is 4 mg taken orally three times a day.

Dosage forms: Cyproheptadine HCl syrup I.P., Cyproheptadine HCl tablets I.P., Cyproheptadine tablets B.P.

2. Azatadine

6,11-Dihydro-11-(1-methyl-4-piperidyllidene)-5H-benzo-[5,6]-cyclohepta-9-[1,2-6] pyridine

Synthesis
Route I. From: 2-Chloro-3-phenethylpyridine

Route II. From: Phenylacetonitrile

Properties and uses: Azatadine is a potent, long-acting antihistaminic with antiserotonin activity. In early testing, azatadine exhibited more than three times the potency of chlorpheniramine in the isolated guinea pig ileum screening and more than seven times the oral potency of chlorpheniramine in the protection of guinea pig against a double lethal dose of intravenously administered histamine.

Azatadine is an aza isostere of cyproheptadine in which the 10, 11-double bond is reduced. It has low sedative effect.

I. g. Miscellaneous
1. Antazoline (Antistine)

N-Benzyl-*N*-((4,5-dihydro-1*H*-imidazol-2-yl)methyl)benzenamine

Synthesis

Benzyl aniline → (−HCl) → Antazoline

Properties and uses: Antazoline hydrochloride is a white crystalline powder, sparingly soluble in water, soluble in alcohol, and slightly soluble in methylene chloride. The phosphate salt is soluble in water, bitter taste. It is used for the treatment of rhinitis and conjunctivitis.

Assay: Dissolve the sample in alcohol and titrate against 0.1 M alcoholic potassium hydroxide using phenolphthalein as indicator.

Dose: Usual dose is 50–100 mg per day.

I. h. Newer agents
1. Ketotifen Fumarate (Zaditen)

4-(1-Methyl-4-piperidylidene)-4*H*-benzo[4,5]cyclohepta[1,2-b]thiophen-10(9*H*)

Synthesis

Properties and uses: Ketotifen fumarate is a white to brownish-yellow crystalline powder, sparingly soluble in water, slightly soluble in methanol and in acetonitrile. The recommended dose of ketotifen solution is one drop instilled into each affected eye every 8–12 hr. Most frequently used for conjuctival infection, and rhinitis. Ketotifen solution should be used with caution during pregnancy or during nursing. This is an analogue of the tricyclic H_1-receptor antagonist and serotonin receptor antagonist. It has only minor anticholinergic and antiserotonergic activity. It has been used in the prophylactic treatment of asthma.

Assay: Dissolve the sample in a mixture of anhydrous acetic acid and acetic anhydride and titrate against 0.1 M perchloric acid. Determine the end point potentiometrically.

Dose: Usually, the dose is 1 mg orally two times a day.

II. H$_1$-Antagonists with nonclassical structure
1. Astemizole (Histalong)

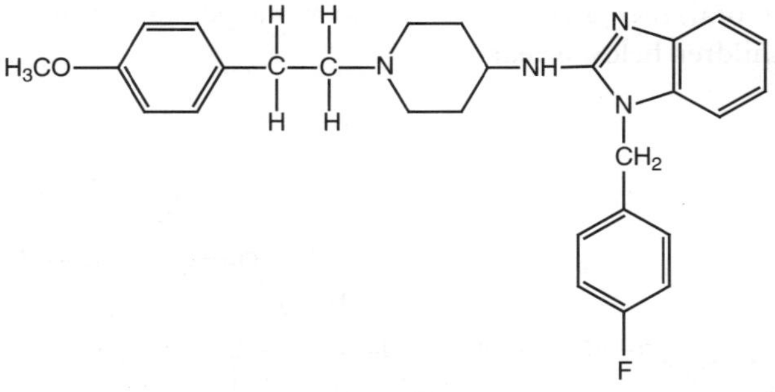

1-(4-Fluorobenzyl)-N-(1-(4-methoxyphenethyl)piperidin-4-yl)-1H-benzo[d]imidazol-2-amine

Synthesis

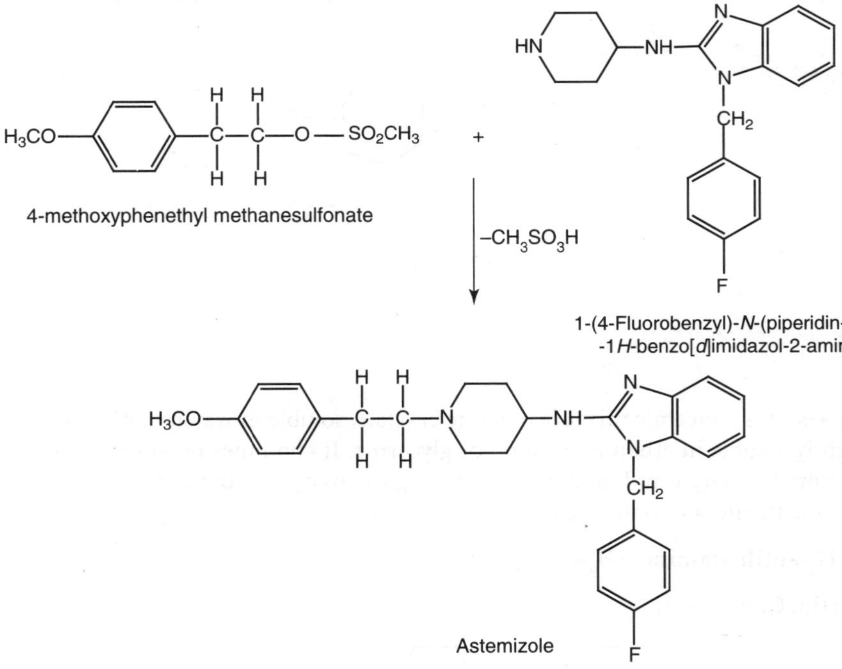

4-methoxyphenethyl methanesulfonate + 1-(4-Fluorobenzyl)-N-(piperidin-4-yl)-1H-benzo[d]imidazol-2-amine

$-CH_3SO_3H$

→ Astemizole

Properties and uses: Astemizole is a white powder, practically insoluble in water, soluble in methylene chloride, methanol, and in alcohol. The drug is found to be more potent and possesses longer duration of action than the terfenadine. It has a slow onset, is long acting, and nonsedating piperidine antihistaminic having practically little anticholinergic activity. It is indicated for seasonal allergic rhinitis and chronic utricaria. It is an effective antiallergic agent giving protection against asthma, hay fever, and chronic utricaria. It does not exhibit any noticeable CNS activity.

Assay: Dissolve the sample in a mixture of anhydrous acetic acid and methyl ethyl ketone, and titrate against 0.1 M perchloric acid using naphtholbenzein solution as an indicator.

Dose: Usual dose is 10 mg (oral) increased, if required, to 30 mg per day for upto 7 days 1 h before meals. It is not recommended for children below 6 years.

2. Tazifylline

Properties and uses: Tazifylline is proved for its successful antiallergic activity, with no significant occurrence of side effects (dryness of mouth and sedation) and long duration of action.

3. Azelastine

Properties and uses: It is a racemic mixture of white crystals, soluble in water, methanol or propylene glycol, but only slightly soluble in ethanol, octanol, or glycerine. It combines potent H_1-receptor antagonism with a negligible anticholinergic and moderate serotonergic activity. It is used in the treatment of itching of the eyes associated with allergic conditions.

III Nonsedative H_1-antihistamines (H_1-antagonists)

1. Cetirizine (Zirtin, Cetin, Cetzine)

2-(2-(4-((4-Chlorophenyl)(phenyl)methyl)piperazin-1-yl)ethoxy)acetic acid

Synthesis
Route I. From: 1-[4-Chlorophenyl (1-phenylmethyl)]-piperazine

Route II. From: hydroxyzine
Cetirizine is an acid metabolite formed by the oxidation of primary alcohol of antihistamine hydroxyzine.

Properties and uses: Cetirizine hydrochloride is a white powder, soluble in water, practically insoluble in acetone and methylene chloride. This is the principal metabolic product of hydroxyzine, the polar acid group prevents its penetration into the CNS. It is used as an antihistamine to treat various allergic conditions. Cetrizine is one of the most widely prescribed H_1-antihistamines. It is highly selective in its interaction with various hormonal binding sites and highly potent as well. Other effects of this drug include fatigue, dry mouth, pharyngitis, and dizziness.

Assay: Dissolve the sample in a mixture of water and acetone (1:7) and titrate against 0.1 M sodium hydroxide to the second point of inflexion and determine the end point potentiometrically.

Dose: Usual dose is 5–10 mg thrice/day.

2. Loratadine (Alaspan, Lorfast)

4-(8-Chlor-5,6-dihydro-benzocyclohepta pyridine-11-ylidene)-1-piperidine carboxylic acid ethylester

Synthesis

8-Chloro azatidine → (i) CNBr (ii) C_2H_5OCOCl → Loratidine

Metabolism: It is a nonsedative antihistaminic drug. The metabolite is desloratidine (descarboethoxy loratidine) is associated with potentially cardiotoxic effect.

Loratadine →[CYP3A4 / CYP2D6]→ [intermediate] → desloratidine

The metabolic conversion of loratidine to descarboethoxy loratidine occurs via oxidative process and not via hydrolysis, and both CYP2D6 and CYP3A4 are to be the isoenzyme catalyzing this oxidative metabolism.

Properties and uses: Loratadine is a white crystalline powder, practically insoluble in water, soluble in acetone and methanol. Loratadine is an azo isomer of cyproheptadine. The replacement of methyl group of azatadine (piperidine nitrogen) by corresponding carbomate and introduction of 8-chloro substitution preserve the antihistaminic action and reduces the CNS effect. The potency of loratidine is comparable with that of astemizole and greater than of terfenadine.

Assay: Dissolve the sample in glacial acetic acid and titrate against 0.1 M perchloric acid. Determine the end point potentiometrically.

3. Epinastine

Properties and uses: This is structurally related to the antidepressant and nonsedative H_1-receptor antagonist mianserin. Introduction of an amidine moiety preserve the antihistamine action and reduce the CNS effect (sedation).

4. Rocastine

2-(2-(Dimethylamino)ethyl)-4-methyl-3,4-dihydro pyrido[3,2-f][1,4]oxazepine-5(2H)-thione

Properties and uses: It is a rapid acting, nonsedating H_1-antagonist. The R-enantiomer was at least 300 times more potent than S-enantiomer.

IV. Inhibition of histamine release (mast cell stabilizer)
i. Cromolyn sodium

ii. Nedocromil sodium

PROBABLE QUESTIONS

1. What is histamine? What are its biological effects? Mention the different histamine receptors.
2. What are allergens? What is the importance of antihistamines in combating various types of allergic conditions? Mention suitable examples to support your answer.
3. Classify the histamine H_1-receptor antagonists. Write the structure, chemical name, and uses of one drug from each category.
4. What are the side effects of classical antihistamines?
5. Outline the synthesis of the following: Diphenhydramine, Chlorpheniramine maleate and Triprolidine.
6. Name any three ethylenediamines being used as antihistamines. Outline the synthesis of any one of them.
7. Write the chemical structure, chemical name, and uses of the following and describe the synthesis of any one drug.
   (a) Mepyramine maleate (b) Tripelenamine hydrochloride
8. Outline the synthesis of the following drugs and mention their uses.
   (a) Promethazine hydrochloride (b) Antazoline (c) Methdilazine hydrochloride.
9. Phenindamine tartarate and chlorpheniramine maleate are two important antihistamines. Describe the synthesis of any one drug in detail.
10. Write a brief account of the following:
    a. Drugs used in the prevention of histamine release
    b. Newer antihistamines
11. Write a comprehensive account of the following:
    a. SAR of H_1-receptor blockers
    b. Mode of action of antihistamines
12. What are nonsedative antihistamines? Enumerate them with the chemical structure and write the synthesis of any one of them.

SUGGESTED READINGS

1. Abraham DJ (ed). *Burger's Medicinal Chemistry and Drug Discovery* (6th edn). New Jersey: John Wiley, 2007.
2. *British Pharmacopoeia*. Medicines and Healthcare Products Regulatory Agency. London, 2008.

3. Bruntan LL, Lazo JS, and Parker KL. *Goodman and Gilman's: The Pharmacological Basis of Therapeutics* (11th edn). New York: McGraw Hill, 2006.
4. Burn JH. 'Antihistamines'. *Br Med J* 4(1): 1357–359, 1955.
5. Gennaro AR. *Remington's: The Science and Practice of Pharmacy* (21st edn). New York: Lippincot Williams and Wilkins, 2006.
6. Idson B. 'Antihistamine drugs'. *Chem Rev* 47: 307–527, 1950.
7. *Indian Pharmacopoeia*. Ministry of Health and Family Welfare. New Delhi, 1996.
8. Hunter RB and Dunlop DM. 'A review of antihistamine drugs'. *Q J Med* 25: 271–90, 1948.
9. Landsteiner K. *The Specificity of Serological Reactions*. New York: Dover Publications, 1962.
10. Lemke TL and William DA. *Foye's Principle of Medicinal Chemistry* (6th edn). New York: Lippincott Williams and Wilkins, 2008.
11. Lednicer D and Mitscher LA. *The Organic Chemistry of Drug Synthesis*. New York: John Wiley, 1995.
12. Orange RP, Kaliner MA, and Austen KF. In *Biochemistry of the Acute Allergic Reaction*, Austen KF and Becker EL (eds). Oxford: Blackwell, 1971.

Chapter 2

Prostaglandins

INTRODUCTION

Prostaglandins (PGs) occur virtually in all mammalian tissues and possess numerous and diverse pharmacological actions. They are comprised of a large number of unsaturated hydroxy, lipids like acids containing 20 carbon atoms. Since they were extracted from prostate gland and seminal vesicles of several animal species, including that of human semen, the term prostaglandin was used for them. It is isolated and purified as hydroxy fatty acid fraction from lipid extracts of seminal vesicles and from it the two biologically active substances, that is, PG E and F, were isolated. Some active compounds were derived from oxygenation of arachidonic acid, a precursor released from membrane phospholipids. The anti-inflammatory and analgesic effects of aspirin and the related nonsteroidal anti-inflammatory drugs (NSAIDs) are due to their inhibitory effects on PG formation.

They are also reported to be present in significant quantities in the reproductive tissues, developing foetus and deciduals, umbilical cord, amniotic fluid, endometrium, menstrual fluid, epidermis, thymus, thyroid, and nerves. Further, in most of the organs, except for genital tissue, the PG is present as prostaglandin E (PGE) and prostaglandin F_2 (PGF_2). Therapeutic potential of PGs are in the treatment of blood pressure, bronchial functions, atherosclerosis, heart attack, inhibition of blood clot formation, childbirth, abortions, stomach ulcers, and other related syndromes.

FUNCTIONS OF PGs

There are varieties of physiological effects including the following:

1. Blood clots are formed when a blood vessel is damaged. A type of PGs called thromboxane (TxA_2) stimulates constriction and clotting of platelets. Conversely, PGI_2 have the opposite effect on the walls of blood vessels.
2. Certain PGs are involved in the induction of labour and other reproductive processes. PGE_2 causes uterine contractions and has been used to induce labour.

Nomenclature

Prostanoic acid

PGs are considered as analogues of poly unsaturated fatty acids. It is a 20 carbon carboxylic acid containing a five-member ring. The PGs (Table 2.1) are classified according to the nature of:

A. Cyclopentane ring.
B. Two side chain.
C. Configuration of newly introduced functional group.

Table 2.1 Various types of PGs.

A- type PGA		10, 11-Unsaturated-9-Keto function
B- type PGB		8, 12-Unsaturated-9-Keto function
C- type PGC		11, 12-Unsaturated-9-Keto function
D- type PGD		11-Keto-9-hydroxy function
E- type PGE		β-hydroxyl ketone with keto moiety at C-9 and α-OH at C-11
F- type PGF		1,3-Diols

The main classes are further subdivided according to the number of double bonds in the side chain. This is indicated by the subscripts 1, 2, or 3 and refers to the fatty acid precursor in most instances.

Examples: PGE_2 and $PGF_2\alpha$.

Two side chains are attached to the cyclopentane ring at C-8 and C-12. The upper chain, having a carboxylic acid group at the terminal, is α-side chain and the lower chain, having OH group at C-15 position, is a β side chain. The α and β chains are in *trans* configuration in the prostanoic acid. The chiral centre C-15 is a δ nature (PGE). The OH group at C-11 in the E series has the α configuration, however, in unnatural configurations the 11-OH is called 11-epi PGs, having arms fused C to each other and are named as iso prostaglandins.

BIOSYNTHESIS

PGs are found in virtually all the tissues and organs. They are autocrine and paracrine lipid mediators that act on platelet endothelium, uterine tissues, and mast cells among others. The biosynthesis of PGE and PGF has been thoroughly established and both of them are derived from arachidonic acid. Two types of pathways have been proposed and are designated as follows:

1. Cyclooxygenase pathway
2. Lipoxygenase pathway

CYCLOOXYGENASE PATHWAY

Arachidonic acid is derived from dietary linoleic acid. It is present as a conjugated component of the phospholipid matrix of the most cellular membrane. Release of free arachidonic acid is due to the stimulation of phospholipase enzyme in response to some traumatic events (tissues damage, toxin, exposure, and hormonal stimulation). The first step in this pathway is the interaction of arachidonic acid with PGH synthase, a haemoprotein, that catalyses both the addition of oxygen and subsequent reduction (peroxide activity) of the 15th position of hydroperoxide to 15(s) configuration alcohol prostaglandin H_2

(PGH$_2$). PGH synthase is also called as cyclooxygenase I (COX-1) or cyclooxygenase II (COX-2). NSAIDs inhibit PGs synthesis; leading to relief of the pain, fever, and inflammation.

PGH$_2$ serves as a substrate for specific enzymes, leading to the production of various PGs, TXA$_2$, and PGI$_2$. While PGE$_2$ is formed by the action of endoperoxide isomerase on PGH$_2$ and PGD$_2$ by the action of isomerase or glutathione-s-transferase on PGH$_2$. PGF$_2$ is formed from PGH$_2$ via endoperoxidase reductase. Thromboxane synthetase acts on PGH$_2$ to produce thromboxane A$_2$.

LIPOXYGENASE PATHWAY

Lipoxygenase are a group of enzymes that oxidize polyunsaturated fatty acid possessing two *cis* double bond separated by a methylene group to produce lipid peroxides. Arachidonic acid is metabolized to form a number of hydroperoxy eicosatetraenoic acid (HPETE) derivatives. These enzymes differ in the position at which they peroxidize arachidonic acid and in the tissues specificity. For example, platelets possess only 12-lipoxygenase, whereas leukocytes possess both 12-lipoxygenase and 5-lipoxygenase. Leukotriens are products of the 5-lipoxygenase pathways and are divided into major classes.

Hydroxylate eicosotetraenoic acid (LTs) is represented by lymphotoxin β_4 (LTB_4) and peptido leukotrienes (PLTs), such as leukotriene C4 (LTC_4), leukotriene D4 (LTD_4) and LTE_4. Lipoxygenase produces leukotrienase from 5-HPETE. Lysine epsilon-aminotransferase (LAT) synthetase converts 5-HPETE to unstable epoxide termed leukotriene A4 (LTA_4) that may be converted by the enzymes into the leukotriene, LTB_4 or by LTC_4 to other leukotrienes (e.g. LTD_4, LTE_4, and LTF_4), and reconjugation with glycine and glutamic acid, respectively.

SAR of PGs

In the upper chain: Methyl esters (misoprostol), sulphonamide (sulprostone), and hydroxyl group (rioprost) possess greater activity than natural PGs.

In the cyclopentane ring: Variation in the cyclopentane ring results in a reduction in the PG activity. Enlargement of the ring or reduction of the ring leads to inactive compounds. Replacement of the carbon atom of cyclopentane ring by O, S, and N also leads to inactive compounds. Replacement of 9-keto group with =CH_2 group gives active (metenprost) PG.

In the lower chain: C-15 hydroxyl group is protected (from metabolism) by the introduction of methyl group at C-15 and gem dimethyl group at C-16. The shifting of C-15 hydroxyl to C-16 position increases the metabolic stability of alkoxy, phenoxy (enprostil, sulprostone) analogues, and they are more active than natural PGs. Introduction of acetylinic group at C-13 and C-14 increase the leuteolytic activity.

SYNTHESIS AND DRUG PROFILE

i. Prostaglandin E_1 (PGE_1)

(*E*)-7-(3-hydroxy-2-(3-hydroxydec-1-enyl)-5-oxocyclopentyl)heptanoicacid

Drugs Acting on Inflammation/Allergy

Synthesis

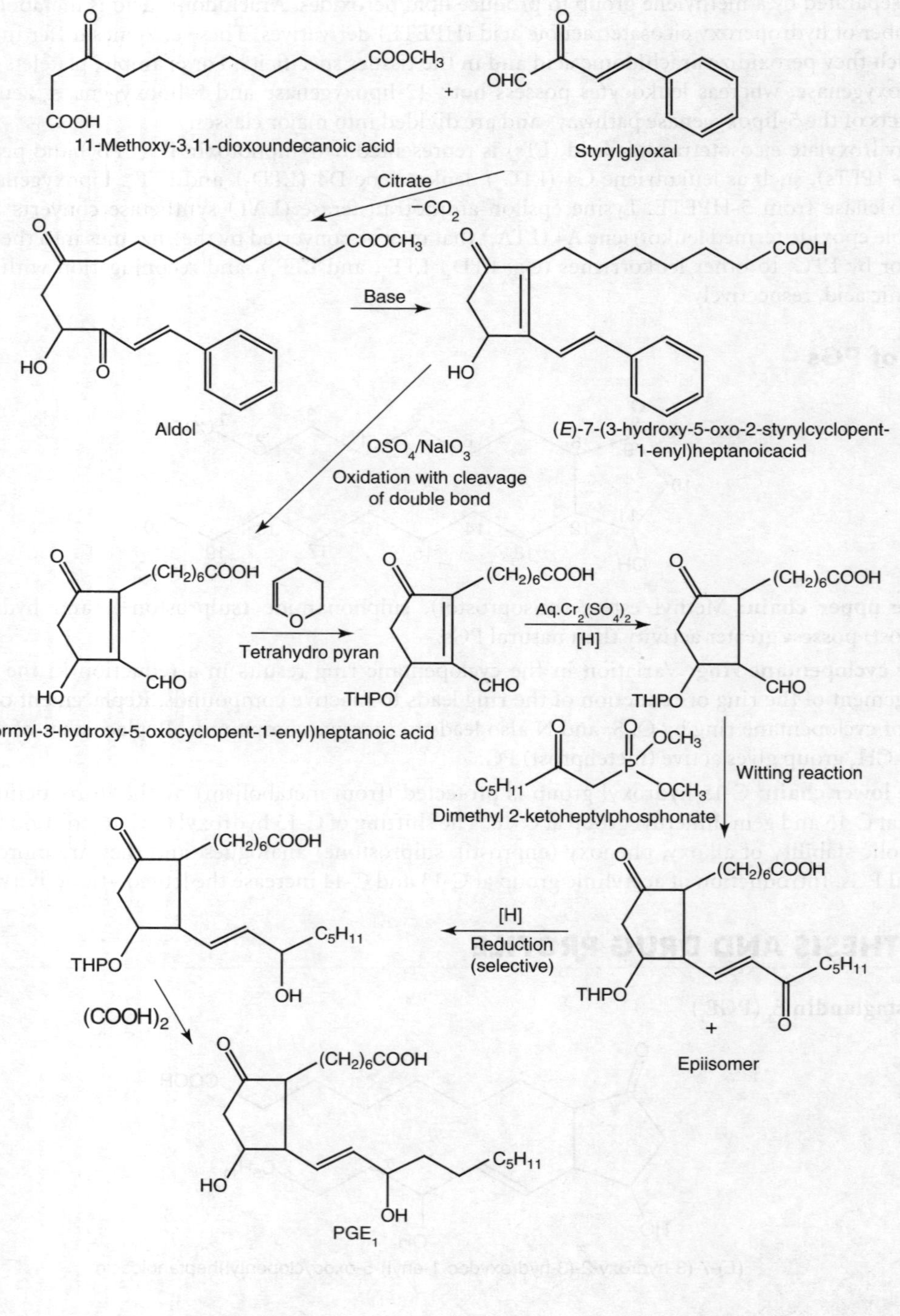

11-Methoxy-3,11-dioxoundecanoic acid + Styrylglyoxal

Citrate, $-CO_2$ → Aldol

Base → (E)-7-(3-hydroxy-5-oxo-2-styrylcyclopent-1-enyl)heptanoic acid

OsO_4/$NaIO_3$, Oxidation with cleavage of double bond →

7-(2-Formyl-3-hydroxy-5-oxocyclopent-1-enyl)heptanoic acid

Tetrahydro pyran →

Aq.$Cr_2(SO_4)_2$ [H] →

Dimethyl 2-ketoheptylphosphonate, Witting reaction →

[H] Reduction (selective) → + Epiisomer

$(COOH)_2$ →

PGE_1

Dose: A dose of misoprostol, 200 μg three times a day for acute duodenal ulcer and comparable with cimetidine.

ii. Prostaglandin D$_2$ [PGD$_2$]

(Z)-7-(5-Hydroxy-2-((S,E)-3-hydroxyoct-1-enyl)-3-oxocyclopentyl)hept-5-enoic acid

Synthesis

PGF₂α

(E)-7-((1R,3R,5S)-3,5-dihydroxy-2-((E)-3-hydroxyoct-1-enyl)cyclopentyl)hept-5-enoic acid

Synthesis

Metabolism: PGs are rapidly metabolized and inactivated by various oxidative and reductive pathways. The initial step involves rapid oxidation of the 15 α-OH group to the corresponding ketone by the PG-specific enzyme called PG 15 α-OH dehydrogenase. This is followed by a reduction of the C-13 and C-14 double bond by PG Δ^{13}-reductase to the corresponding dihydroketone, which represent the major metabolite in plasma. Subsequently, enzymes normally involved in 13 and ω oxidation of fatty acids more slowly cleave the α-chain and oxidize the C-20 terminal methyl group to the carboxylic acid derivative, respectively.

PROBABLE QUESTIONS

1. What are PGs? Classify them with their chemical structure.
2. Write the SAR of PGs.
3. Write the nomenclature of different types of PGs.
4. Write the structure, chemical name, synthesis, and uses of the following compounds.
   (a) PGE_1 (b) PGD_2
5. Explain the role of PGs and eicosanoids to combat the following diseases:
   (a) Gastric ulceration (b) Management of congenital heart disease

SUGGESTED READINGS

1. Abraham DJ (ed). *Burger's Medicinal Chemistry and Drug Discovery* (6th edn). New Jersey: John Wiley, 2007.
2. Axen U, Pike JE, and Schneider WP. 'The total synthesis of prostaglandins'. In *The Total Synthesis of Natural Products*, Vol. I, J Apsimon (ed), pp. 81–142. New York: John Wiley, 1973.
3. Bruntan LL, Lazo JS, and Parker KL. *Goodman and Gilman's: The Pharmacological Basis of Therapeutics* (11th edn). New York: McGraw Hill, 2006.
4. Bailey JM (ed). *Prostaglandins, Leukotrienes and Lipoxins*. New York: Plenum Press, 1985.
5. Davis-Bruno KL and Halushka PV. 'Molecular pharmacology and therapeutic potential of thromboxane A2 receptor'. *Adv Drug Res* 25: 173–202, 1994.
6. Flower RJ. 'Eicosanoids: The nobel prize'. *Trends in Pharmacol Sci* 4: 1–2, 1983.
7. Gennaro AR. *Remington's The Science and Practice of Pharmacy* (21st edn). New York: Lippincot Williams and Wilkins, 2006.
8. Lednicer D and Mitscher LA. *The Organic Chemistry of Drug Synthesis*. New York: John Wiley, 1995.
9. Lemke TL and William DA. *Foye's Principle of Medicinal Chemistry* (6th edn). New York: Lippincott Williams and Wilkins, 2008.
10. Reynolds EF (ed). *Martindale the Extra Pharmacopoeia* (31st edn). London: The Pharmaceutical Press, 1997.
11. Roberts SM and Scheinmann F. *New Synthetic Routes to Prostaglandins and Thromboxanes*. London: Academic Press, 1982.
12. Vane JR and Grady J (eds). *Therapeutic Application of Prostaglandins*. Boston: Edward Arnold, 1993.

Chapter 3

Analgesics, Antipyretics, and NSAIDs

INTRODUCTION

Nonsteroidal anti-inflammatory drugs (NSAIDs) are used primarily to treat inflammation, mild-to-moderate pain, and fever. Specific uses include the treatment of headache, arthritis, sports injuries, and menstrual cramps. Aspirin is used to inhibit the clotting of blood and prevent strokes and heart attacks in individuals at high risk. NSAIDs are also included in many cold and allergic preparations.

NSAIDs are associated with a number of side effects. The frequency of side effects varies according to the drugs; the most common side effects are gastro intestinal tract (GIT) disturbances, such as nausea, diarrhoea, constipation, vomiting, decreased appetite, and peptic ulcer. NSAIDs may also cause fluid retention, leading to oedema; the most serious side effects are kidney failure, liver failure, ulcers, and prolonged bleeding after an injury of surgery. Some individuals are allergic to NSAIDs and may develop shortness of breath when NSAIDs are administered. People with asthma are at a higher risk for experiencing serious allergic reaction to NSAIDs. Use of aspirin in children and teenagers with chicken pox or influenza has been associated with the development of Reye's syndrome. Therefore, aspirin and salicylate should not be used in children and teenagers with suspected or confirmed chicken pox or influenza.

Antipyretics are the drugs that reduce the elevated body temperature. Anti-inflammatory agents are used to cure or prevent inflammation caused by prostaglandin (PGE_2). These drugs are widely utilized for the alleviation of minor aches, pains, fever, and symptomatic treatment of rheumatic fever, rheumatoid arthritis, and osteoarthritis. The biosynthetic pathway of prostaglandins (PGs) is depicted in Figure 3.1.

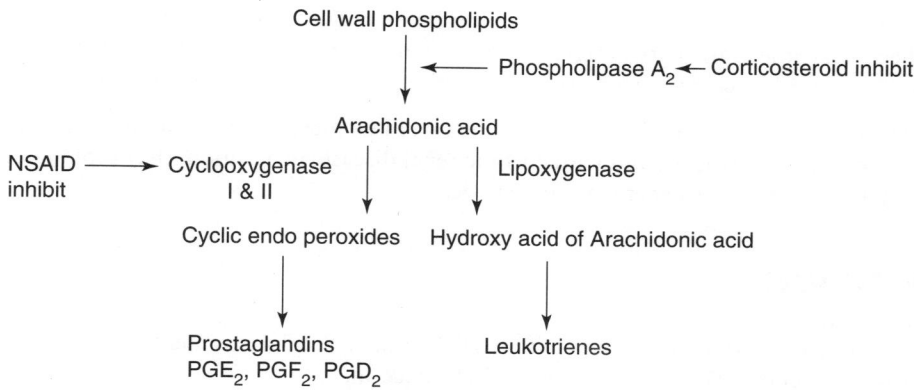

Figure 3.1 Biosynthetic pathway of PGs.

General Structure of PG

PG is a naturally occurring 20-carbon cyclopentano fatty acid derivative, derived from arachidonic acid.

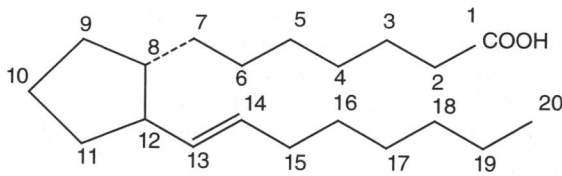

Mode of action: NSAIDs inhibit cycloxygenase (COX), the enzyme that catalyses the synthesis of cyclic endoperoxides, from the arachidonic acid to form PGs. The two COX isoenzymes are COX-1 and COX-2. The function of COX-1 is to produce PGs that are involved in normal cellular activity, (protection of gastric mucosa, maintenance of kidney function). While, COX-2 is responsible for the production of PGs at the inflammation sites. Most NSAIDs inhibit both COX-1 and COX-2 with varying degree of selectivity. Selective COX-2 inhibitor may eliminate the side effects associated with NSAIDs due to COX-1 inhibition, such as gastric and renal effect.

Side Effects

In stomach: Biosynthesis of PGs, especially PGE_2 and PGI_2, serves as cytoprotective agents in gastric mucosa; these PGs inhibit acid secretion by the stomach, enhance mucosal blood flow, and promote the secretion of cytoprotective mucus in the GIT. Inhibition of the PGs synthesis may make the stomach more susceptible to damage and lead to gastric ulcer.

In platelets: Platelet's function get disturbed because NSAIDs prevent the formation of Thromboxane A_2 (TXA_2) in platelets, as TXA_2 is a potent platelet-aggregating agent. This accounts for the tendency of these drugs to increase the bleeding time and this side effect has been exploited in the prophylactic treatment of thromboembolic disorder.

In uterus: NSAIDs prolong gestation because of the inhibition of PGF_2 in uterus. PGF_2 is a potent uterotropic agent and their biosynthesis by uterus increase dramatically in the hours before parturition. Accordingly, some anti-inflammatory drugs have been used as a colytic agent to inhibit preterm labour.

In kidney: NSAIDs decrease renal blood flow and the rate of glomerular filtration in patients with congestive heart failure, hepatic cirrhosis, and with chronic renal disease, in addition, they prolong the retention of salt and water, this may cause oedema in some patients.

CLASSIFICATION

I. Salicylic acid derivatives: Aspirin, Diflunisal, Salsalate, Sulphasalazine.
II. p-Amino phenol derivatives: Paracetamol, Phenacetin.
III. Pyrazolidine dione derivatives: Phenyl butazone, Oxyphenbutazone, Sulphin-pyrazone.
IV. Anthranilic acid derivatives: Mefenemic acid, Flufenemic acid, Meclofenamate.
V. Aryl alkanoic acid derivative.
   a. Indole acetic acid: Indomethacin.
   b. Indene acetic acid: Sulindac.
   c. Pyrrole acetic acid: Tolmetin, Zormipirac.
   d. Phenyl acetic (propionic) acid: Ibuprofen, Diclofenac, Naproxen, Caprofen, Fenoprofen, Keto-profen, Flurbiprofen, Ketorolac, Etodaolac.
VI. Oxicams: Piroxicam, Meloxicam, Tenoxicam.
VII. Selective COX-2 inhibitors: Celecoxib, Rofecoxib, Valdecoxib.
VIII. Gold compounds: Auronofin, Aurothioglucose, Aurothioglucamide, Aurothiomalate sodium.
IX. Miscellaneous: Nabumetone, Nimesulide, Analgin.
X. Drug used in gout: Allopurinoll, Probenecid, sulphinpyrazone.

I. Salicylates

Salicylates not only posses antipyretic, analgesic, and anti-inflammatory properties, but also other actions that have been proven to be therapeutically beneficial because salicylates promote the excretion of uric acid and they are useful in the treatment of gouty arthritis. More attention has been given to the ability of salicylates (aspirin) to inhibit platelet aggregation, which may contribute to heart attack and strokes, and hence, aspirin reduces the risk of myocardial infarction. In addition, a recent study suggested that aspirin and other NSAIDs might be protective against colon cancer.

Structural Activity Relationship (SAR) of Salicylates

- The active moiety of salicylates is salicylate anion, side effects of aspirin, particularly GIT effects appear to be associated with the carboxylic acid functional group.
- Reducing the acidity of the carboxy group results in a change in the potency of activity. Example—the corresponding amide (salicylamide) retain the analgesic action of salicylic acid, but is devoid of anti-inflammatory properties.
- Substitution on either the carboxyl or phenolic hydroxyl group may affect the potency and toxicity. Benzoic acid itself has only week activity.
- Placement of the phenolic hydroxyl group at meta or para to the carboxyl group abolish the activity.

- Substitution of halogen atom on the aromatic ring enhances potency and toxicity.
- Substitution of aromatic ring at the 5th position of salicylic acid increase anti-inflammatory activity (diflunisal).

Metabolism of salicylic acid derivatives: The initial route of metabolism of these derivatives is their conversion to salicylic acid, which is excreted in urine as free acid (10%) or undergoes conjugation with either glycine to produce the major metabolites of salicylic acid (75%) or with glucuronic acid to form glucuronide (15%). In addition, small amount of metabolites resulting from microsomal aromatic hydroxylation leads to gentisic acid.

i. Aspirin (Emipirin, Bufferin)

2-Acetoxybenzoic acid (or) Acetyl salicylate

Synthesis

Salicylic acid + $(CH_3CO)_2O$ $\xrightarrow{H^+}$ Aspirin

Properties and uses: Aspirin is a white crystalline powder, slightly soluble in water and soluble in alcohol, indicated for the relief of minor aches and mild-to-moderate pain in the conditions such as arthritis and related arthritic condition. Also used in myocardial infarction prophylaxis.

Assay: Dissolve the sample in alcohol and add 0.5 M sodium hydroxide. Allow to stand and titrate against 0.5 M hydrochloric acid using phenolphthalein as an indicator. Perform a blank titration.

Dose: Usual adult dose: 300 to 650 mg every 3 or 4 h orally or 650 mg to 1.3 g as the sustained-release tablet every 8 h; rectal, 200 mg to 1.3 g three or four times a day.

Dosage forms: Aspirin tablets I.P., B.P., Dispersible aspirin tablets B.P., Effervescent soluble aspirin tablets B.P., Gastro-resistant aspirin tablets B.P., Aspirin and Caffeine tablets B.P., Co-codaprin tablets B.P., Dispersible co-codaprin tablets B.P.

ii. Sodium salicylate

Sodium 2-hydroxybenzoate

Synthesis

$$2 \text{ Salicylic acid} + Na_2CO_3 \longrightarrow 2 \text{ Sodium salicylate} + H_2O + CO_2$$

Properties and uses: Sodium salicylate is a white crystalline powder, soluble in water, sparingly soluble in alcohol. It is used for fever and for the relief of pain. It also possesses anti-inflammatory actions similar to aspirin and symptomatic therapy of gout.

Assay: Dissolve the sample in anhydrous acetic acid and titrate against 0.1 M perchloric acid. Determine the end-point potentiometrically.

iii. Salsalate (Disalacid, Saloxium)

2-(2-Hydroxybenzoyloxy)benzoic acid

Synthesis

Benzyl salicylate + Benzyloxy benzoyl chloride

$-H_2O$ ↓

Debenzylation
H^+/catalyst

Salsalate

Properties and uses: Salsalate or salicylsalicylic acid is a dimer of salicylic acid. It is insoluble in gastric juice, but is soluble in the small intestine where it is partially hydrolyzed into two molecules of salicylic acid and absorbed. It does not cause GI blood loss. It has antipyretic, analgesic, and anti-inflammatory properties similar to those of aspirin. It is employed in the treatment of rheumatoid arthritis and other rheumatic disorders.

Dose: Usual adult dose is 325–1000 mg 2–3 times a day, orally.

iv. Sulphasalazine (Azultidine, Azaline)

Properties and uses: Sulphasalazine is a bright yellow or brownish-yellow fine powder, practically insoluble in water and methylene chloride, very slightly soluble in alcohol, soluble in dilute solutions of alkali hydroxides. Sulphasalazine is a mutual prodrug. In large intestine, it is activated to liberate 5-amino salicylic acid, which in turn inhibits PG synthesis and the sulphapyridine is useful for the treatment of infection. Hence, sulphasalazine is used in the treatment of ulcerative colitis.

Synthesis

Assay: Dissolve and dilute the sample in 0.1 M sodium hydroxide and add 0.1 M acetic acid and measure the absorbance at the maxima of 359 nm using ultraviolet spectrophotometer. Prepare a standard solution at the same time and in the same manner, using sulphasalazine reference standard.

Dose: Dose orally is initially 3–4 g daily, followed by 500 mg four times a day for maintenance.

Dosage forms: Sulphasalazine tablets B.P.

v. Diflunisal

5-(2, 4-Diflurophenyl) salicylic acid

Synthesis

2,4 Difluro nitro biphenyl →
(i) Reduction
(ii) Diazotisation
(iii) Δ with HCl
→ (4'-fluoro-2'-fluoro-4-hydroxybiphenyl)

Carboxylation | K_2CO_3 / CO_2

→ Diflunisal

Properties and uses: Diflunisal is a white crystalline powder, practically insoluble in water, soluble in alcohol, and dilute solutions of alkali hydroxides. It is more potent than aspirin, but produces fewer side effects, and has a biological half-life 3–4 times greater than that of aspirin. It is a nonselective cyclooxygenase inhibitor used as antipyretic, analgesic, and anti-inflammatory.

Assay: Dissolve the sample in methanol, add water, and titrate against 0.1 M sodium hydroxide using phenol red as indicator, until the colour changes from yellow to reddish-violet.

II. *p*-Amino phenol derivatives

These derivatives possess analgesic and antipyretic action, but lack anti-inflammatory effects. Acetanilide was introduced into the therapy in 1886 as an antipyretic–analgesic agent. However, it was subsequently found to be too toxic, having been associated with methemaglobinemia and jaundice.

Phenacetin was introduced in the following year and was widely used but was withdrawn recently because of its nephrotoxicity. Acetaminophen (paracetamol) was introduced in 1893 and it remains the only useful agent of this group used as an antipyretic and an analgesic agent.

Acetanilide | Phenacetin | Paracetamol

Metabolism of para aminophenol derivatives: These drugs undergo hydrolysis to yield aniline derivatives that produce directly or through their conversion to hydroxylamine derivatives, such as Acetaminophen that undergoes rapid first pass metabolism in the GIT to *o*-sulphate conjugate. The *N*-hydroxylamine is then converted into a reactive toxic metabolite, acetiminoquinone, which produce toxicity to the kidney and liver in conjugation with hepatic glutathione to form mercapturic acid or cysteine conjugates.

SAR of *p*-amino Phenol Derivatives

1. Etherification of the phenolic function with methyl or propyl groups produces derivatives with greater side effects than ethyl derivatives.
2. Substituents of the nitrogen atom, which reduce the basicity, also reduce activity unless the substituent is metabolically labile. Example—acetyl groups.
3. Amides derived from aromatic acid. Example—*N*-phenyl benzamides that are less active or inactive.

i. Phenacetin (Acetophenetidin)

C_2H_5O—⟨benzene ring⟩—$NHCOCH_3$

p-Ethoxy acetanilide

Synthesis

Route I. From: *p*-nitro phenol

P-Nitro phenol $\xrightarrow[\text{NaOH, }-HBr]{C_2H_5-Br \text{ under pressure}}$ P-Ethoxy nitro benzene $\xrightarrow[(H)]{Fe/HCl}$ P-Ethoxy amino benzene $\xrightarrow[\text{Acetylation }(CH_3CO)_2O]{CH_3COOH}$ Phenacetin

Route II. From: aniline

Aniline $\xrightarrow[\text{(ii) KOH}]{\text{(i) }H_2SO_4}$ *p*-aminophenol $\xrightarrow[CH_3COOH]{\text{Acetylation }(CH_3CO)_2O}$ *p*-hydroxyacetanilide $\xrightarrow[\text{Ethylation}]{C_2H_5Br}$ Phenacetin

Route III. From: chlorobenzene

Chlorobenzene $\xrightarrow[H_2SO_4]{\text{Nitration }HNO_3}$ *p*-nitrochlorobenzene $\xrightarrow[-NaCl]{C_2H_5ONa}$ *p*-ethoxynitrobenzene $\xrightarrow[(H)]{Fe/HCl}$ *p*-ethoxyaminobenzene $\xrightarrow[\text{Acetylation }(CH_3CO)_2O]{CH_3COOH}$ Phenacetin

Properties and uses: It exists as a white glistering powder with a bitter taste, sparingly soluble in water and soluble in chloroform. It is an analgesic and an antipyretic with similar effectiveness as an aspirin. It has a greater potential for toxicity (hemolytic anaemia and methemoglobinaemia) than paracetamol.

Dose: Usual dose as oral for adults is 300 mg to 2 g per day.

ii. Paracetamol (Metacin, Tylenol, Tapar, Calpol)

Para-acetamino phenol

Synthesis

Para-nitro phenol $\xrightarrow[\text{Reduction}]{[H]}$ Para-amino phenol $\xrightarrow[\text{Glacial acetic acid}]{(CH_3CO)_2O}$ Paracetamol

Properties and uses: Paracetamols exist as white crystalline powder, sparingly soluble in water, soluble in alcohol, and very slightly soluble in methylene chloride. Paracetamols produce antipyresis by acting on the hypothalamic heat-regulating centre and analgesia by elevating the pain threshold. Hepatic necrosis and death have been observed following over dosage; hepatic damage is likely in an adult who takes more than 10 g in a single dose or if a 2-year old child takes more than 3 g.

Assay: Dissolve the sample in a mixture of water and dilute sulphuric acid (1:3), reflux, cool, and dilute with water. Add dilute hydrochloric acid and titrate against 0.1 M cerium sulphate using ferroin as an indicator until a greenish-yellow colour is obtained. Perform a blank titration.

Dose: Usual oral adult dose is 500 mg to 1 g for three or four times a day.

Dosage forms: Paracetamol tablets I.P, B.P., Paracetamol syrup I.P., Co-codamol tablets B.P., Effervescent Co-codamol tablets B.P., Co-dydramol tablets B.P., Co-proxamol tablets B.P., Paracetamol capsules B.P., Paediatric paracetamol oral solution B.P., Paracetamol oral suspension B.P., Paracetamol suppositories B.P., Dispersible paracetamol tablets B.P., soluble paracetamol tablets B.P.

III. 3, 5-Pyrazolidinediones

Name	R	R₁
Phenyl butazone	–H	–C_4H_9
Oxyphenbutazone	–OH	–C_4H_9
Sulphin pyrazone	–H	–$(CH_2)_2SOC_6H_5$

SAR of 3, 5-Pyrazolidinediones

- Replacement of one of the nitrogen atom in the pyrazolidinediones with an oxygen atom yields isoxazole analogues, which are as active as pyrazolidinediones derivatives.
- In 3, 5-pyrazolidinedione derivatives, pharmacological activities are closely related to their acidity, the dicarbonyl function at the 3rd and 5th positions enhance the acidity of hydrogen atom at the 4th position.
- Presence of a keto group in the γ-position of the butyl side chain produces the active compound.
- Decreasing or eliminating acidity by removing the acidic proton at 4th position (e.g. 4, 4-dialkyl derivatives) abolishes anti-inflammatory activity. Thus, if the hydrogen atom at the 4th position of phenyl butazone is replaced by substituents, such as a methyl group, antiinflammation activity is abolished.
- If acidity is enhanced too much, anti-inflammatory and sodium-retaining activities decrease while other properties, such as the uricosuric effect increases.
- Introduction of polar function in these alkyl groups give mixed results. The γ-hydroxy-*n*-butyl derivative posseses pronounced uricosuric activity, but give fewer anti-inflammatory effects.
- Substitution of 2-phenyl thio ethyl group at the 4th position produces antigout activity (sulphinpyrazone).
- Presence of both the phenyl groups is essential for neither anti-inflammatory nor analgesic activity.
- *m*-Substitution of aryl rings of the phenyl butazone gives uniformly inactive compounds. *p*-Substitution, such as methyl, chloro, nitro, or OH of one or both rings retains activity.

i. Phenylbutazone (Butazolidin, Busone)

4-^{n}Butyl-1,2 biphenyl-3, 5 pyrazolidinedione

Synthesis
Route I. From: Diethylmalonate

Diethyl malonate $\xrightarrow{\underset{CH_3(CH_2)_3Br}{C_2H_5ONa}}$ butyl diethyl malonate $\xrightarrow{\text{Diphenyl hydrazine (NH-C}_6\text{H}_5, \text{NH-C}_6\text{H}_5)}$ Phenylbutazone

Route II. From: Diethyl-butyl malonate or butyl malonylchloride

Diethyl butyl malonate (C$_4$H$_9$—CH(COOC$_2$H$_5$)$_2$)

(Or)

Butyl malonyl chloride (C$_4$H$_9$—CH(COCl)$_2$) + Diphenyl hydrazine $\xrightarrow[\text{at 0°C pyridine}]{\text{ether solution}}$ Phenylbutazone

Properties and uses: Phenylbutazone is a white crystalline powder, practically insoluble in water, sparingly soluble in alcohol, and soluble in alkaline solutions. It is a pyrazole derivative that has antipyretic, analgesic, and anti-inflammatory actions, because of its toxicity it is not used as a general antipyretic or analgesic. It is a usual practice reserved for use in the treatment of osteoarthrosis, ankylosing spondylitis, arthritis, acute superficial thrombophlebitis, painful shoulder, and Reiter's disease, where less toxic drugs have failed.

Assay: Dissolve the sample in acetone and titrate against 0.1 M sodium hydroxide using bromothymol blue as indicator until a blue colour is obtained, which persists for few seconds. Perform a blank titration.

Dose: The usual dose is 100–600 mg per day.

ii. Oxyphenbutazone (Tandearil, Oxaril)

Synthesis
Route I. From aniline

Route II. From: Diethyl butyl malonate

[Reaction scheme: Diethyl butyl malonate + 1-benzoyloxy-4-(2-phenylhydrazinyl)benzene derivative → (condensation, cyclization, –C₂H₅OH, C₂H₅ONa in absolute ethanol) → benzoylated phenylbutazone intermediate → (debenzoylation by hydrolysis) → Oxyphenbutazone]

Properties and uses: It exists as a white to yellowish white, odourless, crystalline powder, soluble in water, alcohol, chloroform, and ether. Used as an analgesic and in arthritis.

Dose: Usual oral adult dose for antirheumatic is 100 or 200 mg three times daily; for maintenance the dose is 100 mg one to four times a day; for the treatment of gout 400 mg initially as a loading dose, then 100 mg every 4 h.

IV. Anthranilic acid derivatives (Fenamates)

The anthranilic acid class NSAIDs result from the application of classic medicinal chemistry bioisosteric drug design concepts as these derivatives are nitrogen isoteres of salicylic acid.

[Structure: N-phenylanthranilic acid — benzene ring with COOH and NH-phenyl substituents ortho to each other]

SAR of Anthranilic Acid Derivatives (Fenamates)

- The position of the carboxyl function is important for the activity of anthranilic acid derivatives that are active, whereas the 3 and 4 amino benzoic acid analogues are not active.
- Replacement of carboxylic acid function with the isosteric tetrazole results in the retention of anti-inflammatory activity.
- Placement of substitution on the anthranilic acid ring generally reduces the activity.
- Substitution on the N-aryl ring can lead to conflicting results. In the ultraviolet erythema assay for anti-inflammatory activity, the order of activity was generally 3′ > 2′ > 4′ for mono substitution with CF_3 group (flufenamic acid) being particularly potent. The opposite order of activity was observed in rat paw oedema assay, the 2′–Cl derivatives being more potent than 3′–Cl analogues.
- In disubstituted derivatives, where the nature of the two substitutes is the same 2′, 3′-disubstitution appears to be the most effective (mefenemic acid).
- The NH moiety of anthranilic acid is essential for the activity as the replacement of NH function with O, CH_2, S, SO_2, N-CH_3, or $NCOCH_3$ functionalities significantly reduced the activity.

i. Flufenamic Acid (Arlef, Tarlef)

N (α,α,α-Trifluoro-m-tolyl) Anthranilic acid

Synthesis

o-Iodo benzoic acid + m-Trifluoro methyl aniline → (Copper-bronze Ullman condensation) → Flufenamic acid

Properties and uses: Flufenamic acid is a pale yellow crystalline powder or needles. It has analgesic, anti-inflammatory, and antipyretic actions; it is employed in the treatment of rheumatic disorder and dysmenorrhoea.

Dose: 400–600 mg per day in divided doses.

ii. Mefenamic acid

2-(2,3-Dimethylphenylamino)benzoic acid

Synthesis

2-Chlorobenzoic acid + 2,3-Dimethylbenzenamine → (Copper-bronze Ullmann condensation) → Mefenamic acid

An analogues approach by reaction of *o*-chloro benzoic acid with 2,3-dimethyl aniline.

Metabolism: Its metabolism occurs through regioselective oxidation of 3-methyl group and glucuronidation of mephanamic acid. Majority of the 3-hydroxy methyl metabolite and dicarboxylic acid products are excreted.

Uses: Used as an analgesic and anti-inflammatory agent.

iii. Meclofenamate Sodium

Sodium 3-(2,6-dichloro-3-methylphenylamino)benzoate

Synthesis: It is obtained by Ullman condensation employing 2, 6 dichloro 3-methyl aniline.

V. Arylalkanoic acids

General structure

SAR of Arylalkanoic Acids

1. The centre of acidity is usually located one carbon atom adjacent to a flat surface represented by an aromatic or hetero aromatic ring.
2. The distance between these centres is critical because increasing this distance to two or three carbons generally decreases activity.
3. All agents possess a centre of acidity, which can be represented by a carboxylic acid and hydroxamic acid, a sulphonamide or a terazole.
4. Substitution of a methyl group on the carbon atom separating the aromatic ring leads to enhancement of anti-inflammatory activity.

a. Indole acetic acid derivatives
i. Indomethacin (Indocin, Indocid)

1-(p-Chloro benzoyl)-5-methoxy-2 methyl indole-3-acetic acid.

Synthesis

Metabolism: It is converted into inactive metabolites, that is, 50% of single dose is 5-O-demethylated and 10% conjugated with glucuronic acid. Nonhepatic enzymes hydrolyze indomethacin to N-deacetylated metabolite.

Properties and uses: It is a white or yellow crystalline powder, insoluble in water and sparingly soluble in alcohol. Indomethacin is more effective than aspirin. The most frequent side effects are gastric distress and headache. It also has been associated with peptic ulceration, blood disorders, and possible death (these side effects appear to be closely related and sometimes can be minimized by reducing the dose). It is not recommended for use in children because of possible interference with the resistance to infection. Used as anti-inflammatory and analgesic in rheumatic arthritis, spondylitis, and to lesser extent in gout.

Assay: Dissolve the sample in acetone and pass nitrogen for 15 min and titrate with 0.1 M sodium hydroxide using phenolphthalein as indicator.

Dose: In gout, usual adult dose orally is 100 mg initially, followed by 50 mg three times a day until pain is relieved. As an antirheumatic by oral route, the dose is 50 mg two or three times a day. And as an antipyretic, the dose is orally 25–50 mg three times a day.

Dosage forms: Indometacin capsules I.P., B.P., Indometacin Suppositories I.P., B.P.

V. b. Indeneacetic acid derivatives
i. Sulindac (Clinoril)

5 Fluoro-2-methyl-1[(4 methyl sulphinyl) phenyl methylene] Indene-3-acetic acid

Metabolism: It is a prodrug to form active metabolites of sulphite. In addition to it, sulindac is oxidized to corresponding sulphone and other sulphone-glucuronide conjugates.

Properties and uses: Suindac is a yellow crystalline powder, very slightly soluble in water, soluble in methylene chloride, and dilute solutions of alkali hydroxides, sparingly soluble in alcohol. The (Z) isomer of sulindac showed much more potent anti-inflammatory activity than the corresponding (E)-isomer. The more polar and inactive sulphoxide is virtually the only form excreted. It has analgesic, antipyretic, and anti-inflammatory properties. It is usually employed in the treatment of rheumatic and muscular skeletal disorders, acute gouty arthritis, and osteoarthritis.

Synthesis
Route I. From: 3-(4-fluorophenyl)-2-methyl propanoic acid

Synthesis
Route II. From *p*-Fluoro benzaldehyde

p-Flouro benzaldehyde → [(CH₃CH₂CO)₂O, C₂H₅COONa] → fluoro cinnamic acid derivative → [Pd–C, H₂] → fluoro phenyl propionic acid → [Phosphoric acid, 95°C, –H₂O] → **6-Fluoro-2-methyl Indanone** → [CN CH₂ COOH, CH₃COONH₄, –H₂O] → cyano-carboxylic indanylidene → [–CO₂] → CH–CN indanylidene → [equilibrium] → CH₂CN indene → [(i) KOH (ii) HCl] → CH₂COOH indene → [NaOCH₃, *P*-Thiomethyl benzal (H₃C-S-C₆H₄-CHO)] → Z-Isomer predominate (thiomethyl benzylidene indene acetic acid) → [NaIO₄, [O]] → **Sulindac**

Assay: Dissolve the sample in methanol and titrate against 0.1 M sodium hydroxide. Determine the end point potentiometrically.

Dose: Usual adult oral dose is 150 mg twice a day with food.

Dosage forms: Sulindac tablets B.P.

SAR of Indole Acetic Acid Derivatives

1. Placement of other acidic functionalities instead of the carboxyl group decreases activity and the amide derivatives are inactive.
2. Substituents of R^1 useful for increasing anti-inflammatory activity are ranked as $C_6H_4CH_2$ > alkyl > H.
3. Acylation of the indole nitrogen with aryl/alkyl carboxylic acids results in the decrease of activity.

4. Presence of substituents on the *N*-benzoyl derivatives in the *p*-position with F, Cl, CF$_3$, or S-CH$_3$ groups provide greatest activity.
5. X substituents activity are ranked as 5-OCH$_3$ > N (CH$_3$)$_2$ > CH$_3$ > H.
6. The presence of indole ring nitrogen is not essential for activity because the corresponding 1-benzylidenylindene analogue (sulindac) is also active.
7. Alkyl groups especially methyl group at 2nd position is much active than aryl substituted analogues.
8. Substitution of a methyl group at the α position of the acetic acid side chain leads to equiactive analogues.
9. Anti-inflammatory activity was displayed only by the dextrorotatory enantiomer with similar absolute configuration; it has 25 times the activity of phenylbutazone.

SAR of Pyrrole Acetic Acid Derivative

V. c. Pyrrole acetic acid derivative

Replacement of the *p*-tolyl group with a *p*-chloro benzoyl moiety produced little effect on activity, whereas introduction of a methyl group in the 4th position and 5-*p*-chloro benzoyl analogues (zomeapirac) proved to be four times potent as tolmetin.

i. Tolmetin Sodium (Tolectin)

Sodium 2-(1-methyl-5-(4-methylbenzoyl)-1*H*-pyrrol-2-yl)acetate

Synthesis
From: 1-Methyl pyrrole

Metabolism: It is metabolized extensively first pass, involving hydroxylation of *p*-methyl group to primary alcohol, which is subsequently oxidized to dicarboxylic acid.

Properties and uses: It is a light yellow, crystalline powder, soluble in water, slightly soluble in alcohol. It has antipyretic, analgesic, and anti-inflammatory actions. It is employed in the treatment of rheumatic and musculoskeletal disorders. The drug is, however, comparable to indomethacin and aspirin in the control and management of disease activity.

Dose: Adult oral dose initially is 400 mg three times a day, subsequently adjusted as per patient's response.

ii. Zomepirac (Zomax)

1, 4. Dimethyl-5-(*p*-chloro benzoyl) pyrrole-2-acetic acid

Properties and uses: A greater degree of analgesia for severe pain is claimed for Zomepirac. It is used as an analgesic and an ant-inflammatory drug. It is four times as potent as tolmetin.

Dose: Dose is 400 to 600 mg of zomepirac daily (zomepirac sodium 1.2 g is approximately equivalent to 1 g of zomepirac).

Synthesis
Route I. From Chloro acetone

Route II. From: Enol of ethyl acetone dicarboxylate

[Reaction scheme showing synthesis of Zomepirac from enol of ethyl acetone dicarboxylate, via reaction with CH_3NH_2, then CH_3COCH_2Cl, followed by (i) NaOH, (ii) Δ, (iii) C_2H_5OH/H^+, then (i) Cl-C$_6$H$_4$-COCl, (ii) NaOH to yield Zomepirac]

V. d. Aryl and heteroaryl acetic/propionic acid derivatives

i. Ibuprofen (Brufen, Motrin)

[Structure of ibuprofen]

2 (*p*-Iso butyl-phenyl) propionic acid

Synthesis
Route I. From Isobutyl benzene

[Reaction scheme: Isobutyl benzene → (HCl/HCHO, ZnCl₂, Chloromethylation) → p-isobutyl benzyl chloride → (NaCN) → p-isobutyl benzyl cyanide → (NaNH₂) → sodium salt of nitrile → (CH₃I) → α-methyl nitrile → (H⁺) → Ibuprofen]

Route II. From: Isobutyl benzene

[Reaction scheme: Isobutyl benzene → ((CH₃CO)₂O, Acetylation) → p-Isobutyl acetophenone → (HCN) → Cyanohydrin derivative → ((i) HI reduction, (ii) Hydrolysis) → Ibuprofen]

Metabolism: Oxidative metabolite of ibuprofen and unchanged drugs are excreted in urine. Oxidation involves ω, ω_1, and ω_2 oxidation of the para isobutyl side chain, followed by alcohol oxidation, resulting from ω oxidation to corresponding carboxylic acid.

Properties and uses: Ibuprofen is a white crystalline powder or colourless crystals, practically insoluble in water, soluble in acetone, methanol, methylene chloride, and dilute solutions of alkali hydroxides and carbonates. The precursor Ibufenac, which was abandoned owing to hepatotoxicity, was less potent. Moreover, the activity resides in the (s)–(+) isomer, not only in Ibuprofen but also throughout the arylacetic acid series. Furthermore, these isomers are the more potent inhibitors of PG synthetase. It is an anti-inflammatory drug that possesses antipyretic and analgesic action and is used for the treatment of rheumatoid arthritis and osteoarthritis.

Assay: Dissolve the sample in methanol and titrate against 0.1 M sodium hydroxide using phenolphthalein as indicator, until red colour is obtained. Perform a blank titration

Dose: Usual oral adult dose as an analgesic (dysmenorrhoea) is 200–400 mg four to six times a day; in rheumatoid arthritis and osteoarthritis. The dose is 300–400 mg three or four times a day.

Dosage forms: Ibuprofen tablets I.P., B.P, Ibuprofen cream B.P., Ibuprofen gel B.P., Ibuprofen oral suspension B.P.

ii. Ibufenac

2-(p-Isobutyl-phenyl) acetic acid

Synthesis

Isobutyl benzene → (Friedal–Craft's acylation, CH₃COCl, AlCl₃, –HCl) → P-Isobutyl acetophenone → (Willgerodt oxidation) → Ibufenac

Properties and uses: It was formerly employed in the rheumatic conditions, but was found to cause hepatotoxicity. It has analgesic, antipyretic, and anti-inflammatory actions.

iii. Diclofenac (Voltaren, Voveran)

o-(2, 6-Dichloro anilino) Phenyl acetic acid

Metabolism: There are four major metabolites that are produced by aromatic hydroxylation, that is, 4-hydroxy derivative, 5-hydroxy, 3-hydroxyl, and 4,5-dihydroxy metabolites. Remaining metabolites are excreted as sulphate conjugates.

Properties and uses: Diclofenac sodium is a white or slightly yellowish crystalline slightly hygroscopic powder, sparingly soluble in water, soluble in methanol and alcohol, slightly soluble in acetone. Used in the treatment of rheumatic arthritis.

Assay: Dissolve the sample in anhydrous acetic acid and titrate against 0.1 M perchloric acid. Determine the end point potentiometrically.

Dose: The usual dose is 20–50 mg three times a day. It can also be given as a suppository.

Dosage forms: Diclofenac tablets I.P., Diclofenac injection I.P., Prolonged-release diclofenac tablets B.P., Gastro-resistant diclofenac tablets B.P., Prolonged-release diclofenac injection B.P., Prolonged-release diclofenac capsules B.P.

Synthesis

[Synthesis scheme: 2,6-Dichlorodiphenylamine → (COCl–COCl, –HCl) → N-acyl intermediate → (Cyclization, AlCl₃) → isatin-like intermediate → (NH₂–NH₂, KOH (H)) Wolf-Kishner reduction → Indane derivative → (i) KOH (ii) HCl → Diclofenac]

iv. Naproxen (Naprosyn)

(±)2-(6-Methoxy-2-naphthyl) propionic acid

Metabolism: It is converted to 6-O-desmethyl metabolite and then to glucuronide conjugate.

Properties and uses: Naproxen is a white crystalline powder, practically insoluble in water, soluble in ethanol and in methanol. The drug is fairly comparable to aspirin both in the management and control of disease symptoms. Nevertheless, it has relatively lesser frequency and severity of nervous system together with milder GI-effects. It possesses analgesic, anti-inflammatory, and antipyretic actions, and it is used in the treatment of rheumatic arthritis, dysmenorrhea, and acute gout.

Assay: Dissolve the sample in a mixture of water and methanol (1:3) and titrate against 0.1 M sodium hydroxide, using 1 ml of phenolphthalein solution as indicator.

Dose: For adult in rheumatoid arthritis, 250–375 mg as initial dose two times a day; in acute gout, 750 mg as loading dose followed by 250 mg three times a day until relieved.

Dosage forms: Naproxen oral suspension B.P., Naproxen suppositories B.P., Naproxen tablets B.P., Gastro-resistant naproxen tablets B.P.

Synthesis

[Scheme: Synthesis of (S)-Naproxen starting from 2-Methoxy naphthalene]

2-Methoxy napthalene →(CH₃COCl, AlCl₃)→ 6-methoxy-2-acetylnaphthalene →(Willgerodt-Kindler reaction, HN(morpholine), S)→ thiomorpholide intermediate →(H₂SO₄)→ CH₂COOH derivative →(CH₃OH/H⁺)→ CH₂COOCH₃ derivative →((i) NaH, (ii) CH₃I)→ CH(CH₃)COOCH₃ derivative →(NaOH)→ (±)-2-(6-methoxynaphthalen-2-yl)propionic acid →(Resolved with cinchonidine)→ (S)-Naproxen

v. Fenoprofen (Nalton)

[Structure: 2-(3-Phenoxy phenyl) propionic acid]

Synthesis

1-(4-Phenoxyphenyl)ethanone →(i) NaBH₄ (Reduction); (ii) PBr₃ (Bromination)→ 1-(4-phenoxyphenyl)ethyl bromide →(NaCN)→ nitrile intermediate →(H⁺)→ Fenoprofen

Metabolism: It is metabolized through glucuronide conjugation with a parent drug and CYP2C9 to 4-hydroxy metabolites.

Properties and uses: Fenoprofen calcium is a white crystalline powder, slightly soluble in water and soluble in ethanol. Fenoprofen calcium has anti-inflammatory (antiarthritic) and analgesic properties. It has been shown to inhibit PG synthetase. It is known to reduce joint-swelling, decrease the duration of morning stiffness, and relieve pain. It is also indicated for acute flares and exacerbations and in the long-term management of osteoarthritis and rheumatoid arhrtitis.

Assay: Dissolve the sample in anhydrous acetic acid and titrate against 0.1 M perchloric acid. Determine the end point potentiometrically. Perform a blank titration.

Dose: Dose is 50–100 mg twice daily with food.

Dosage forms: Fenoprofen tablets B.P.

vi. Ketoprofen (Orudis)

2-(3-Benzoyl phenyl) propionic acid

Synthesis
Route I. From: α-Methylene substituted *m*-benzyl phenyl acetic acid

α-Methylene m-benzyl phenyl acetic acid

Ketoprofen

Route II. From: 2-(4-Aminophenyl) propanoic acid

[Scheme: 2-(4-Aminophenyl)propanoic acid → (i) Diazotization, (ii) Thiophene-Potassium xanthate → 4-mercaptophenyl propanoic acid intermediate → +2-iodobenzoic acid, –HI → thioether diacid intermediate → Friedel-Craft's cyclization, –H₂O → thioxanthone propanoic acid → Raney Ni Desulfuration → Ketoprofen]

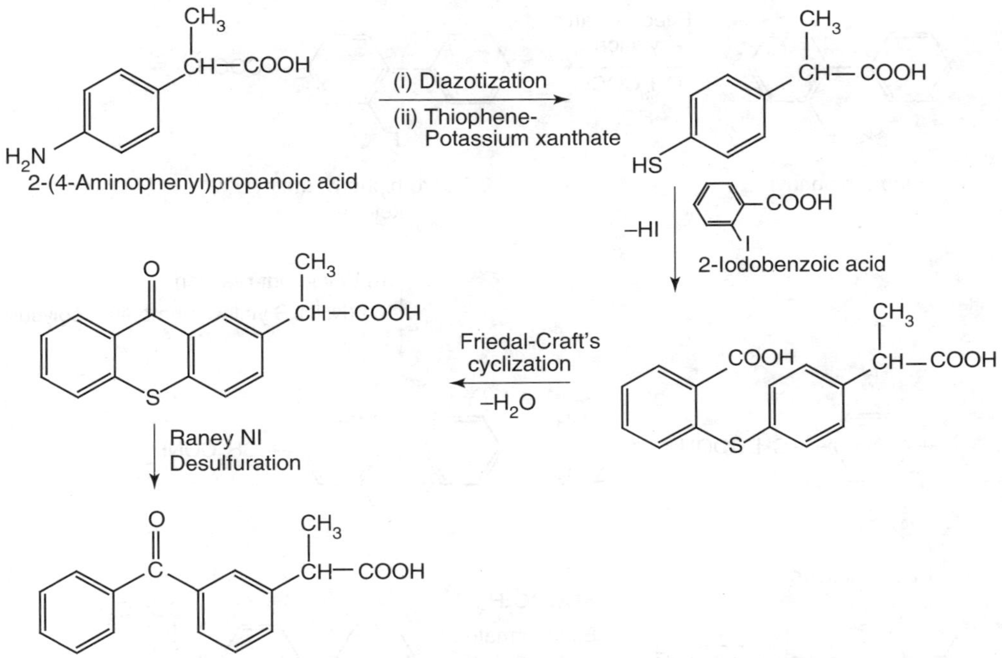

vii. Ketoprofen

Metabolism: It is metabolized by glucuronidation of carboxylic acid, CYP3A4, and CYP2C9 hydroxylation of benzoyl ring and reduction of keto function.

Properties and uses: Ketoprofen is a white crystalline powder, practically insoluble in water, soluble in acetone, in ethanol, and in methylene chloride. It is closely related to fenoprofen in structure, properties, and indications and has a low incidence of side effects and has been approved for counter sale. It is used in the treatment of rheumatoid arthritis and osteoarthritis

Assay: Dissolve the sample in ethanol and dilute with water and titrate against 0.1 M sodium hydroxide. Determine the end point potentiometrically.

Dose: Usual adult oral dose for rheumatoid arthritis is 600 mg four times daily; for osteoarthritis the dose is 300–600 mg four times a day.

Dosage forms: Ketoprofen capsules I.P., B.P., Ketoprofen gel B.P.

viii. Flurbiprofen (Ansaid)

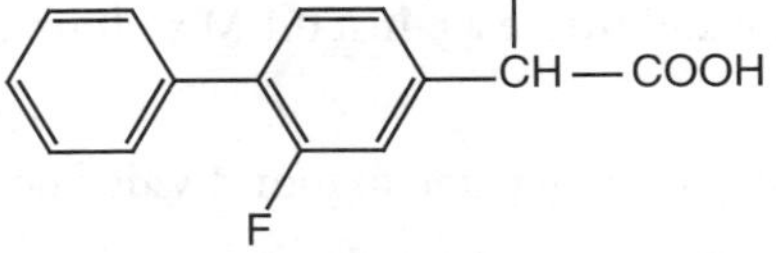

[Structure of Flurbiprofen]

(±) -2-(2-Fluoro-4-biphenyl)-propionic acid

Synthesis

2-Fluoro-biphenyl → (Friedal-Craft's acylation, CH_3COCl, $-HCl$) → **2-Fluoro-biphenyl methyl ketone** (COCH₃)

↓ (i) Willgerodt reaction
(ii) $(NH_4)_2S$ yellow ammonium polysulphate

[biphenyl-F]–CH₂CONH₂ → ($-NH_3$, Δ, H_2O) → [biphenyl-F]–CH₂COOH

↓ Esterification

[biphenyl-F]–CH₂COOC₂H₅ → ($HCOOC_2H_5$ Ethyl formate, C_2H_5ONa) → [biphenyl-F]–CH(COOC₂H₅)₂

↓ Methylation, CH_3I, $-HI$

[biphenyl-F]–C(CH₃)(COOC₂H₅)₂

↓ (i) Acid hydrolysis
(ii) Decarboxylation

[biphenyl-F]–CH(CH₃)–COOH

Properties and uses: Flurbiprofen is a white crystalline powder, practically insoluble in water, soluble in alcohol, in methylene chloride, and aqueous solutions of alkali hydroxides and carbonates. The drug is structurally and pharmacologically related to fenoprofen, ibuprofen, and ketoprofen. Another hydrotropic acid analogue that is used in the acute or long-term management of rheumatoid arthritis and osteoarthritis, it posses analgesic, anti-inflammatory, and antipyretic activities.

Assay: Dissolve the sample in alcohol and titrate against 0.1 M sodium hydroxide. Determine the end point potentiometrically.

Dose: Usual adult dose is 150–200 mg a day in three to four divided doses.

Dosage forms: Flurbiprofen tablets I.P., B.P, Flurbiprofen suppositories B.P.

viii. Caprofen

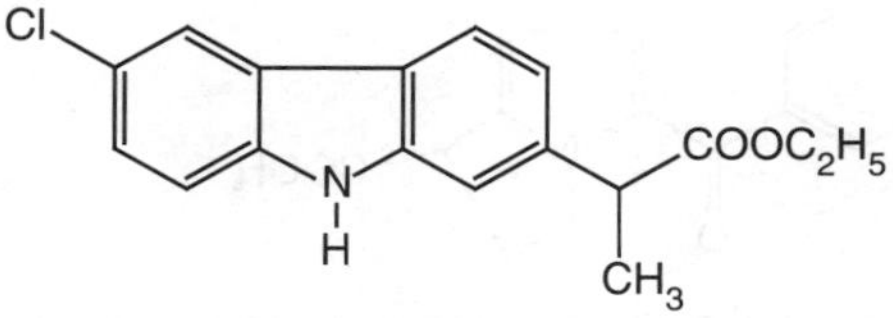

6-Chloro–α-methylcarbazole-2-acetic acid ethyl ester

Synthesis

From: 1-(4-chlorophenyl) hydrazine

1-(4-chlorophenyl)hydrazine + (3-oxocyclohexyl)propanoic acid

↓

6-chloro-2,3,4,9-tetrahydro-1H-carbazole-2-acetic acid derivative

↓ H^+/C_2H_5OH

ethyl ester intermediate

↓ Xylene, P-Chloranil

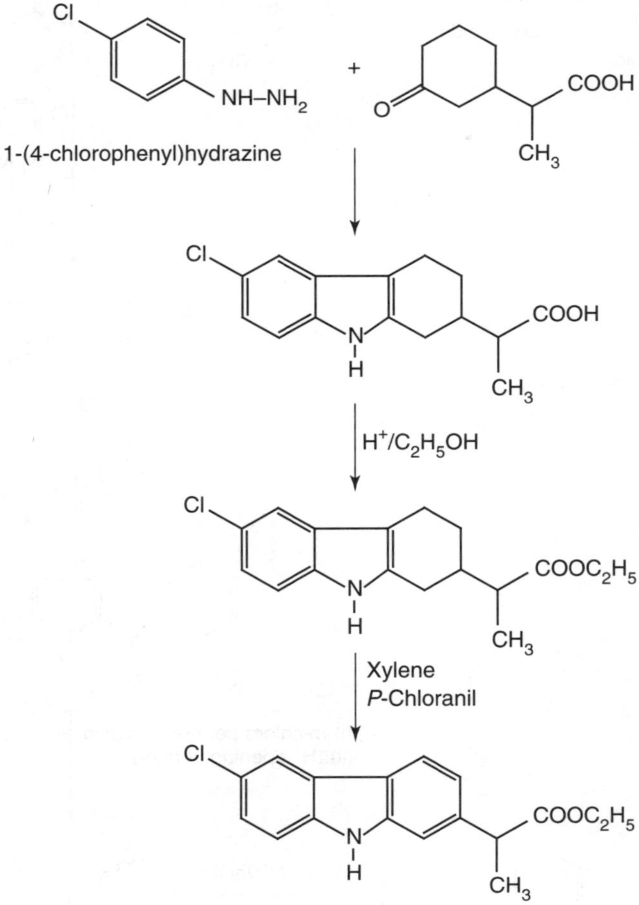

Caprofen

Uses: Used as an analgesic and anti-inflammatory agent.

ix. Ketorolac (Acular, Ketodrops, Ketlur)

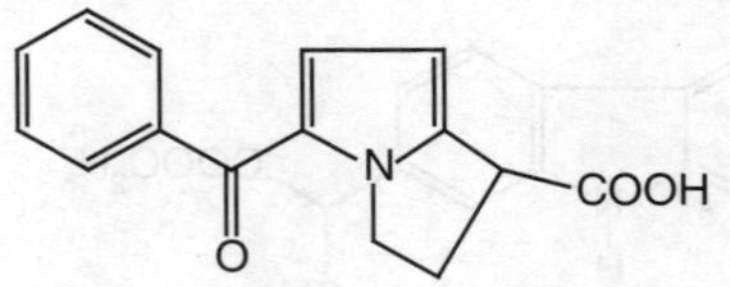

5-Benzoyl-2,3-dihydro-1H-pyrrolizine-1-carboxylic acid

Synthesis

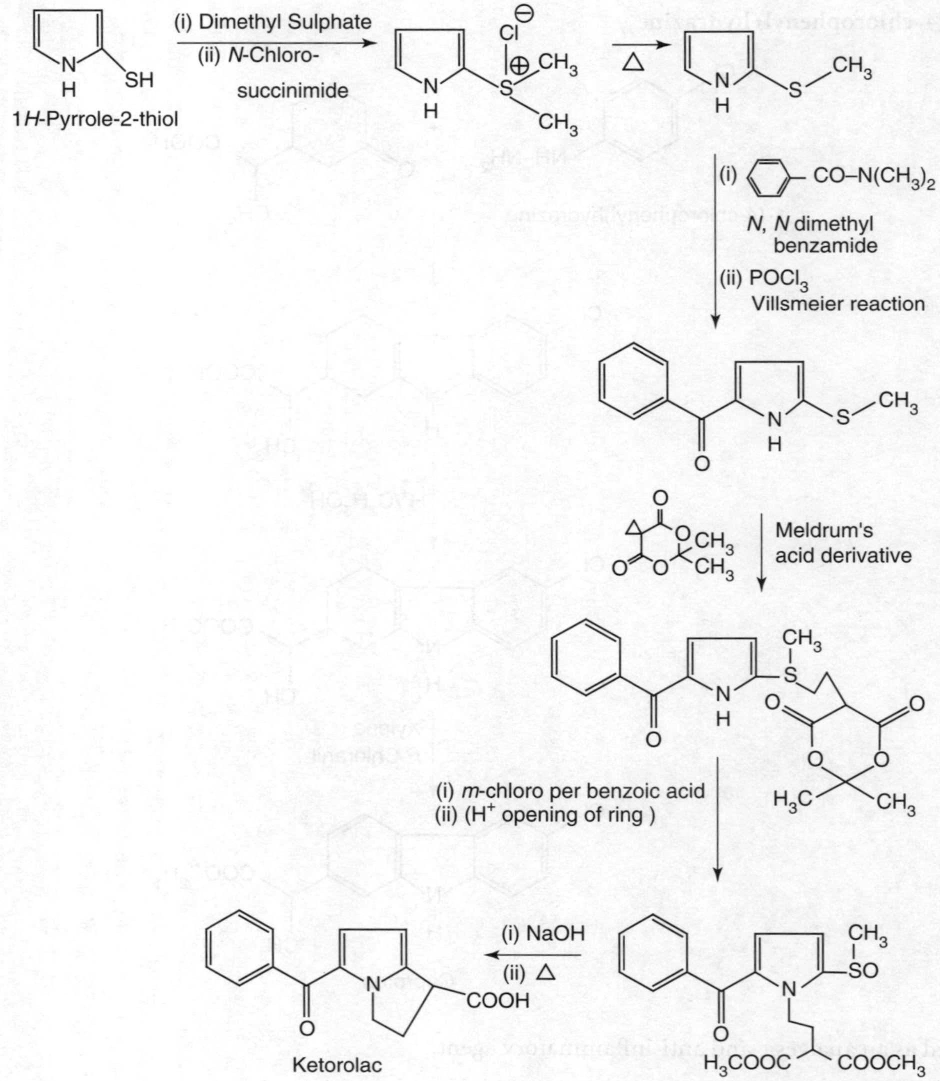

1H-Pyrrole-2-thiol

(i) Dimethyl Sulphate
(ii) N-Chloro-succinimide

Δ

(i) C₆H₅—CO—N(CH₃)₂
N,N dimethyl benzamide
(ii) POCl₃
Villsmeier reaction

Meldrum's acid derivative

(i) m-chloro per benzoic acid
(ii) (H⁺ opening of ring)

(i) NaOH
(ii) Δ

Ketorolac

Properties and uses: Ketorolac is a white crystalline powder, soluble in water and in methanol, slightly soluble in ethanol, practically insoluble in methylene chloride. Ketorolac is a potent analgesic indicated for the treatment of moderately severe and acute pain.

Assay: Dissolve the sample in anhydrous acetic acid and titrate against 0.1 M perchloric acid. Determine the end point potentiometrically.

Dose: The dose for ocular itching, which is associated with seasonal allergic conjunctivitis, for reduction of ocular pain, and for photophobia in patients undergoing incisional refractive sugery, instil one drop of a 0.5% solution into the affected eyes four times daily.

x. Etodolac

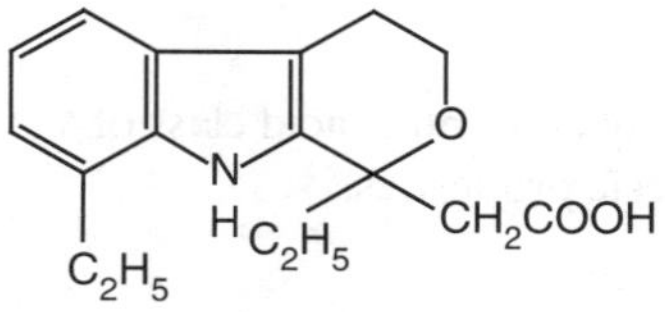
N
H
O
C_2H_5
CH_2COOH
C_2H_5

Synthesis

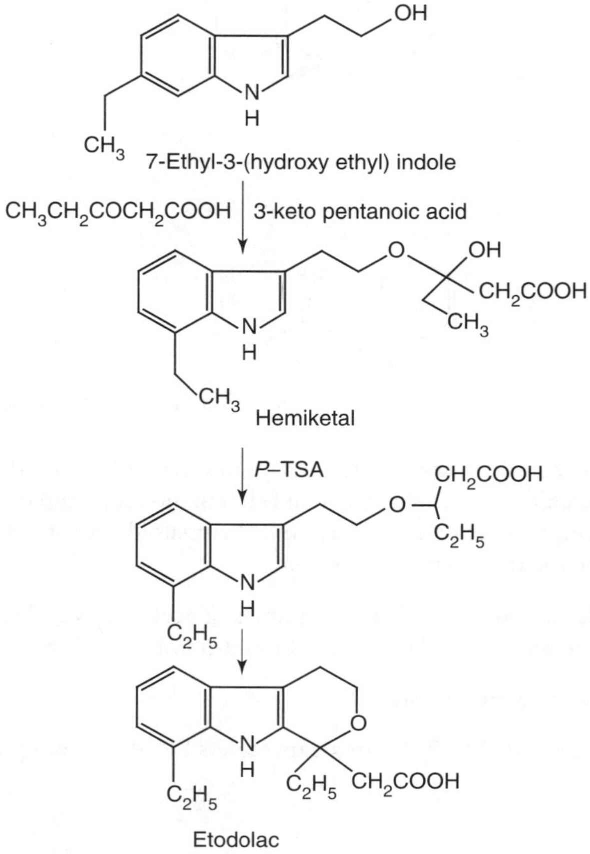
OH
N
H
CH_3
7-Ethyl-3-(hydroxy ethyl) indole
$CH_3CH_2COCH_2COOH$
3-keto pentanoic acid
O
OH
CH_2COOH
CH_3
N
H
CH_3
Hemiketal
P–TSA
CH_2COOH
O
C_2H_5
N
H
C_2H_5
O
N
H
C_2H_5
C_2H_5
CH_2COOH
Etodolac

Metabolism: It is metabolized to 3-hydroxylated metabolite and to glucuronide conjugates.

Properties and uses: Etodolac is a white crystalline powder, practically insoluble in water, soluble in acetone and in ethanol. It has anti-inflammatory activity and inhibits cyclooxygenase. It is used in the treatment of osteoarthritis and rheumatoid arthritis. Gastrointestinal irritation and ulceration is less with this drug than with other drugs.

Assay: Dissolve the sample in methanol and titrate against 0.1 M tetrabutylammonium hydroxide. Determine the end point potentiometrically. Perform a blank titration.

Dosage forms: Etodolac capsules B.P., Etodolac tablets B.P.

VI. Oxicams

The term oxicam described the relatively new enolic acid class of 4-hydroxyl -1,2 benzothiazine carboxamide with anti-inflammatory and analgesic properties.

i. Piroxicam

4-Hydroxy-2-methyl-*N*-2 pyridinyl-1,2 benzothiazine-3 carboxamide-1,1-dioxide

Properties and uses: Piroxicam is a white or slightly yellow crystalline powder, practically insoluble in water, soluble in methylene chloride, and slightly soluble in ethanol. It is employed for acute and long-term therapy for the relief of symptoms of osteoarthritis and rheumatoid arthritis. It also possesses uricosuric action and has been used in the treatment of acute gout.

Assay: Dissolve the sample in a mixture of equal volumes of acetic anhydride and anhydrous acetic acid and titrate against 0.1 M perchloric acid. Determine the end-point potentiometrically.

Dose: Usual adult oral dose is 20 mg per day.

Dosage forms: Piroxicam capsules I.P., B.P., Piroxicam tablets I.P., Piroxicam gel B.P.

Synthesis

[Scheme: Saccharin → (ClCH₂COOCH₃, Methyl chloro acetate) → N-CH₂COOCH₃ intermediate → (Ring expansion reaction, NaOCH₃) → benzothiazine COOCH₃ with NH → (CH₃I, NaOH) → N-CH₃ derivative → (H₂N-pyridine) → **Piroxicam**]

The two more closely related analogues are obtained by varying the heterocyclic amine used in the last step. 2-Amino thiazole thus leads to sudoxicam, while 3-amino-5-methylisoxazole affords isoxicam.

ii. Tenoxicam (Tobitil)

[Structure of Tenoxicam: thieno-benzothiazine with OH, C(=O)-NH-pyridyl, NH, SO₂]

Properties and uses: Tenoxicam is a yellow crystalline powder, practically insoluble in water, sparingly soluble in methylene chloride, very slightly soluble in ethanol, and soluble in solutions of acids and alkalis. Used as cyclooxygenase inhibitor, analgesic, and anti-inflammatory agent.

Assay: Dissolve the sample in anhydrous formic acid, add anhydrous acetic acid, and titrate against 0.1 M perchloric acid. Determine the end point potentiometrically.

Synthesis

[Reaction scheme: Ethyl 4-(chlorosulfonyl)thiophene-2-carboxylate + CH$_3$NHCH$_2$COOC$_2$H$_5$ (Ethyl N-Methyl glycinate) → sulfonamide intermediate → (Base, Claisen condensation) → hydroxy thienothiazine ester → (H$_2$N-pyridyl) → Tenoxicam]

Dose: Dose in the case of musculoskeletal and joint disorders—such as ankylosing spondylitis, osteoarthritis and rheumatoid arthritis— and short-term management of soft tissue injury for adult is 20 mg as a single daily dose given for 7 days in acute cases. For musculoskeletal disorders and other related illnesses, the dose is a maximum of 4 mg a day up to 14 days in severe cases (short-term use).

Dosage forms: Tenoxicam injection B.P., Tenoxicam tablets B.P.

iii. Meloxicam

4-Hydroxy-2-methyl-*N*-(5 methyl-2-thiazolyl)-2H-1, 2-benzothiazine-3-carboxamide-1, 1-dioxide

Metabolism: This category of drugs undergoes aromatic hydroxylation at several positions of aromatic benzothiazine ring. Sudoxicam undergoes primary hydroxylation of thiazole ring, followed by ring opening, whereas isoxicam undergoes primary cleavage reaction of benzothiazine ring

Properties and uses: Meloxicam is a pale yellow powder, practically insoluble in water, slightly soluble in acetone, soluble in dimethylformamide, very slightly soluble in ethanol and in methanol. Used as cyclooxygenase inhibitor, analgesic, and anti-inflammatory.

Assay: Dissolve the sample in a mixture of anhydrous acetic acid and anhydrous formic acid (10:1) and titrate against 0.1 M perchloric acid. Determine the end point potentiometrically.

Dosage forms: Meloxicam tablets B.P.

SAR of Oxicams

- The most active analogues have substituents CH_3 on the nitrogen and electron withdrawing substituents on the anilide phenyl groups, such as Cl and CF_3.
- The introduction of heterocyclic ring in the amide chain significantly increases the anti-inflammatory activity. Example—2-thiazolyl derivative sudoxicam is more potent than indomethacin.
- The most active benzothiazine have acidities in the pKa range of 6–8.

VII. Selective COX-2 inhibitor

The PG that mediates inflammation, fever, and pain are produced solely via COX-2 (highly inducible by inflammatory response), and the PGs that are important in GIT, platelets, uterus, and adrenal function are produced solely via COX-1 (constitutively expressed). Selective COX-2 inhibitors (Celecoxib, Rofecoxib, and Valdecoxib) are devoid of side effects, such as gastric ulcer. It does not affect the normal functioning of platelets, uterus, and renal system.

i. Celecoxib (Celact, Cobix, Revibra)

4-[5-(4-Methyl phenyl)-3-(trifluoro)-1H-pyrazo-lyl]-benzene sulphonamide.

Metabolism: Metabolism of celecoxib occurs in the liver, involves hydroxylation of 4-methyl group to primary alcohol, which is subsequently oxidized to its corresponding carboxylic acid.

Properties and uses: It exists as pale yellow crystals, sparingly soluble in water. Celecoxib is used to treat arthritis, pain, menstrual cramps, and colonic polyps, and also for the relief of pain, fever, swelling, and tenderness caused by osteoarthritis, rheumatoid arthritis and ankylosing spondylitis.

Synthesis

P-Methyl acetophenone + CF$_3$COOC$_2$H$_5$ (Ethyltrifluoro acetate) $\xrightarrow[-C_2H_5OH]{\text{Reflux NaOCH}_3}$ 4-CH$_3$-C$_6$H$_4$-COCH$_2$COCF$_3$

+ 4-Sulphonamidophenyl hydrazine (H$_2$NO$_2$S-C$_6$H$_4$-NH-NH$_2$)

$\xrightarrow[C_2H_5OH]{\text{Reflux}}$ Celecoxib

Dose: For osteoarthritis, the adult dose is 200 mg as a single dose or in two divided doses that may be increased to 200 mg two times a day, if necessary. For rheumatoid arthritis, the adult dose is 100–200 mg two times a day. For elderly people the dose is 100 mg two times a day. For dysmenorrhoea, initially the dose is 400 mg by 200 mg, if necessary, on the 1st day and maintenance dosage is 200 mg two times a day.

ii. Rofecoxib

4-[4-(Methyl sulphinyl) phenyl]-3-phenyl-2-furanone

Synthesis

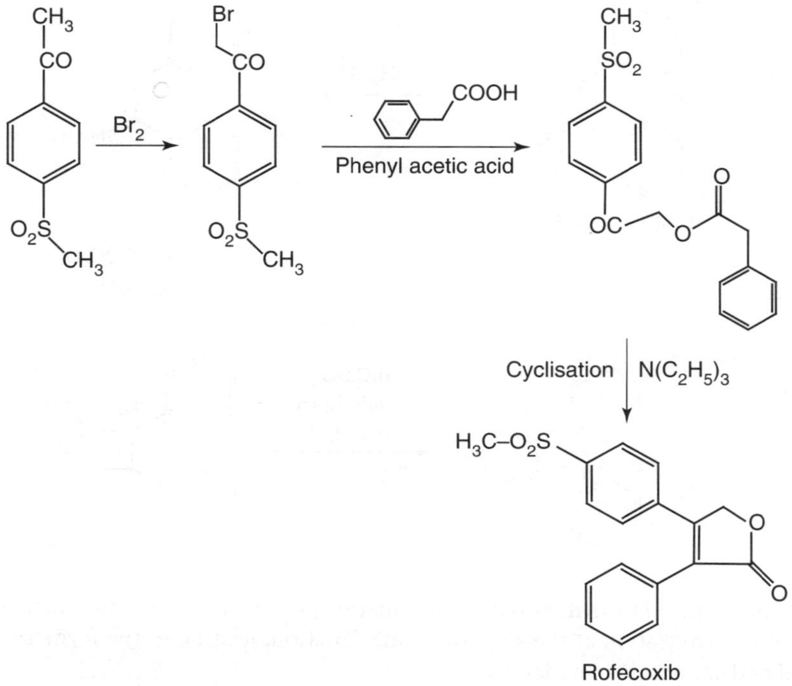

[Scheme: 4-(methylsulfonyl)acetophenone → (with Br₂) α-bromo-4-(methylsulfonyl)acetophenone → (with phenyl acetic acid) ester intermediate → (Cyclisation, N(C₂H₅)₃) → Rofecoxib]

Rofecoxib

Metabolism: The metabolic route of Rofecoxib appears to follow the reduction of dihydrofuranone ring system by cystolic enzyme to *cis* and *trans* hydroxy derivatives.

Properties and uses: It exists as white to light yellow powder, sparingly soluble in acetone, methanol, very slightly soluble in 1-octanol. It is a COX-2 inhibitor with greater potency and a longer half-life than celecoxib. Rofecoxib is used to relieve the pain, tenderness, inflammation (swelling), and stiffness caused by arthritis, and to treat painful menstrual periods and pain from other causes.

iii. Valdecoxib

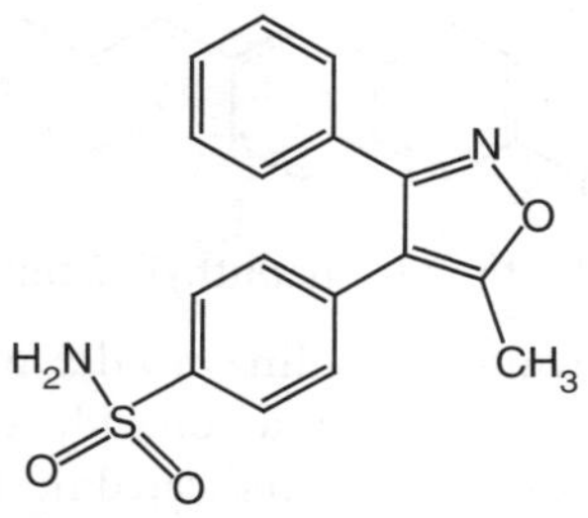

[Structure of Valdecoxib]

4-[5-Methyl-3-phenyl isoxazol-4-yl]-benzene sulphonamide

Synthesis

[Synthesis scheme: 1,2-Diphenylethanone reacts with NH₂OH to form the oxime; then with CH₃COOC₂H₅ (−C₂H₅OH); then (i) ClSO₃H, (ii) NH₄OH, (iii) −H₂O to give the final sulfonamide-substituted isoxazole.]

Metabolism: It is metabolized by hydroxylation of 5-methyl group and it is further metabolized to inactive carboxylate and N-Hydroxylation at the sulphonamide function, leading to the formation of corresponding sulphinic acid and suphomic metabolites.

Properties and uses: It is soluble in most organic solvents, insoluble in water. It is a NSAID drug that exhibits anti-inflammatory, analgesic, and antipyretic activities.

Dose: For dysmenorrhoea the dose is 20 mg twice a day. For osteoarthritis and rheumatoid arthritis the dose is 10 mg once daily.

IX. Miscellaneous

i. Nabumetone (Nabuflam, Niltis)

[Structure of 4-(6-Methoxy-2-naphthyl)-2-butanone]

4-(6-Methoxy-2-naphthyl)-2 butanone

Properties and uses: Nabumetone is a white crystalline powder, practically insoluble in water, freely soluble in acetone, and slightly soluble in methanol. It is a nonacidic compound and because of this nature, it produces minimum gastrointestinal side effect. It is indicated in the treatment of acute and chronic treatment of osteoarthritis and rheumatoid arthritis.

Synthesis

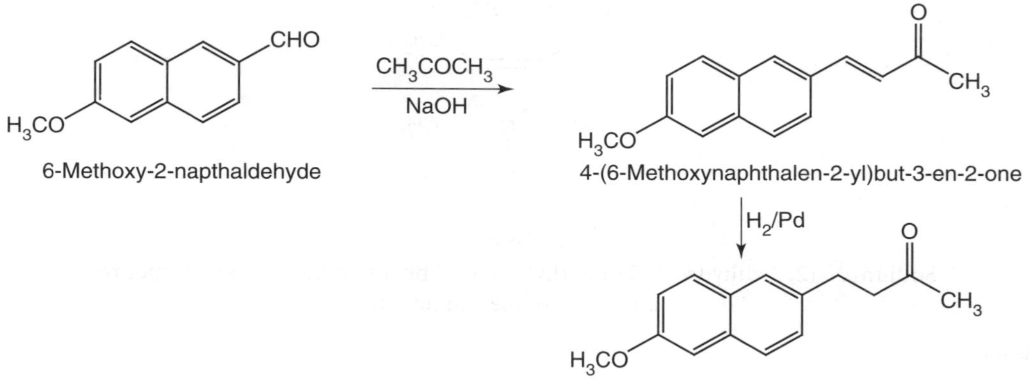

[Scheme: 6-Methoxy-2-napthaldehyde + CH₃COCH₃ / NaOH → 4-(6-Methoxynaphthalen-2-yl)but-3-en-2-one → (H₂/Pd) → Nabumetone]

6-Methoxy-2-napthaldehyde

4-(6-Methoxynaphthalen-2-yl)but-3-en-2-one

Dose: For pain and inflammation associated with osteoarthritis and rheumatoid arthritis adult dose is 1 g as a single dose in the evening followed by 0.5–1 g in the morning.

Dosage forms: Nabumetone oral suspension B.P., Nabumetone tablets B.P.

Assay: It is assayed by adopting liquid chromatography technique.

ii. Nimesulide

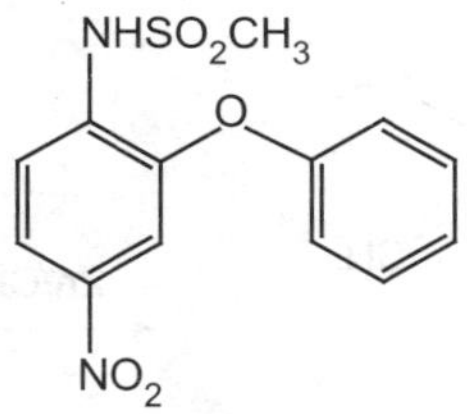

4-Nitro-2-phenoxy methane sulphonamide

Synthesis

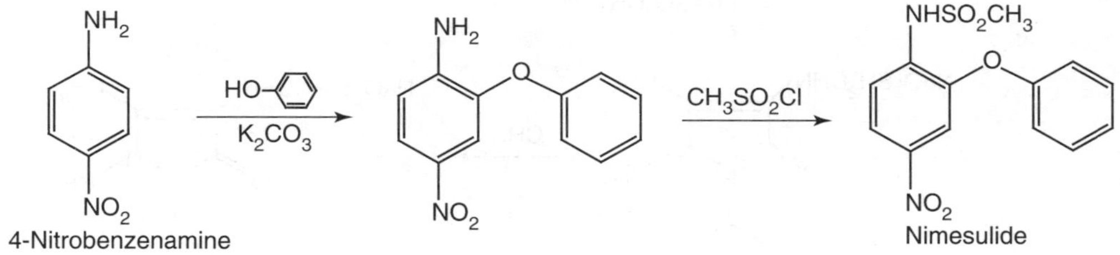

[Scheme: 4-Nitrobenzenamine + HO-phenyl / K_2CO_3 → intermediate + CH_3SO_2Cl → Nimesulide]

4-Nitrobenzenamine

Nimesulide

Properties and uses: Nimesulide is a yellowish crystalline powder, practically insoluble in water, soluble in acetone, and slightly soluble in anhydrous ethanol. It contains a sulphonamide moiety as an acidic group rather than a carbonic acid. It shows moderate incidence of gastric side effects because it exhibits significant selectivity towards COX-2, used as analgesic and anti-inflammatory agent.

iii. Analgin

Sodium N-(2, 3-dihydro-1, 5 dimethyl-3-oxo-2 phenyl-pyrazol-4-yl)-N-methyl amino methane sulphonate

Synthesis

Uses: Used as an analgesic and anti-inflammatory agent.

X. Drugs used in the treatment of gout

An acute attack of gout occurs as a result of anti-inflammatory reaction to crystals of sodium ureate (the end product of purine metabolism in human beings) that is deposited in the joint tissues. Drugs used to treat gout may act in the following ways:

- By inhibiting uric acid synthesis: Allopurinol.
- By increasing uric acid excretion: Probenecid, Sulphinpyrazone.
- Miscellaneous: Colchicines (alkaloid obtained from *Colchicum autumnale*).

i. Allopurinol (Zyloprim)

Pyrazolo pyrimidine-4-one

Synthesis

2-(Ethoxymethylene)malononitrile

Allopurinol

Mode of action: In human beings, uric acid is formed primarily by the xanthine oxidase-catalyzed oxidation of hypoxanthine and xanthine. At low concentrations, allopurinol is a substrate for and competitive inhibitor of the enzyme at high concentrations; it is a noncompetitive inhibitor.

$$\text{Adenine} \xrightarrow[\text{Deaminase}]{\text{Adnine}} \text{Hypoxanthine} \xrightarrow{\text{Xanthine oxidase}} \text{Xanthine} \xrightarrow{\text{Xanthine oxidase}} \text{Uric acid}$$

Allopurinol inhibits this two stages

Metabolism: It is rapidly metabolized via oxidation and numerous ribonucleoside derivatives are formed. The major metabolites are alloxanthine or oxypurinol.

Properties and uses: Allopurinol is a white powder, very slightly soluble in water, in alcohol and in dilute solutions of alkali hydroxides. It is used in the treatment of gout and prevention of urate deposition in patients with leukaemia receiving anticancer drugs, which cause increasing serum uric acid levels.

Assay: It is assayed by adopting liquid chromatography technique.

Dose: Usual adult oral dose for gout is 100–200 mg two or three times a day.

Dosage forms: Allopurinol tablets I.P., B.P.

ii. Probenecid (Benemid)

Synthesis

Metabolism: The metabolite is glucuronide conjugates of carboxylic acid, ω oxidation of N-propyl side chain, and subsequent oxidation, resulting in alcohol to carboxylic acid derivative. ω Oxidation of N-propyl side chain and N-dealkylation are the process steps in the metabolism of probenacid.

Properties and uses: Probenecid exists as white crystalline powder or small crystals, practically insoluble in water, soluble in acetone, and sparingly soluble in ethanol. Probenecid is uricosuric agent that increases the rate of excretion of uric acid and used in the treatment of chronic gout. The oral administration of probenecid in conjugation with penicillin G results in higher and prolonged concentration of the antibiotic in the plasma than when penicillin is given alone.

Assay: Dissolve the sample in alcohol, shaking and heating slightly, if necessary, and titrate against 0.1 M sodium hydroxide. Determine the end point potentiometrically.

Dose: Adult oral dose is 500 mg–2 g per day; usually 250 mg two times a day for one week, then 500 mg twice a day thereafter.

Dosage forms: Probenecid tablets I.P., B.P.

iii. Sulphinpyrazone (Anuturane)

Synthesis

Metabolism: The metabolic product results from sulphoxide reduction, sulphur, and aromatic oxidation and C-glucuronidation of heterocyclic ring. The metabolite resulting from para hydroxylation of phenyl ring posseses uricosuric effect.

Properties and uses: Sulphinpyrazone is a white powder, very slightly soluble in water, sparingly soluble in alcohol, soluble in dilute solutions of alkali hydroxides and used as uricosuric agent.

Assay: Dissolve the sample in acetone and titrate against 0.1 M sodium hydroxide using bromothymol blue as an indicator, until the colour changes from yellow to blue.

Dose: Initial oral dose is 100–200 mg per day, taken with meals or milk.

Dosage forms: Sulphinpyrazone tablets B.P.

PROBABLE QUESTIONS

1. Explain schematically, the biosynthetic pathway of PGs and describe how does the NSAIDs act as antipyretics and analgesics?
2. Outline the synthesis of the following NSAIDs: Paracetamol, Phenylbutazone, and Indomethacin.
3. Classify the NSAIDs and write the structure, chemical name, and uses of at least one compound from each category.
4. Write the names of three drugs belonging to the category of aniline and para aminophenol analogues. Outline the synthesis of one of them.
5. What is cyclooxygenase II? Name the drugs that selectively inhibit the cyclooxygenase II along with the synthesis of any one of them.
6. Explain how the salicylic acid analogues act as potent antipyretics and analgesics. Mention suitable examples to support your answer.
7. Write the metabolism of para amino phenol derivatives with their chemical structure and indicate the metabolic product responsible for hepatotoxic.
8. The metabolite of phenylbutazone is a more effective drug. Outline its synthesis and the important uses.
9. Name a sulphur containing pyrazolidine drug used as an antipyretic and analgesic, and write its synthesis.
10. Structural analogues of *N*-aryl anthranilic acid yielded some potent antipyretics, analgesics, and anti-inflammatory compounds. Justify the statement with two examples and write their synthesis.
11. Outline the synthesis of the following NSAIDs: Ibuprofen, Diclofenac, and Nabumetone.
12. Explain the mode of action of antipyretics and analgesics by citing the examples of some typical drugs, which you have studied.
13. Write in detail about antipyretics and analgesics.
14. What are salicylates? Enumerate the derivatives of salicylic acid used as NSAIDs with their chemical structure. Describe the SAR and metabolism of salicylates.
15. Outline the synthesis and uses of the following NSAIDs: Piroxicam, Sulindac, and Zomepirac sodium.
16. Write a brief note on arylactic acid derived from NSAIDs.
17. What are the major side effects of NSAIDs? Explain how the GIT disturbances can be corrected.
18. Explain the mode of action of antigout drugs and outline the synthesis, metabolism, and uses of any two of them.

SUGGESTED READINGS

1. Abraham DJ (ed). *Burger's Medicinal Chemistry and Drug Discovery* (6th edn). New Jersey: John Wiley, 2007.
2. *British Pharmacopoeia*. Medicines and Healthcare Products Regulatory Agency, London, 2008.

3. Bruntan LL, Lazo JS, and Parker KL. *Goodman and Gilman's: The Pharmacologica Basis of Therapeutics* (11th edn). New York: McGraw Hill, 2006.
4. *Indian Pharmacopoeia*. Ministry of Health and Family Welfare. New Delhi, 1996.
5. Lednicer D and Mitscher LA. *The Organic Chemistry of Drug Synthesis*. New York: John Wiley, 1995.
6. Lemke TL and William DA. *Foye's Principle of Medicinal Chemistry* (6th edn). New York: Lippincott Williams and Wilkins, 2008.
7. Gennaro AR. *Remington's The Science and Practice of Pharmacy* (21st edn). New York: Lippincot Williams and Wilkins, 2006.
8. Reynolds EF (ed). *Martindale the Extra Pharmacopoeia* (31st edn). London: The Pharmaceutical Press, 1997.

SECTION II

DRUGS ACTING ON RESPIRATORY SYSTEM

1 Expectorants and Antitussives — 109

Chapter 1

Expectorants and Antitussives

INTRODUCTION OF RESPIRATORY SYSTEM

There are many drugs acting on respiratory system, that is, antitussives, antiasthmatics, expectorants, and mucolytics. There are some drugs that act centrally for suppression of cough through the inhibition of mechano or chemoreceptors. Normally, cough is beneficial for expelling all the dust particles that enter into the respiratory tract. However, when the cough becomes severe due to any inflammation in the respiratory tract or in the lungs, it is necessary to treat with some drugs, such as mucolytics, antiasthmatics, or any expectorants.

The drugs that are used for bronchial asthma are $ß_2$ adrenergic agonists because it is caused due to the irregulation of autonomic control towards these receptors in the lungs and respiratory tract, which produces constriction. Therefore, the difficulty in breathing persists and can be treated, especially, with $ß_2$ adrenergic agonists. For example, salmeterol, terbutaline, formeterol, and some methyl xanthines (caffeine, theophylline) as well as anticholinergics (ipratropium bromide, tiotropium bromide). The inflammation persisting may be treated better with corticosteroids. Bronchial asthma may also be due to the hypersensitive reactions, due to the release of histamine and acetylcholine in the tracheo-bronchial regions. These can be treated by using some mast cell stabilizers called sodium chromglycate and leukotriene antagonists, that is, montelukast and zafirlukast.

Antitussives are the drugs that act in the central nervous system (CNS) to raise the threshold of cough centre or act peripherally in the respiratory tract to reduce tussual impulse, example, opioids and non-opioids.

Mucolytics are the drugs that depolymerize the mucopolysaccharides and they break the network of tenacious sputum. These events mark the expulsion of sputum with the help of ciliary movement. Examples: bromohexine, adothoda vasaka.

Expectorants are the drugs that increase the bronchial secretion and reduce the viscosity of sputum for removal by coughing. Sodium and potassium citrate and ammonium chloride are used as expectorants.

EXPECTORANTS AND ANTITUSSIVES

Antitussives are drugs that reduce coughing. Coughing may be diminished by reducing respiratory secretion, eliminating a source of irritation, or decreasing the sensitivity of irritant receptors within the respiratory tract. Antitussives can act either by raising the threshold of the cough centre or by reducing the number of impulses transmitted to the centre from the peripheral receptors. The antitussives are divided into two main classes:

1. Centrally active antitussives that affect the cough centre in the medulla.
2. Peripherally active antitussives that act at the receptor level in the respiratory tract.

Pharyngeal demulcents sooth the throat and reduce the afferent impulse from the inflamed/irritated mucosa. Expectorants are drugs that increase the secretion of bronchus and reduce the viscosity, thereby removing cough and sputum. The drugs usually used as expectorants are salts of sodium, potassium, and ammonium compounds. Guaiphenesin, vasaka, and balsam of tolu are plant products. These also enhance the mucociliary movement. Ammonium salts are nauseating and reflexly increase the respiratory secretion. Antitussives acts centrally and relieve the cough. They act on the cough centre in the medulla oblongata and increase the threshold to cough. These drugs control the cough rather than eliminate it. The drugs that are used as antitussives are codeine, an opium alkaloid, and selective drugs are also there for the action on the cough centre, but it may produce respiratory depression at higher dosage. In non-opioids, noscapine and dextromethorphan are usually used. Noscapine is an opium alkaloid of benzoisoquinoline series. It depresses cough, but has no narcotic, analgesic, or dependence effects. Dextromethorphan is a synthetic compound and it is a d-isomer and used as antitussives.

CLASSIFICATION

I. Centrally active antitussive agents

i. Dextromethorphan HBr

ii. Levopropoxyphene napsylate

iii. Noscapine

iv. Pholcodine

v. Codeine Phosphate

II. Peripherally acting antitussives

i. Benzonatate

H₃C(H₂C)₃HN—C₆H₄—C(=O)—O—(OCH₂CH₂)₉OCH₃

ii. Carbetapentane

1-phenylcyclopentyl-COO(CH₂)₂O(CH₂)₂N(C₂H₅)₂

iii. Caramiphen

1-phenylcyclopentyl with C_6H_5 and COOCH₂CH₂N(C₂H₅)₂

iv. Chlophedianol hydrochloride

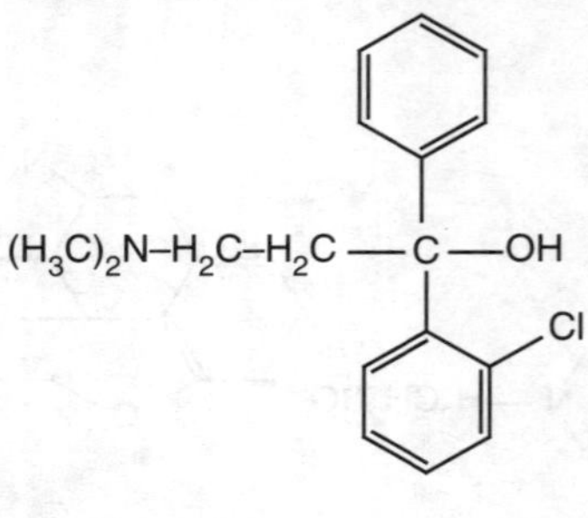

v. Isoaminile

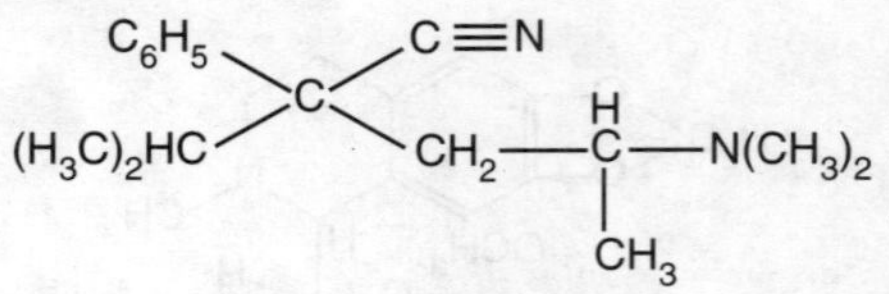

SYNTHESIS AND DRUG PROFILE

I. Centrally acting antitussive agents

i. Dextromethorphan HBr

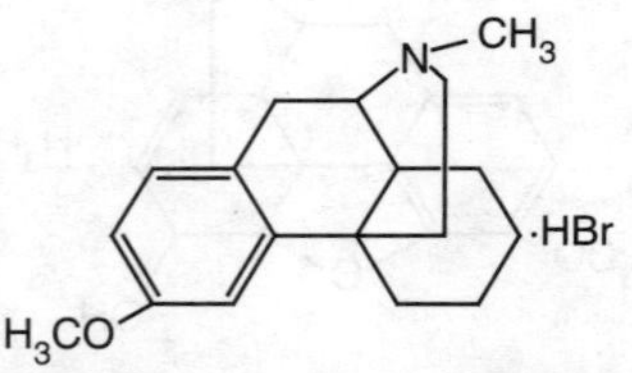

3-Methoxy-17-methyl-9 α, 13 α, 14 α,-morphinan hydrobromide

Synthesis

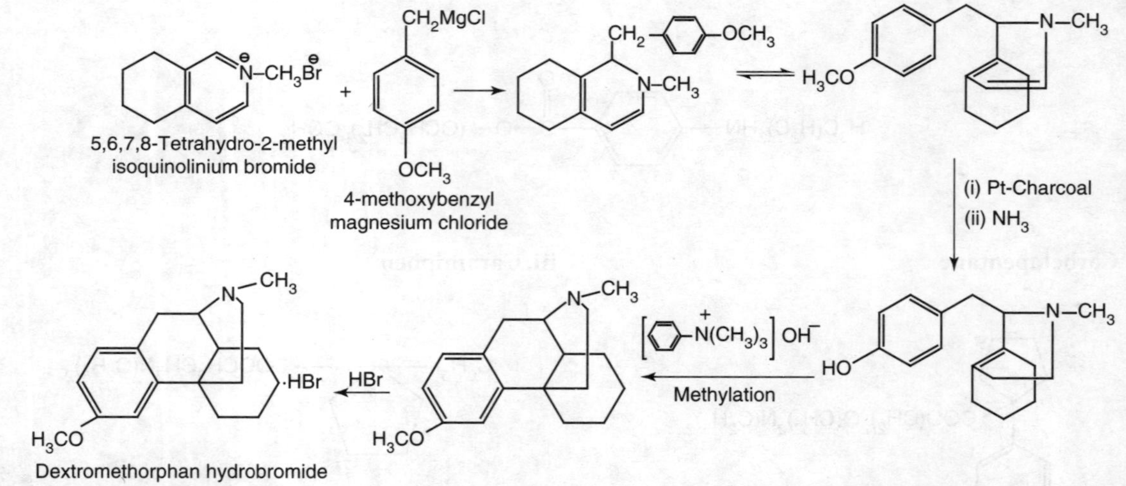

5,6,7,8-Tetrahydro-2-methyl isoquinolinium bromide

4-methoxybenzyl magnesium chloride

(i) Pt-Charcoal
(ii) NH_3

Methylation

Dextromethorphan hydrobromide

Properties and uses: Dextromethorphan hydrobromide (HBr) is a white crystalline powder, sparingly soluble in water, and soluble in alcohol. It is a substituted dextro isomer of the opioid levomethorphan.

It is not an analgesic or an addictive. Dextromethorphan HBr should not be given to patients who are on monoamine oxidase inhibitors therapy. It is an opioid receptor agonist used as a cough suppressant.

Assay: Dissolve the sample in a mixture of 0.01 M hydrochloric acid and alcohol (1:4) and titrate against 0.1 M sodium hydroxide. Determine the end point potentiometrically. Read the volume added between the two points of inflexion.

ii. Levo proproxyphene napsylate (Novrad)

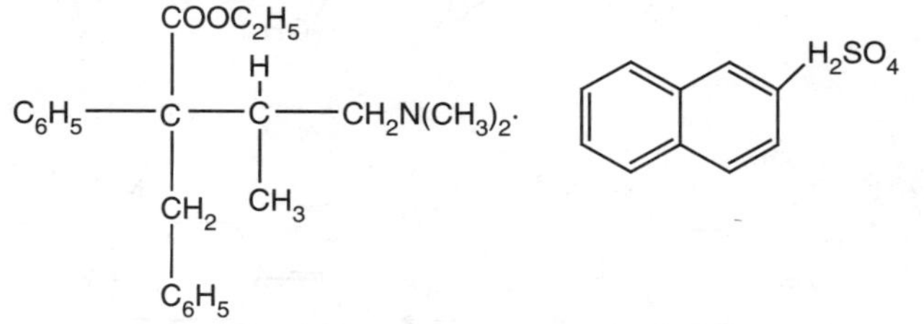

(-) α [(2-Dimethylamino)-1-methyl ethyl]-α-phenyl phenylethyl propionate(1:1)monohydrate-2-napthalene.sulphonic acid salt

Properties and uses: It is a white, bitter, crystalline powder, odourless, soluble in water, alcohol, or chloroform. It has little or no analgesic activity. It has been found to be relatively less potent than codeine in the treatment of cough reflexes. The (−)-isomer of the drug showed greater antitussive activity in comparison to either the (+)-isomer or the racemic mixture.

Dose: Usually 50–100 mg after every 4 h.

Synthesis

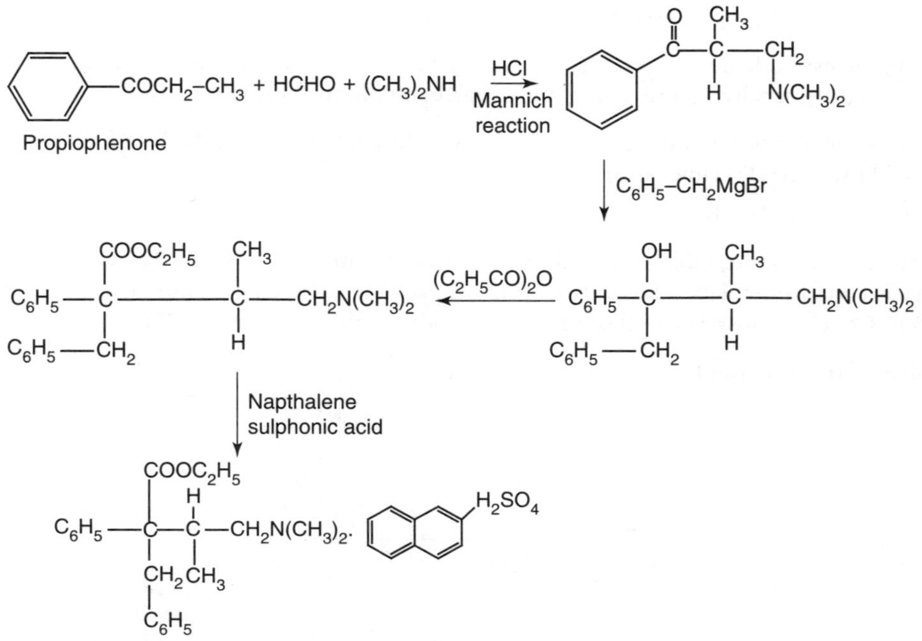

Levoproxyphene Napsylate

iii. Codeine phosphate (Zenodyl)

Synthesis

Properties and uses: Codeine phosphate is a white crystalline powder, soluble in water, and slightly soluble in ethanol. This drug acts by suppression of the cough centre in the brain stem.

Assay: Dissolve the sample in a mixture of anhydrous acetic acid and dioxan (1:2) and titrate against 0.1 M perchloric acid using crystal violet as indicator.

Dose: 10–20 mg every 4 to 6 h.

Dosage forms: Co-codamol tablets B.P., Effervescent co-codamol tablets B.P., Co-codaprin tablets B.P., Dispersible co-codaprin tablets B.P., Codeine linctus, paediatric Codeine linctus B.P., Codeine phosphate injection B.P., Codeine phosphate oral solution B.P., Codeine phosphate tablets B.P.

iv. Pholcodine (Ethnine, Simplex)

Synthesis

Morphine + O(CH₂CH₂)₂NCH₂CH₂Cl (morpholinylethyl chloride), −HCl → Pholcodine

Properties and uses: Pholcodine is a white crystalline powder, sparingly soluble in water, soluble in acetone, alcohol, and dilute mineral acid. It is as effective as codeine. It is a cough suppressant with mild sedative, but practically negligible analgesic action. It is employed for the relief of unproductive cough.

Assay: Dissolve the sample in anhydrous acetic acid, warm gently and titrate against 0.1 M perchloric acid. Determine the end point potentiometrically at the second point of inflexion.

Dose: The dose for adults is 5–15 mg, for children over 2 years 5 mg, for children below 2 years 2.5 mg.

Dosage forms: Pholcodine linctus B.P., Strong pholcodine linctus B.P.

II. Peripherally acting antitussives

i. Benzonatate (Tessalon)

$H_3C(H_2C)_3HN$—C₆H₄—C(=O)—O—$(CH_2CH_2O)_9OCH_3$

Synthesis

Ethyl-*p*-(butylamino)benzoate + Polyethylene glycol monoethyl ether n=9 → Benzonatate

Properties and uses: It is a long-chain polyglycol derivative chemically related to tetracaine and benzocaine. It is a potent antitussive agent. It usually acts by inhibiting the transmission of impulses of the cough reflex in the vagal nuclei of the medulla and predominately depresses polysynaptic spinal reflexes. It is regarded as a cough suppressant acting both centrally and peripherally.

Dose: The usual dose is 100 mg three times daily.

ii. Carbetapentane (Toclase)

2-(2-(Diethylamino)ethoxy)ethyl 1-phenylcyclopentanecarboxylate

Structure: cyclopentyl-phenyl-C-COO(CH$_2$)$_2$O(CH$_2$)$_2$N(C$_2$H$_5$)$_2$

Synthesis

1-Phenylcyclopent-anecarbonyl chloride (Ph-C(cyclopentyl)-COCl) + OH(CH$_2$)$_2$O(CH$_2$)$_2$N(C$_2$H$_5$)$_2$ [2-(2-(Diethylamino)ethoxy)ethanol] →(Condensation)→ Carbetapentane [Ph-C(cyclopentyl)-COO(CH$_2$)$_2$O(CH$_2$)$_2$N(C$_2$H$_5$)$_2$]

Properties and uses: It is a cough suppressant and is reported to reduce bronchial secretions. It is found to be effective in acute coughs associated with common upper respiratory infections.

Dose: The usual dose is 25–150 mg per day in divided doses.

iii. Caramiphen

2-(diethylamino)ethyl-1-phenylcyclopentanecarboxylate

Structure: phenyl-cyclopentyl-C-COOCH$_2$CH$_2$N(C$_2$H$_5$)$_2$

Synthesis

2-phenylacetonitrile (Ph-CH$_2$CN) →[Br(CH$_2$)$_4$Br]→ Ph-C(cyclopentyl)-CN →[NaOH, H$_2$O]→ Ph-C(cyclopentyl)-COOH →[SOCl$_2$]→ Ph-C(cyclopentyl)-COCl →[OHCH$_2$CH$_2$N(C$_2$H$_5$)$_2$]→ Ph-C(cyclopentyl)-COOCH$_2$CH$_2$N(C$_2$H$_5$)$_2$ (Caramiphen)

Uses: It is a cough suppressant, less active than codeine, but with longer duration of action. It has little effect on respiration and no tolerance of dependence develops.

iv. Isoaminile

$$\text{(H}_3\text{C)}_2\text{HC}-\underset{\underset{\text{CH}_2-\underset{\underset{\text{CH}_3}{|}}{\overset{\overset{H}{|}}{C}}-\text{N(CH}_3)_2}{|}}{\overset{\overset{C_6H_5}{|}}{C}}-C\equiv N$$

Uses: Used for control and management of cough, it is also a bronchodilator.

PROBABLE QUESTIONS

1. Define and classify the expectorants and antitussive agents. Support your answer with the help of two examples from each category along with the chemical structure.
2. Write a brief account of the stimulant expectorants. Outline the synthesis of guaiphensin.
3. Outline the synthesis of the following drugs: (a) Benzonatate (b) Carbetapentane citrate
4. Name two drugs that act as centrally acting antitussive agents and are analogues of morphine. Outline the synthesis of one such compound.
5. Mannich reaction of propiophenone yields levopropoxphene napsylate. Describe the synthetic route to yield the final product.
6. Write the structure and chemical name of the five important drugs that are used abundantly in suppressing cough.
7. What are sedative expectorants? Classify them and give the structure, chemical names and uses of one compound from each group.
8. Centrally acting antitussive agents act by depressing medullary cough centre in the CNS to suppress cough reflexes. Justify the statement by citing at least three potent drugs.

SUGGESTED READINGS

1. Abraham DJ (ed). *Burger's Medicinal Chemistry and Drug Discovery* (6th edn). New Jersey: John Wiley, 2007.
2. Boyd EM. 'Expectorants and respiratory tract fluids'. *Pharmacol Rev* 6(4): 521–42, 1954.
3. Bruntan LL, Lazo JS, and Parker KL. *Goodman and Gilman's: The Pharmacological Basis of Therapeutics* (11th edn). New York: McGraw Hill, 2006.
4. Lemke TL and William DA. *Foye's Principle of Medicinal Chemistry* (6th edn). New York: Lippincott Williams and Wilkins, 2008.
5. Lednicer D and Mitscher LA. *The Organic Chemistry of Drug Synthesis*. New York: John Wiley, 1995.
6. Gennaro AR. *Remington's The Science and Practice of Pharmacy* (21st edn). New York: Lippincot Williams and Wilkins, 2006.

SECTION III

DRUGS ACTING ON DIGESTIVE SYSTEM

| 1 | Antiulcer Agents | 121 |
| 2 | Antidiarrhoeals | 137 |

Chapter 1

Antiulcer Agents

INTRODUCTION

Antiulcer agents are drugs that are used in the treatment of peptic and gastric ulcers. These are classified on the basis of mechanism of action.

CLASSIFICATION

I. Reduction of gastric acid secretion.
   a. H_2-antihistamines: Cimetidine, Ranitidine, and Famotidine.
   b. Proton pump inhibitors: Omeprazole, Lansoprazole, and Pantoprazole.
   c. Anticholinergics: Pirenzepine, Propantheline, and Oxyphenonium.
   d. Prostaglandin analogues: Misoprostol.

II. Neutralization of gastric acid (Antacids).
   a. Systemic: $NaHCO_3$ and Sodium citrate.
   b. Nonsystemic: $Mg(OH)_2$, $CaCO_3$, Aluminium hydroxide gel and Magnesium trisilicate.

III. Ulcer protectives: Sucralfate, Colloidal Bismuthsubcitrate (CBS).

IV. Anti-*Helicobacter pylori* drugs: Amoxicillin, Clarithromycin, Metronidazole, Tinidazole, and Tetracycline.

CHEMICAL STRUCTURES OF GASTRIC ACID SECRETION INHIBITORS

Ia. H_2-antihistamines

i. Nizatidine

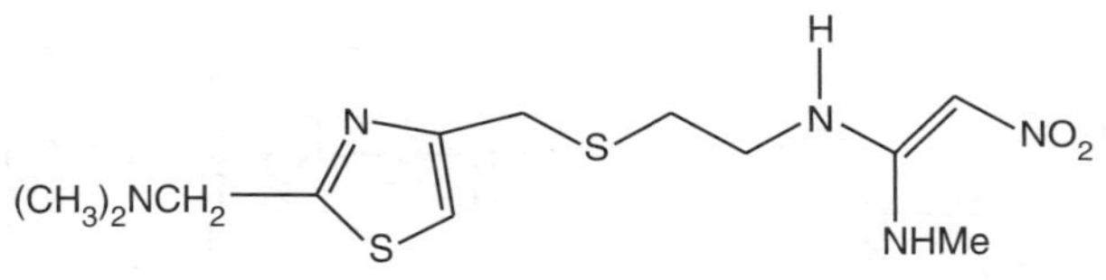

122 Drugs Acting on Digestive System

ii. Cimetidine

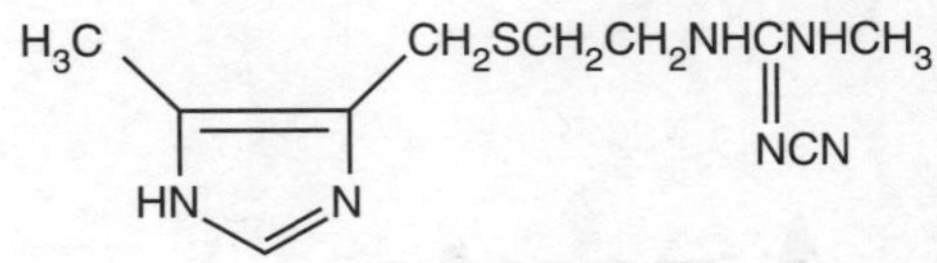

iii. Roxatidine

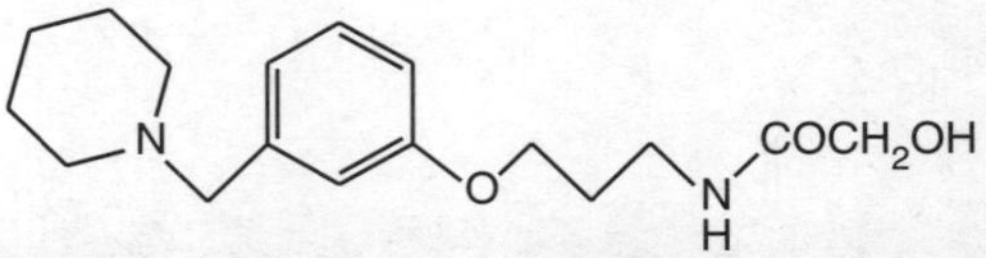

iv. Famotidine

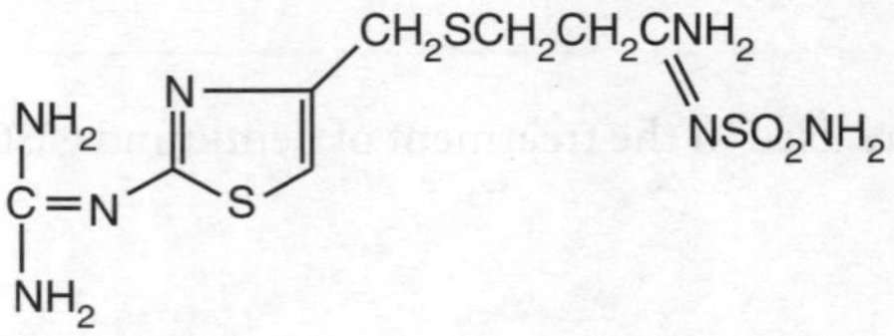

v. Ranitidine

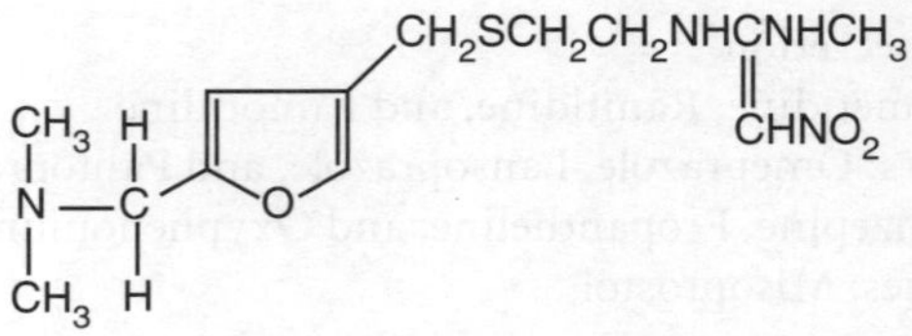

vi. Oxmetidine

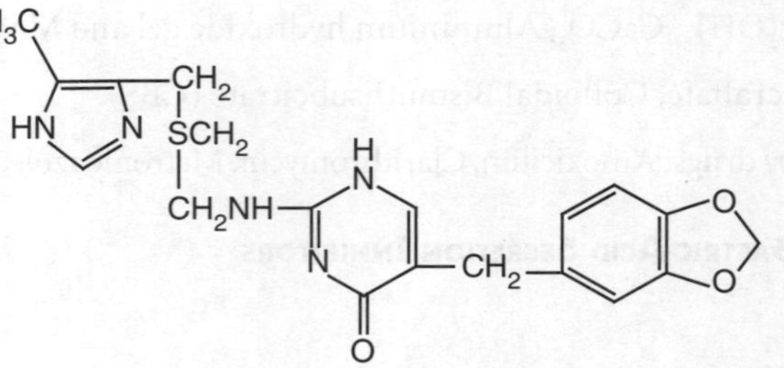

vii. Etintidine

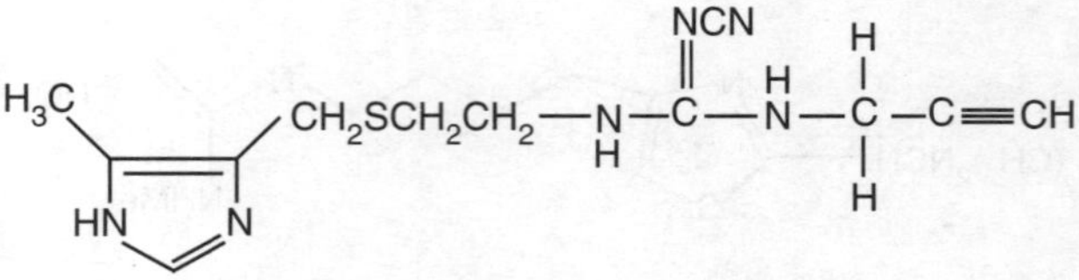

Antiulcer Agents

viii. Lupitidine

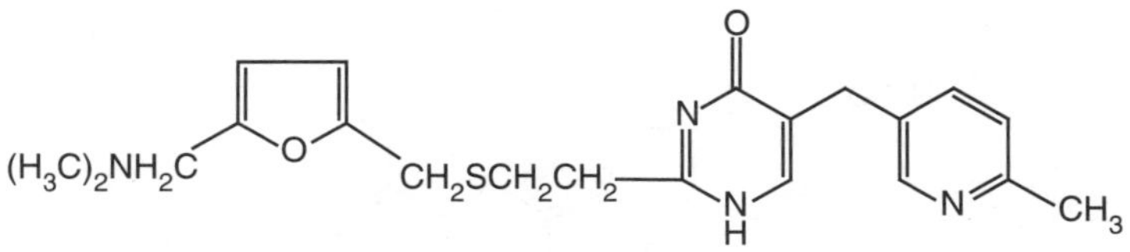

ix. Tiotidine

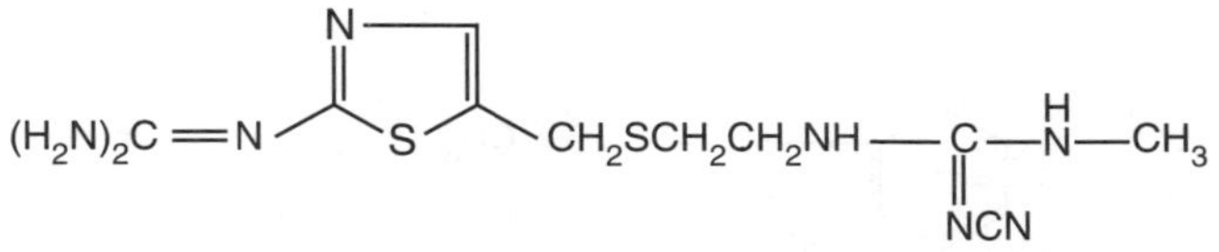

Lamitidine analogues

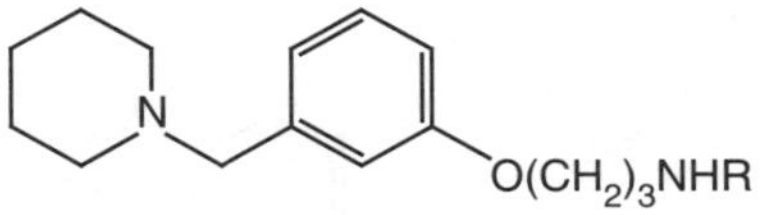

Name	R
Lamitidine	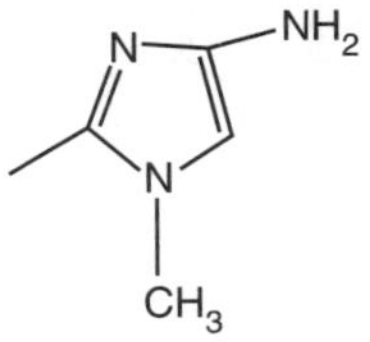 4-amino-2-methyl-1-methylimidazol-5-yl (imidazole with NH$_2$, CH$_3$, and N–CH$_3$)
Pifatidine	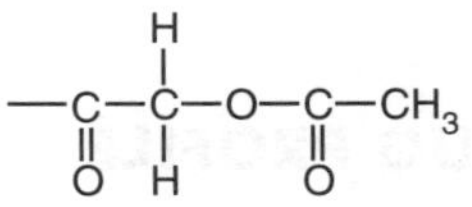 –C(=O)–CH(H)(H)–O–C(=O)–CH$_3$
Loxtidine	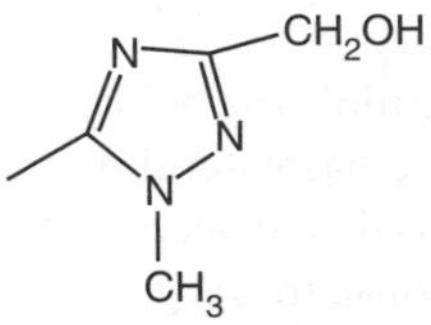 3-(hydroxymethyl)-5-methyl-1-methyl-1,2,4-triazole (triazole with CH$_2$OH, CH$_3$, N–CH$_3$)

I b. Proton pump inhibitors

i. Omeprazole

ii. Lansoprazole

iii. Pantoprazole

iv. Rabeprazole

SYNTHESIS AND DRUG PROFILE

Ia. H_2-receptor antagonists

Mode of action: These drugs inhibit the acid production by reversibly competing with histamine for the binding with H_2-receptor on the basolateral membrane of parietal cells. The most predominant effect of H_2-receptor antagonist is on basal acid secretion. Histamine on H_2-receptors produces cAMP-dependent protein kinase to elicit the response in the gastrointestinal tract (GIT). The H_2-antagonists reversibly bind the H_2-receptors and reduce the cAMP formation, which is responsible for the activation of proton pump and subsequently reduces the gastric acid formation in the GIT.

i. Cimetidine (Tagamet)

Synthesis

Route I. From: Ethyl-5-methyl-imidazole-4-carboxylate

Ethyl 5-methyl-1*H*-imidazole-4-carboxylate → (i) H⁺ / (ii) [H] → (5-methylimidazol-4-yl)methanol + HSCH₂CH₂NH₂ → (−H₂O) → 5-methyl-4-(CH₂SCH₂CH₂NH₂)-imidazole → (−CH₃SH, (CH₃S)₂C=NCN) → intermediate CH₂SCH₂CH₂NHCSCH₃ (=NCN) → (CH₃NH₂, −CH₃SH) → Cimetidine

Route II: From: Ethyl-2-chloro acetoacetate

Ethyl-2-chloro acetoacetate → enol form (H₃C–C(OH)=C(Cl)–COOC₂H₅) → 2 HCONH₂ (Addition elimination sequence) → diformamido intermediate → (−Formate) → ethyl 5-methyl-imidazole-4-carboxylate → LiAlH₄ [H] → (5-methylimidazol-4-yl)methanol + HSCH₂CH₂NH₂ → HCl → 4-(CH₂SCH₂CH₂NH₂)-5-methylimidazole → (CH₃S)₂C=NCN, −CH₃SH → CH₂SCH₂CH₂NHCSCH₃ (=NCN) intermediate → CH₃NH₂, −CH₃SH → Cimetidine

Properties and uses: Cimetidine hydrochloride is a white crystalline powder, soluble in water, and sparingly soluble in ethanol. It is a H_2-receptor antagonist that not only inhibits gastric acid secretion, but also prevents other actions of histamine mediated by H_2-receptors. It is used in the treatment of peptic ulceration. Cimetidine has a weak antiandrogenic effect. Gynaecomastia may occur in patients treated for a month or more.

Assay: Dissolve the substance in a mixture of 0.01 M HCl and alcohol (1:10) and titrate against 0.1 M sodium hydroxide. Determine the end point potentiometrically.

Dose: Oral dose is 200 mg thrice a day with meals and 400 mg at night.

ii. Famotidine (Famocid, Famtac)

Synthesis

Properties and uses: Famotidine is a white or yellowish-white crystalline powder or crystals, very slightly soluble in water, soluble in anhydrous ethanol and glacial acetic acid, but practically insoluble in ethyl acetate. It acts as a competitive, reversible H_2-antagonist with a slow onset of equilibrium. This type of blockade is called nonequilibrium antagonism. It is used in the treatment of duodenal and gastric ulcers, Zollinger–Ellison syndrome, and heart burn.

Assay: Dissolve the sample in anhydrous acetic acid and titrate against 0.1 M perchloric acid. Determine the end-point potentiometrically.

Dose: The dose for gastric or duodenal ulcer is 40 mg at night for 4–8 weeks. The dose for prophylaxis or relapse is 20 mg at night. Not recommended for usage in children.

Dosage forms: Famotidine tablets B.P.

iii. Ranitidine (Zantac)

Synthesis

Metabolism of cimetidine, ranitidine, and fomotidine: Hydroxylation of the imidazole C-4 methyl group of cimitidine occurs. Ranitidine is excreted largely unchanged, but minor metabolic pathways include N-demethylation as well as N- and S-oxidation. The metabolites are thought not as contributing to the therapeutic properties of parent drugs, with the exception of nizanidine, from which the N-demethyl metabolites retains H_2-antihistamine activity.

Properties and uses: Ranitidine hydrochloride is a white or pale yellow crystalline powder, soluble in water, slightly soluble in anhydrous ethanol and methylene chloride. In Ranitidine, the imidazole ring of cimitidine was replaced by furan in conjugation with some rearrangement of the terminal functionality; the substituted guanidine group has been isosterically modified by utilizing a nitromethenyl moiety to basicity. It is used in the treatment of duodenal ulcer, gastric ulcer, and pathological hypersecretory conditions.

Assay: Dissolve the sample in water and titrate against 0.1 M sodium hydroxide. Determine the end point potentiometrically.

Dose: The dose is 150 mg (as the hydrochloride) two times a day.

Dosage forms: Ranitidine HCl injection I.P., Ranitidine HCl tablets I.P., Ranitidine injection B.P., Ranitidine oral solution B.P., Ranitidine tablets B.P.

iv. Etintidine

Synthesis

Uses: Used as antiulcer and it is twice as active as cimetidine.

v. Oxmetidine

5-(Benzo[*d*][1,3]dioxol-5-yl methyl)-2-(2-((5-methyl-1*H*-imidazol-4-yl)methylthio)ethylamino)pyrimidin-4(1*H*)-one

Synthesis

5-(Benzo[*d*][1,3]dioxol-5-yl-methyl)-2-mercaptopyrimidin-4(1*H*)-one

Oxmetidine

Properties and uses: It shows a time dependent and slow onset of action, which differentiates it from ranitidine. It is reported to have histamine H_2-receptor blocking activity.

vi. Nizatidine

N,N-Dimethyl-4-((2-(1-(methylamino)-2-nitrovinylamino)ethylthio)methyl)thiazol-2-amine

Synthesis

[Reaction scheme: 2-(Dimethylamino)ethanethioamide + Ethyl 3-bromo-2-oxopropanoate → thiazole intermediate → (i) LAH (ii) HSCH₂CH₂NH₂ → intermediate + H₃CS–C(=CHNO₂)NHCH₃ → –CH₃SH → Nizatidine]

Properties and uses: Nizatidine is a white or slightly brownish crystalline powder, sparingly soluble in water, and soluble in methanol. It is used as histamine H_2-receptor antagonist in the treatment of peptic ulcer.

Assay: It is assayed by adopting liquid chromatography techniques.

Dosage forms: Nizatidine intravenous infusion B.P.

vii. Roxatidine (Rotane, Zorpex)

Synthesis

[Reaction scheme: 3-Hydroxybenzaldehyde + Piperidine → Reductive alkylation (NaBH₄) → intermediate → –HBr, Br(H₂C)₃N-phthalimide → phthalimide intermediate → Cleaving phthalimide (NH₂NH₂) → amine intermediate → –HCl, ClOCCH₂OH → Roxatidine]

Dose and uses: Oral dose for peptic ulcer for adults is 150 mg at bedtime or 75 mg twice a day for 4–6 weeks; maintenance dose is 75 mg at bedtime. Dose for gastroesophageal reflux disease/oesophagitis, including erosions and ulcerations for adults is 75 mg twice a day or 150 mg at bedtime for 6–8 weeks. The dose for gastritis for adults is 75 mg once daily in the evening. For Zollinger–Ellison syndrome, the dose for adult is 75 mg twice a day. In anaesthetic premedication for adults, the dose is 75 mg in the evening on the day before surgery and repeated every 2 h before induction of anaesthesia, alternatively, 150 mg once on the night before surgery.

SAR of H_2-receptor Antagonists

The H_2-receptor antagonists were the result of the international modification of the histamine structure and deliberate search for a chemically related substance that would act as competitive inhibitor of the H_2-receptors.

- Imidazole ring is not the only required ring for competitive antagonism of histamine H_2-receptors. Other heterocyclic rings (furan, thiophene, thiazole, etc) that enhance the potency and selectivity of H_2-receptor antagonism can be used.
- The ring and terminal nitrogen should be separated by four carbon atoms for optimum antagonistic activity. The isosteric thioether link is also present in certain drugs.
- The terminal nitrogen group should be polar, nonbasic substituents for maximal antagonist activity. In general, antagonistic activity varies inversely with the hydrophilic character of the nitrogen group (exception ranitidine and nizatidine)

I. b. Proton pump inhibitors

Mode of action: These drugs suppress gastric acid secretion through $H^+ K^+$ ATPase pump, the two major signalling pathways that are present with the parietal cells, that is, cAMP dependent and Ca^{2+}. The respective receptors for the actions are M_3 and H_2. These receptors are modulated through the respective ionic mechanism and elicited by the acetylcholine from M_3 and histamine from H_2 receptor for release of the gastric acid mediated through $H^+ K^+$ ATPase pump. The proton pump inhibitors act on these receptors and inhibit $H^+ K^+$ ATPase, and reduce the activation of parietal cells to release the gastric acid.

i. Omeprazole (Ocid, Omez, Omicap)

5-Methoxy-2-((4-methoxy-3,5-dimethylpyridin-2-yl) methylsulfinyl) benzoimidazole

Synthesis

H₃CO—(benzene ring)—NH₂, NH₂
4-Methoxybenzene-1,2-diamine

(i) CS₂
(ii) C₂H₅ONa

→ 5-methoxy-2-mercapto-1H-benzimidazole (H₃CO-benzimidazole-SH) + 2-(chloromethyl)-3-methyl-4-methoxy-5-methylpyridine (Cl-CH₂-pyridine with CH₃, OCH₃, CH₃ substituents)

NaH ↓

H₃CO-benzimidazole-S-CH₂-pyridine(CH₃, OCH₃, CH₃)

← m-Chloroperbenzoic acid

Omeprazole: H₃CO-benzimidazole-S(=O)-CH₂-pyridine(CH₃, OCH₃, CH₃)

Properties and uses: Omeprazole sodium is a white hygroscopic powder, soluble in water, alcohol, and propylene glycol, very slightly soluble in methylene chloride. It is used in the treatment of duodenal ulcer, gastric ulcer, and pathological hypersecretory conditions.

Assay: Dissolve the sample in water and titrate against 0.1 M HCl. Determine the end-point potentiometrically.

Dose: The oral dose for NSAID-associated duodenal or gastric ulcer, gastroduodenal erosions, and prophylaxis in patients with history of gastroduodenal lesions for adult is 20 mg daily. For prophylaxis of acid aspiration during anaesthesia, the dose for adults, initially, is 40 mg given in the evening before surgery and another dose is 40 mg 2–6 h before the procedure. For acid-related dyspepsia, the dose for adults is 10 or 20 mg daily for 2–4 weeks. For peptic ulcer, the dose for adult is 20 mg daily as a single dose or 40 mg daily in severe cases. Duration of treatment for duodenal ulcers is 4 weeks; gastric ulcers is 8 weeks. Maintenance dose is 10–20 mg once daily. Capsule/tablet should be swallowed whole, do not crush or chew. Eradication of *H. pylori* infection: Dose for this treatment for adults varies with regimen, that is, 20 mg once daily or 40 mg a day as single or in two divided doses, and requires combination therapy with antibiotics.

ii. Lansoprazole (Lancid, Lancus, Lansec)

H₃CO-benzimidazole-S(=O)-CH₂-pyridine(CH₃, OCH₂CF₃)

5-Methoxy-2-((3-methyl-4-(2,2,2-trifluoroethoxy)pyridin-2-yl)methylsulfinyl)-1H-benzo[d]imidazole

Synthesis

Properties and uses: This drug is used to protect the acidic environment in the stomach. It is used in the treatment and prevention of NSAIDs-induced gastric ulcers as well as Zollinger–Ellison syndrome.

Dose: The oral dose for pathological hypersecretory conditions, example, Zollinger–Ellison syndrome, for adults initially is 60 mg daily and adjusted as required, daily doses greater than 120 mg should be given in two divided doses. For acid-related dyspepsia for adults, the dose is 15–30 mg once daily in the morning for 2–4 weeks. For peptic ulcer, the dose for adults is 30 mg once daily in the morning, given for 4 weeks (duodenal ulcer) or for 8 weeks (gastric ulcer). For NSAID-associated ulceration and prevention of NSAID-induced ulcers, the dose for adults is 15–30 mg daily for 4–8 weeks. For the eradication of *H. pylori* infection the dose for adults is 1-week triple therapy, that is, 30 mg two times a day combined with clarithromycin 500 mg two times a day and either amoxicillin 1 g two times a day or metronidazole 400 mg two times a day.

iii. Pantoprazole (Pantop, Pantodac, Pantocid)

5-(Difluoromethoxy)-2-((3,4-dimethoxypyridin-2-yl)methylsulfinyl)-1*H*-benzo[*d*]imidazole

Synthesis

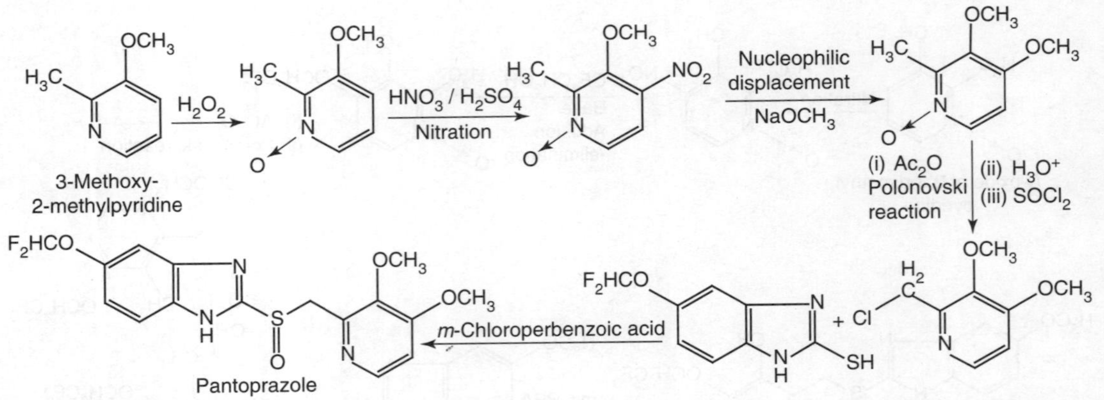

[Scheme: 3-Methoxy-2-methylpyridine → (H₂O₂) N-oxide → (HNO₃/H₂SO₄ Nitration) 4-nitro N-oxide → (Nucleophilic displacement, NaOCH₃) 3,4-dimethoxy-2-methylpyridine N-oxide → (i) Ac₂O Polonovski reaction (ii) H₃O⁺ (iii) SOCl₂ → 2-chloromethyl-3,4-dimethoxypyridine; coupling with 5-(difluoromethoxy)-2-mercapto-1H-benzimidazole → sulfide → (m-Chloroperbenzoic acid) → **Pantoprazole**]

Properties and uses: It is used in the treatment of pathological hypersecretory conditions associated with Zollinger–Ellison syndrome. There is no evidence that any of the pantoprazole metabolites have significant pharmacological activity.

Dose: The oral dose for gastroesophageal reflux disease and oesophagitis, including erosions and ulcerations, for adults is 20–40 mg once daily in the morning for 4 weeks, increased to 8 weeks, if necessary. The maintenance dose is 20–40 mg daily increased to 40 mg each morning, if symptoms return. The dose for peptic ulcer for adults is 40 mg once daily in the morning for 2–4 weeks for duodenal ulceration or 4–8 weeks for benign gastric ulceration. The dose for the eradication of *H. Pylori* infection for adults for triple therapy is 40 mg twice a day combined with clarithromycin 500 mg two times a day and either amoxicillin 1 g twice a day or metronidazole 400 mg twice a day. The dose for prophylaxis of NSAIDs-associated peptic ulcer for adults is 20 mg daily. For Zollinger–Ellison syndrome and other hypersecretory states, the adult dose initially is 80 mg daily, adjusted to individual requirements. Maximum daily dose is 240 mg daily. Daily doses greater than 80 mg should be given in two divided doses.

Intravenous: The intravenous dose for Zollinger–Ellison syndromes and other hypersecretory states for adults is 80 mg (as the Na salt) daily over 2–15 min. Maximum doses are 240 mg daily in divided doses, if rapid control is required. In the cases of peptic ulcer, gastroesophageal reflux disease, oesophagitis, including erosions and ulcerations the adult dose is 40 mg (as the Na salt) daily (over 2–15 min) until the patient can be resumed.

iv. Rabeprazole (Rabeloc, Rabifast, Rabitop)

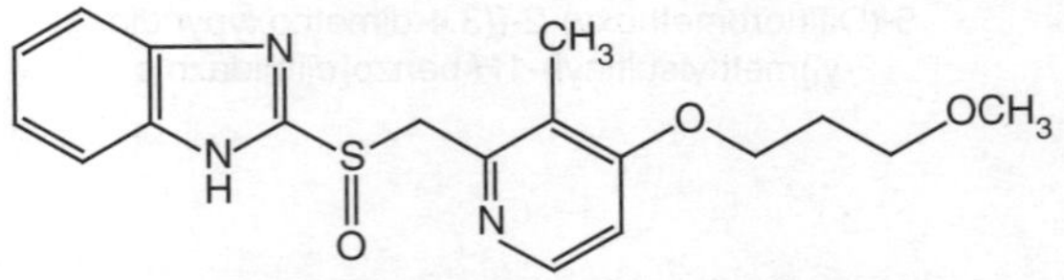

[Structure of Rabeprazole]

2-((4-(3-Methoxypropoxy)-3-methylpyridin-2-yl)
methylsulfinyl)-1H-benzo[d]imidazole

Synthesis

Uses: It is used in gastric hypersecretory disorders.

Dose: The dose for pathological hypersecretory conditions, example, Zollinger–Ellison syndrome, for adults initially is 60 mg daily, adjusted according to response. Maximum dose is 120 mg daily. For active peptic ulcer diseases for adults is 20 mg daily given for 4–8 weeks for duodenal ulcer and 6–12 weeks for gastric ulcer. In the case of eradication of *H. Pylori* infection the dose for adults as a combination with antibacterials is 20 mg twice a day combined with clarithromycin 500 mg twice a day and either amoxicillin 1 g twice a day or metronidazole 400 mg twice a day to be taken for a week.

Metabolism of proton pump inhibitors: Metabolism of omeprazole and other proton pump inhibitors occurs primarily in the liver. The sulphonated, hydroxylated, and O-demethylated metabolites have been reported as products. The oxidative metabolism of omeprazole is catalyzed principally by CYP2C19 (primarily 5'-hydroxylation and to a lesser extent, benzimidazole O-demethylation).

Different proton pump inhibitors depend differently on CYP2C19 for the oxidative metabolism, and the enantiomer show variation of independence on CYP2C19 and other pathways. Pantaprazole and lansoprazole show greater metabolism via CYP2C19. The enantiomer being affected differently than Rabeprazole, which is metabolized only to a small extent by oxidative CYP450 enzyme.

PROBABLE QUESTIONS

1. Define and classify antiulcer agents with one example in each category and write the synthesis and uses of one of them.
2. Write the mode of action of proton pump inhibitors. Outline the synthesis and uses of lansoprazole.
3. What are H_2-receptor antagonists? How does it act as antiulcer agents ? Describe the synthesis, metabolism, and uses of ranitidine.
4. Write a short note on anti-*H. pylori* drugs.
5. Name the thiazole and imidazole containing H_2 blockers and write the synthesis, metabolism, and uses of one of them.

SUGGESTED READINGS

1. Block JH and Beale JM. *Wilson Gisvold's Textbook of Organic Medicinal and Pharmaceutical Chemistry* (11th edn). New York: Lippincott Williams and Wilkins, 2004.
2. *British Pharmacopoeia*. Medicines and Healthcare Products Regulatory Agency. London, 2008.
3. Bruntan LL, Lazo JS, and Parker KL. *Goodman and Gilman's: The Pharmacological Basis of Therapeutics* (11th edn). New York: McGraw Hill, 2006.
4. Gennaro AR. *Remington: The Science and practice of Pharmacy* (21st edn). New York: Lippincot Williams and Wilkins, 2006.
5. *Indian Pharmacopoeia*. Ministry of Health and Family Welfare. New Delhi, 1996.
6. Lednicer D and Mitscher LA. *The Organic Chemistry of Drug Synthesis*. New York: John Wiley, 1995.
7. Lemke TL and William DA. Foye's *Principle of Medicinal Chemistry* (6th edn). New York: Lippincott Williams and Wilkins, 2008.
8. Wolff ME. *Burger's Medicinal Chemistry and Drug Discovery* (5th edn). New York: John Wiley, 1995.

Chapter 2

Antidiarrhoeals

INTRODUCTION

Diarrhoea means loose bowel movements resulting into the frequent passage of watery, uniformed stools with or without mucous and blood. This condition may arise due to the change in the nature of the diet and routine or sometimes due to bacterial infection. The former type of diarrhoea is the mild form while the infective diarrhoea is more powerful and persistent. Organism escapes from gastric acid and other digestive processes reaches the bowel. Their metabolic products irritate the nerve ending of intestinal wall leading to severe diarrhoea. In this condition, to compensate the loss of body fluids, a mixture of salt (sodium chloride or sodium bicarbonate) and water is to be given frequently. The simple type of diarrhoea may be controlled just by using intestinal adsorbents while infected diarrhoea needs the use of intestinal antiseptics.

Adsorbents

These substances have the power of adsorbing gases, bacteria, and toxins without undergoing any chemical reaction. They also posses the protective property apart from their adsorbent action. They form a coating over the intestinal mucosa to reduce its irritation, example of this category are kaolin, calcium carbonate, magnesium trisilicate, and aluminium hydroxide, pectin, bismuth subsalicylate and polycarbophill and various psyllium seed derivatives.

1. Diphenoxylate HCl (Lemotil)

Synthesis

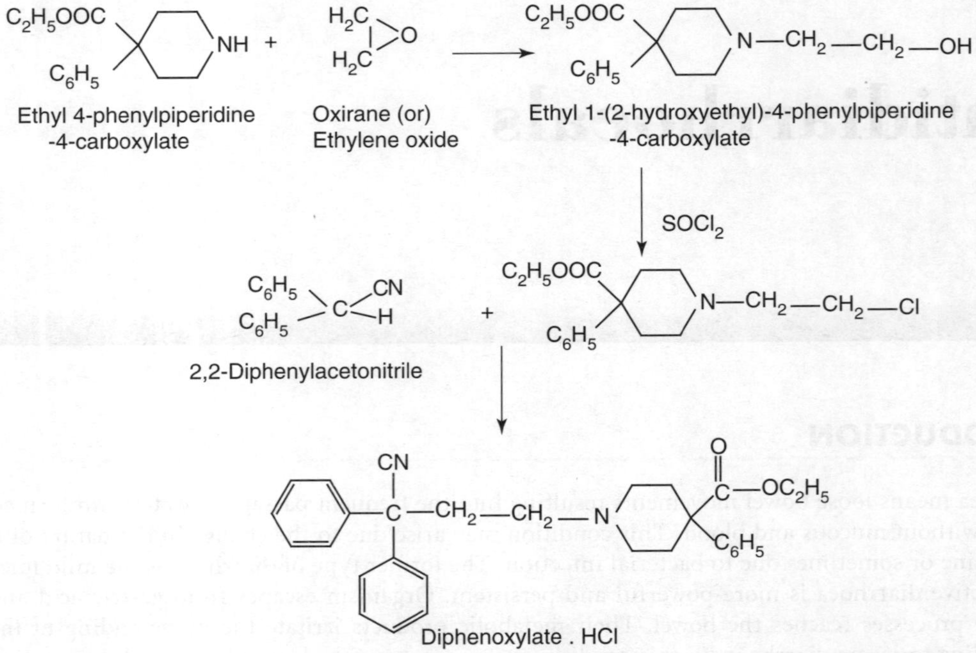

C2H5OOC
C6H5
NH
+
H2C
H2C
O
Ethyl 4-phenylpiperidine -4-carboxylate
Oxirane (or) Ethylene oxide
N—CH2—CH2—OH
Ethyl 1-(2-hydroxyethyl)-4-phenylpiperidine -4-carboxylate
SOCl2
CN
H
2,2-Diphenylacetonitrile
N—CH2—CH2—Cl
C—OC2H5
C—CH2—CH2—N
Diphenoxylate . HCl

Properties and uses: It is a weak meperidine congener lacking analgesic activity. It is used for the symptomatic activity of diarrhoea in patients with mild chronic inflammatory bowel disease and for infectious gastroenteritis.

Dose: The usual adult dose orally is 5 mg four times a day.

2. Loperamide

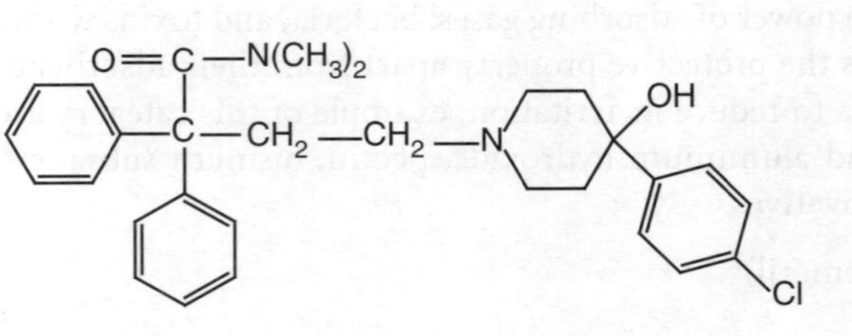

O=C—N(CH3)2
C—CH2—CH2—N
OH
Cl

Properties and uses: It is a synthetic meperidine congener devoid of sedative or respiratory depressant actions. It is orally used as an antidiarrhoeal agent. Loperamide exerts spasmolytic effect on the gastrointestinal tract (GIT) muscle by depressing slow cholinergic phase and rapid prostaglandin mediated phase of smooth muscle contraction. It may act on the intestinal nerve endings or on the ganglia.

Intestinal Antiseptics

These agents are used to treat severe diarrhoeal forms, which are due to microbial infection. They mainly comprise of certain members of the sulphonamides and antibiotics that are poorly absorbable in the GIT, and thus, reach in high concentrations to the small and large bowels. Examples are sulphasalazine, sulphaguanidine, phthalyl sulphathiazole, succinyl sulphathiazole. Various combinations of sulphonamides and antibiotics along with kaolin are available either in the form of cream or suspension. Streptomycin, neomycin, chloramphenicol, tetracyclines and nystatin are the examples of such antibiotics used for this purpose.

1. Antisecretory drugs

i. Sulphasalazine (salicylazosulphapyridine)

Synthesis

Metabolism: It undergoes reductive metabolism by gut bacteria, converting the drug into sulphapyridine and 5-amino salicylic acid, which are the active components.

Reaction scheme: Sulphasalazine (structure with HOOC, HO-phenyl-N=N-phenyl-SO₂-NH-pyridine) undergoes [H] in Gut to give 5-Amino salicylic acid (Mesalamine) + Sulphapyridine.

Properties and uses: Sulphasalazine is a bright yellow or brownish-yellow fine powder, practically insoluble in water and methylene chloride and sparingly soluble in alcohol. It dissolves in dilute solutions of alkali hydroxides and used in the treatment of inflammatory bowel diseases such as ulcerative colitis.

Assay: Dissolve and dilute the sample in 0.1 M sodium hydroxide and add 0.1 M acetic acid and measure the absorbance at the maxima of 359 nm using ultraviolet spectrophotometer.

Dosage forms: Sulphasalazine tablets B.P.

ii. Bismuth subsalicylate

It acts by decreasing prostaglandin synthesis in the intestinal mucosa, thereby reducing Cl^- secretion. It has some prophylatic value in traveller's diarrhoea (probably due to weak antibacterial action also), but it is rather inconvenient to carry and take.

iii. Atropine: Atropinic drugs can reduce bowel motility and secretion, but have poor efficacy in secretory diarrhoeas. They may benefit nervous/drug (neostigmine, metaclopramide, reserpine) induced diarrhoeas and provide some symptomatic relief in dysenteries diverticulitis.

iv. Octreotide: This somatostatin analogue has a long plasma as well as potent antisecretory/antimotility action on the gut. It has been used to control diarrhoea in carcinoid and vasoactive intestinal peptide secreting tumours and for refractory diarrhoea in AIDS patients, but needs to be given by subcutaneous injections.

v. Racecadotril: This recently introduced prodrug is rapidly converted to thiorphan, an enkephalinase inhibitor. It prevents the degradation of endogenous enkephalins, which are mainly δ opioid receptor agonists. Racecadotril decreases intestinal hypersecretion, without affecting motility by lowering mucosal cAMP due to enhanced enkephalins action. It is indicated in the short-term treatment of acute secretory diarrhoeas.

PROBABLE QUESTIONS

1. Define and classify antidiarrhoeal agents with suitable examples. Write the synthesis and uses of any two of them.
2. Write short notes on antisecretary drugs used in diarrhoea.
3. Write the synthesis of loperamide and diphenoxylate.

SECTION IV

DRUGS ACTING ON BLOOD AND BLOOD FORMING ORGANS

| 1 | Coagulants | 145 |
| 2 | Plasma Expanders | 160 |

Chapter 1

Coagulants

INTRODUCTION

Homeostasis is the cessation of blood loss from damaged vessels. Platelets first adhere to macromolecules in the subendothelial regions of injured blood vessels; they aggregate to form the primary haemostatic plug. Platelets stimulate the local activation of plasma coagulation factors, leading to generation of a fibrin clot that reinforces the platelet aggregate. Later, as wound healing occurs, the platelet aggregates and fibrin clots are degraded. Thrombosis is a pathological process in which a platelet aggregates and a fibrin clot occludes blood vessels. Arterial thrombosis may result in ischaemic necrosis of tissues supplied by the artery (e.g. myocardial infarction due to thrombosis of coronary artery). Venous thrombosis may cause tissue drain by the vein to become edematous and inflamed.

Coagulation of blood comprises the formation of fibrin by a series of interactions among a large number of protein factors and other substances. Blood coagulation process requires coagulation factors, calcium, and phospholipids.

- The coagulation factors (proteins) are manufactured by the liver.
- Ionized calcium (Ca^{++}) is available in the blood and from intracellular sources.
- Phospholipids are prominent components of the cellular and platelet membranes. They provide a surface on which the chemical reactions of coagulation can take place. The coagulation factors are numbered in the order of their discovery.

Factor I—Fibrinogen
Factor II—Prothrombin
Factor III—Tissue thromboplastin (tissue factor)
Factor IV—Ionized calcium (Ca^{++})
Factor V—Labile factor or proaccelerin
Factor VI—Unassigned
Factor VII—Stable factor or proconvertin
Factor VIII—Antihaemophilic factor
Factor IX—Plasma thromboplastin component, Christmas factor

Factor X—Stuart–Prower factor
Factor XI—Plasma thromboplastin antecedent
Factor XII—Hageman factor
Factor XIII—Fibrin stabilizing factor

Mechanism of Blood Clotting

Coagulation can be initiated by either of the two distinct pathways (Fig. 1.1):

1. The intrinsic pathway can be initiated by events that take place within the lumen of blood vessels. This requires only elements (clotting factors, Ca^{++} platelet surface, etc) found within or intrinsic to the vascular system.
2. The extrinsic pathway is the other route to coagulation. It requires tissue factor (tissue thromboplastin), a substance that is extrinsic to or not normally cumulating in the vessel. Tissue factor is released when the vessel wall is ruptured.

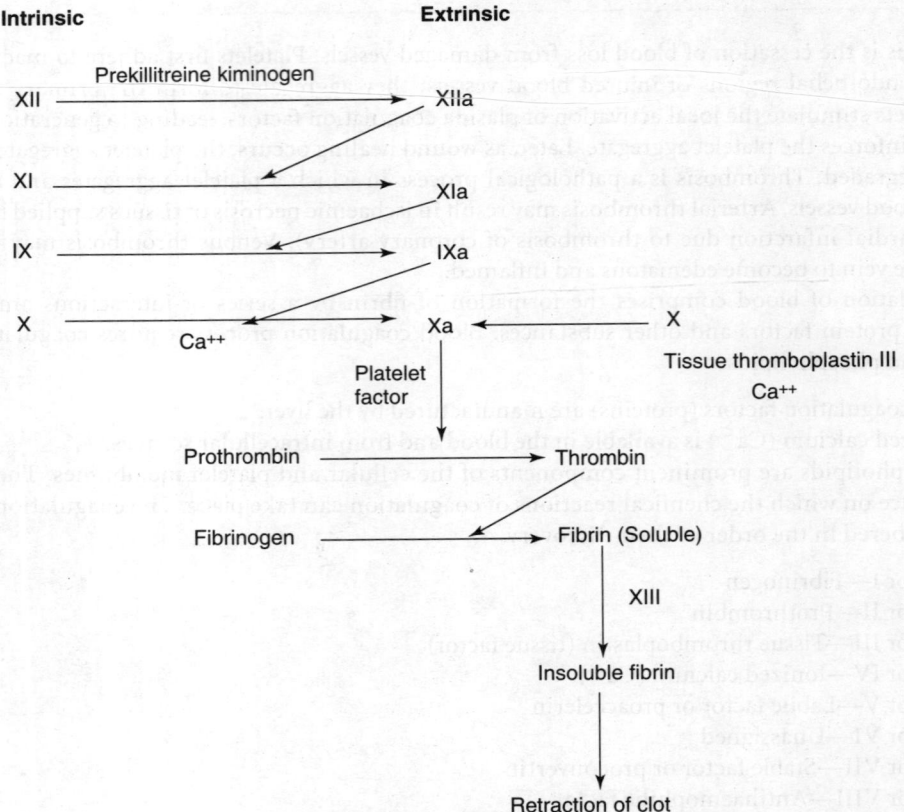

Figure 1.1 Mechanism of blood clotting.

1. Calcium salts: Calcium salts, especially Ca^{++} intravenous injections, are very popular, but it does not help much unless there is deficiency of Ca^{++} in the blood.

2. Vitamin K (Synonym: Vitamin K_1-Phytomenadione)

Properties and uses: Phytomenadione is a clear intense yellow viscous oily liquid, practically insoluble in water, sparingly soluble in ethanol, and miscible with fatty oils. Vitamin K is essential to keep up the prothrombin level in blood by forming prothrombin in the liver. Hence, it is used orally and intramuscular (IM), now water-soluble vitamin K is available for intravenous (IV) administration. This is called methyl naphthaquinone and is very useful in emergency.

Assay: It is assayed by adopting liquid chromatography technique.

Dosage forms: Phytomenadione injection B.P., Phytomenadione tablets B.P.

3. Vitamin K_3 (Menadione)

Properties and uses: Menadione is a pale-yellow crystalline powder, practically insoluble in water, soluble in toluene, sparingly soluble in alcohol and methanol. Used as source of vitamin K and has prothrombogenic property.

Assay: Dissolve the sample in glacial acetic acid and add dilute hydrochloric acid and zinc powder. Allow the mixture to stand and titrate against 0.1 M ammonium cerric nitrate using ferroin as indicator.

Anticoagulants

Anticoagulants are drugs that prevent the clotting of blood. Heparin is a glucosaminoglycan found in the secretory granules of mast cells. It is synthesized from uridine diphosphate sugar precursor as a polymer of alternating D-gluconic acid and N-acetyl-D-glucosamine residue. About 10–15 glucosaminoglycan chains, each containing 200–300 monosaccharide units, are attached to a core protein and yield a proteoglycan with a molecular mass of 750,000–1,000,000 daltons. The glucosaminoglycan then undergoes a series modification, which includes *n*-acetylation and *n*-sulphonation of glucosamine, epimerization of D-gluconic acid to L-iduronic acid, O-sulphation of iduronic and glucoronic acid residues at the C_2 position, and O-sulphation of glucosamine residue at C_3 and C_6 position. Each of these modification reactions is incomplete, yielding variety of oligosaccharide structures. After the heparin proteoglycan has been transported to the mast cell granule, an endo-β-D-glucuronidase degrades the glycosamionoglycan chains to 5000–30,000 dalton fragments over a period of hours.

CLASSIFICATION

Anticoagulants are classified as follows:
  I. In vitro anticoagulants: Heparin, Sodium oxalate, and Sodium citrate.
  II. In vivo anticoagulants.
   1. Heparin: injectable
   2. Oral
      a. Coumarin derivatives: Warfarin, Bishydroxycoumarin.
      b. Indandiones: Phenindione, Diphenadion.

I. In vitro anticoagulants
Heparin, Sodium citrate, Sodium oxalate

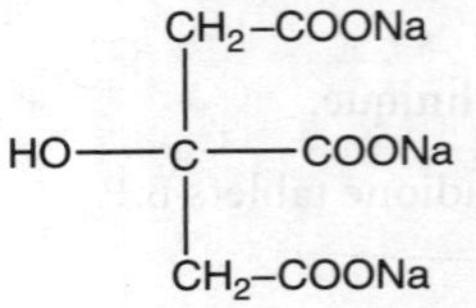

Sodium citrate

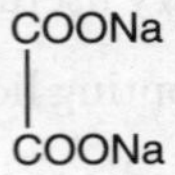

Sodium oxalate

II. In vivo anticoagulants
a. Coumarin derivatives

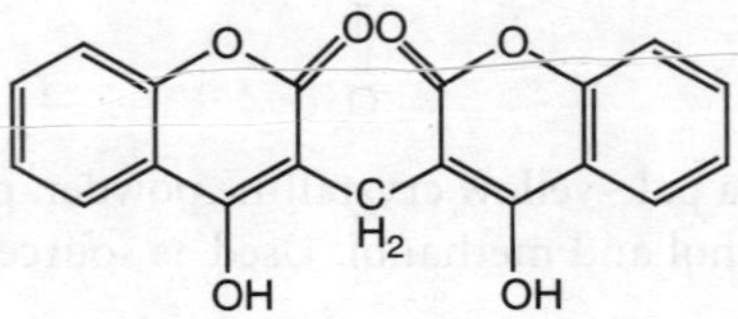

Dicoumarol

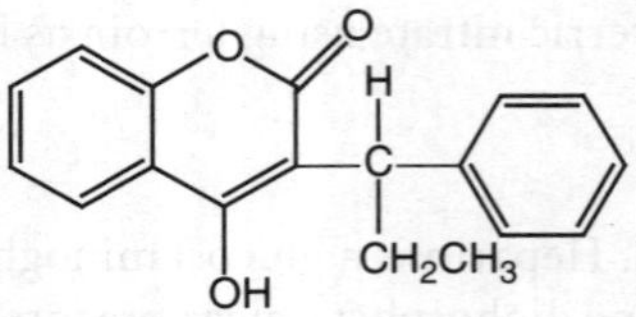

Phenprocoumon

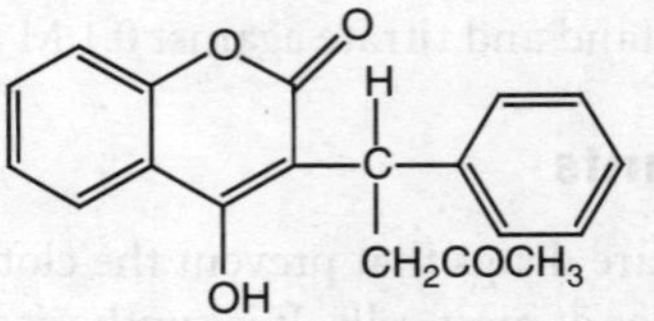

Warfarin

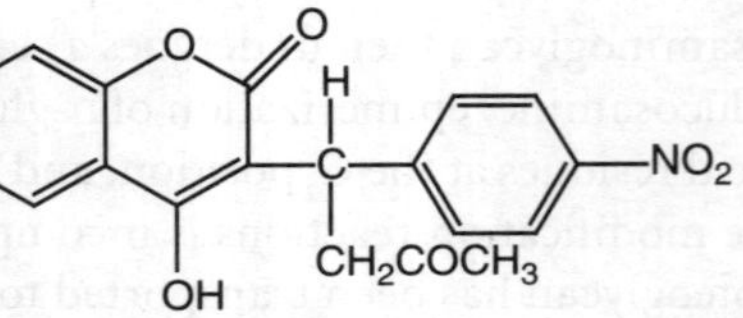

Acenocoumarol

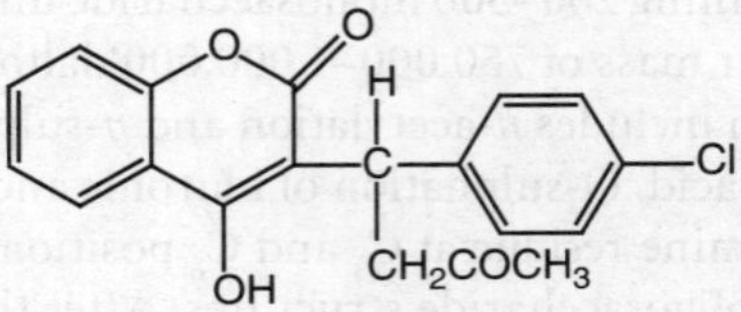

Coumachlor

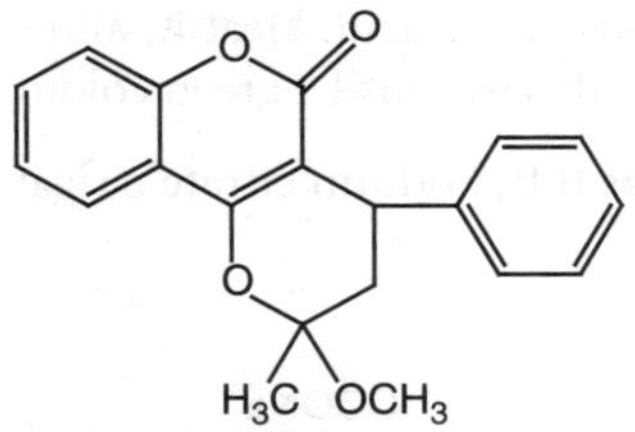

Cyclocoumarol

b. Indandione derivatives

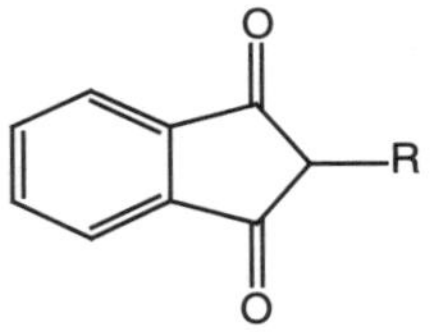

Name	R₁
Phenindione	$-C_6H_5$
Anisindione	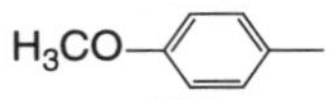 $H_3CO-\langle\text{C}_6H_4\rangle-$
Bromindione	$Br-\langle\text{C}_6H_4\rangle-$
Diphenadione	$-COCH(C_6H_5)_2$

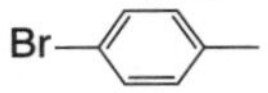

SYNTHESIS AND DRUG PROFILE

I. In vitro anticoagulants

i. Sodium citrate

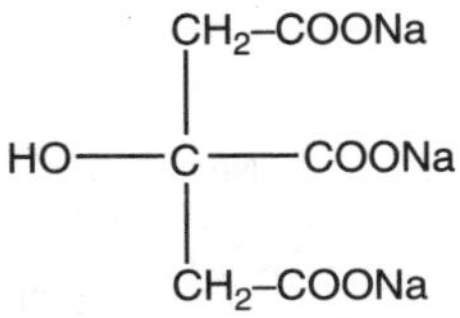

Synthesis

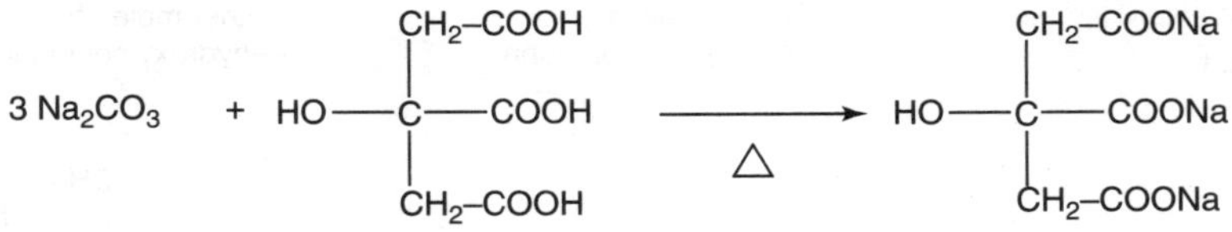

$$3\ Na_2CO_3 + \text{Citric acid} \xrightarrow{\Delta} \text{Sodium citrate}$$

Properties and uses: Sodium citrate exists as white crystalline powder or granular crystals, soluble in water, but insoluble in alcohol and used as systemic alkalinizing substance.

Assay: Dissolve the sample in anhydrous acetic acid. Heat it, allow to cool and titrate against 0.1 M perchloric acid using naphtholbenzein as indicator until a green colour is obtained.

Dosage forms: Sodium citrate eye drops B.P., Sodium citrate irrigation solution B.P.

ii. Sodium oxalate

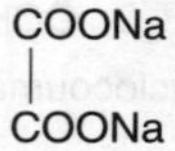

$$\begin{array}{c} COONa \\ | \\ COONa \end{array}$$

Synthesis

$$Na_2CO_3 + \begin{array}{c} COOH \\ | \\ COOH \end{array} \xrightarrow{\Delta} \begin{array}{c} COONa \\ | \\ COONa \end{array}$$

Oxalic acid → Sodium oxalate

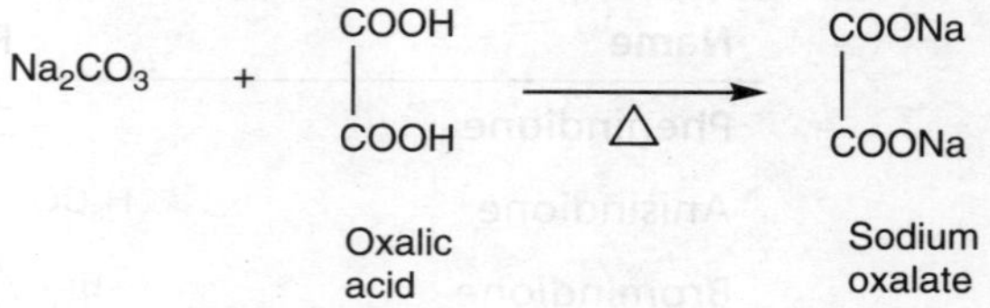

II. In vivo anticoagulants or coumarin derivatives

i. Bishydroxycoumarin (Dicoumarol)

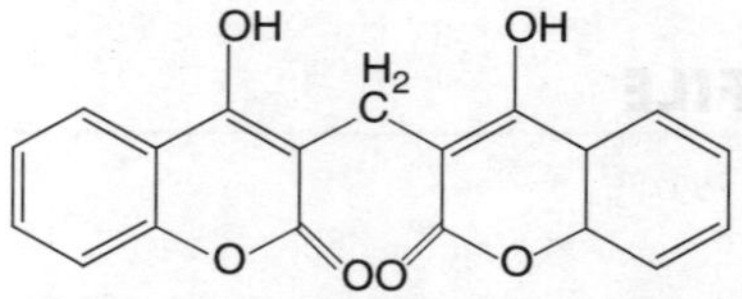

4-Hydroxy-3-((4-hydroxy-2-oxochroman-3-yl)methyl)-2H-chromen-2-one

Synthesis

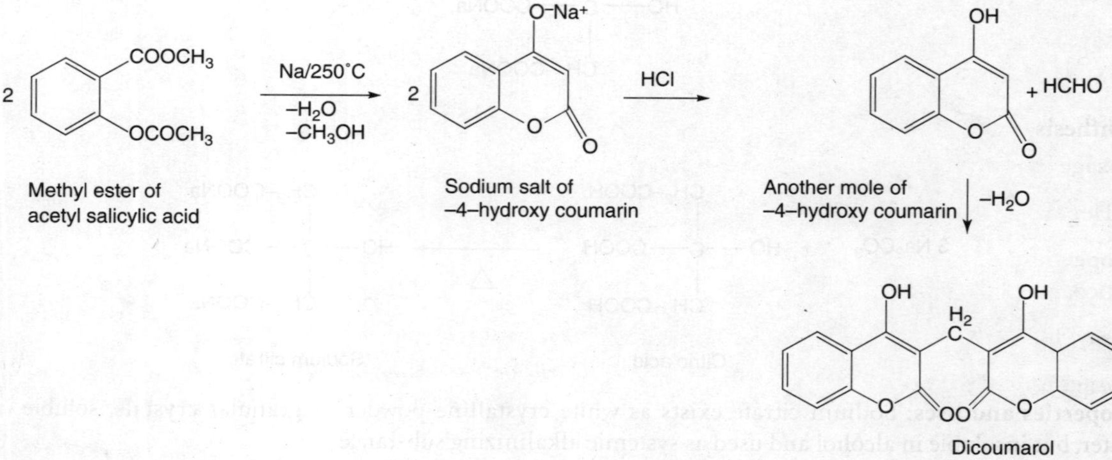

2 [Methyl ester of acetyl salicylic acid] $\xrightarrow[-H_2O, -CH_3OH]{Na/250°C}$ 2 [Sodium salt of –4–hydroxy coumarin] $\xrightarrow{HCl}$ [Another mole of –4–hydroxy coumarin] + HCHO $\xrightarrow{-H_2O}$ Dicoumarol

Properties and uses: It is used in postoperative thrombophlebitis, pulmonary embolus, acute embolic, and thrombolic occlusion of peripheral arteries.

ii. Warfarin (Coumarin, Coumadia)

4-Hydroxy-3-(3-oxo-1-phenylbutyl)-2H-chromen-2-one

Synthesis

Properties and uses: Warfarin sodium is a white hygroscopic powder, soluble in water, alcohol, and acetone, very slightly soluble in methylene chloride. The (−) (S) isomer of warfarin has shown itself to be five to eight times more potent than (+) (R) enantiomer. Warfarin is a synthetic anticoagulant used in patients undergoing orthopaedic surgery.

Assay: Dissolve the sample in 0.01 M sodium hydroxide and measure the absorbance after dilution at the maxima of 308 nm using ultraviolet spectrophotometer.

Dose: The dose for adults is 10–15 mg per day for 2 to 4 days.

Dosage forms: Warfarin tablets I.P., B.P.

ii. Heparin

Properties and uses: Heparin sodium is a white hygroscopic powder, soluble in water and used as an anticoagulant.

Assay: It is assayed by adopting spectrophotometric method.

Dosage forms: Heparin injection B.P.

iii. Ethyl biscoumacetate

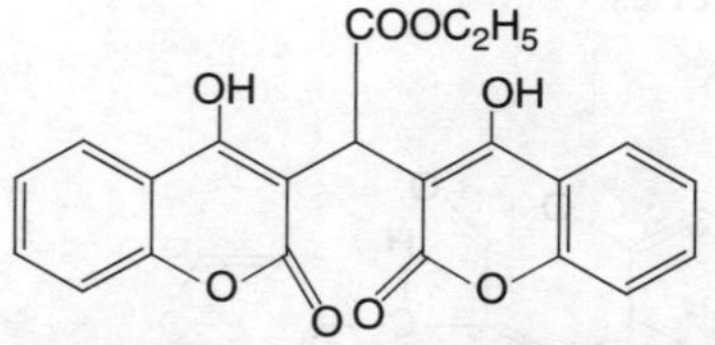
COOC2H5
OH
OH
O
O
O
O

Ethyl 2,2-bis(4-hydroxy-2-oxo-2*H*-chromen-3-yl)acetate

iv. Acenocoumarol

Properties and uses: Acenocoumarol is a white to buff-coloured powder, practically insoluble in water and ether, slightly soluble in ethanol. It dissolves in aqueous solutions of the alkali hydroxides. Used as vitamin K epoxide reductase inhibitor and as oral anticoagulant.

Assay: Dissolve the sample in acetone and titrate against 0.1 M sodium hydroxide using bromothymol blue as indicator.

Dosage forms: Acenocoumarol tablets B.P.

II. b. Indanedione derivatives—General method of preparation

Synthesis of Phenindione, Anisindione, and Bromindione

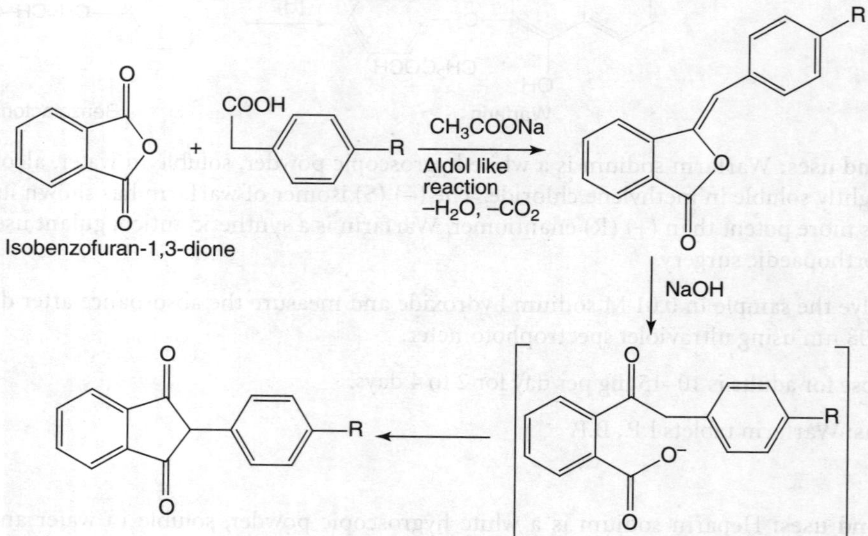
Isobenzofuran-1,3-dione
COOH
R
CH3COONa
Aldol like
reaction
–H2O, –CO2
NaOH
O–

Name	R
Phenindione	–H
Anisindione	$-OCH_3$
Bromindione	–Br

These 1,3-indandiones have been recognized for their anticoagulant activity.

i. Phenindione

Properties and uses: Phenindione exists as white crystalline powder, very slightly soluble in water, slightly soluble in ethanol and ether. Used as oral anticoagulant.

Assay: To the sample, add ethanol and warm it, cool to room temperature, add 10% v/v solution of bromine in ethanol, and allow standing with occasional shaking. Add 2-naphthol and shake until the colour of the bromine is discharged. Add water, and dilute potassium iodide solution and titrate the liberated iodine against 0.1 M sodium thiosulphate using starch mucilage as indicator.

Dosage forms: Phenindione tablets I.P., B.P.

ii. Thrombolytics (Fibrinolytics)

Fibrinolytics are drugs used to lyse thrombi and to recanalize occluded blood vessels mainly coronary artery. Anticoagulants are designed to prevent thrombus formation. A proteolytic enzyme, known as plasmin, which is released by its precursor protein plasminogen causes the destruction or dissolution of a thrombus. Plasminogen activators (e.g. streptokinase, urokinase) bring about this conversion (Fig. 1.2).

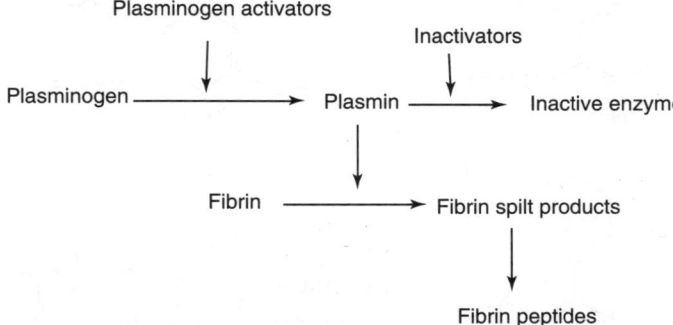

Figure 1.2 Dissolution of thrombus.

Certain other compounds have been found to promote the synthesis of various plasminogen activators. For example, anabolic steroids, act indirectly as fibrinolytic agents. All these agents are useful in the treatment of pulmonary embolic and acute coronary thrombosis. Streptokinase and urokinase are commonly used fibrinolytic agents in the treatment of acute thromboembolic diseases.

a. Streptokinase

Streptokinase is obtained from group-C beta haemolytic *Streptococci*. It is inactive; therefore, to be active it must be converted to plasminogen, which causes proteolysis of plasmin. It is typically used in myocardial infarctions and arterial thrombosis.

b. Urokinase

It is isolated from the human urine, now prepared from the cultures of human renal cells. It is nonantigenic and is a glycosylate serine protease containing 41 amino acid residues. It is a substrate for plasminogen, which is activated to plasmin.

c. Anistrepalse

It is a streptokinase–plasminogen complex in which plasminogen is isolated and acts as a slow released form of plasminogen activator. Coupling of the streptokinase–plasminogen complex to *p*-amidinophenyl-*p*-anisate blocks the catalytic centre of the complex, but allows it to bind to fibrin. As the anisoyl group is slowly hydrolyzed in vivo, the complex is allowed to bind to fibrin prior to activation. It is used in the management of acute myocardial infarction.

d. Aspirin

Synthesis and drug profile is discussed in sec I, NSAIDs.

Antiplatelet drugs (Antithrobocytic drugs)

Platelets provide the initial haemostatic plug at the sites of vascular injury. Platelet aggregation is implicated in thrombus formation in arterial systems and pathogenesis of atherosclerosis. Thus, agents that inhibit platelet aggregation should be able to modify or prevent atherosclerotic disease and thrombosis.

Drugs interfering with platelet functions are as follows:

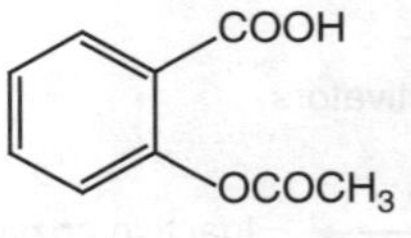

Aspirin

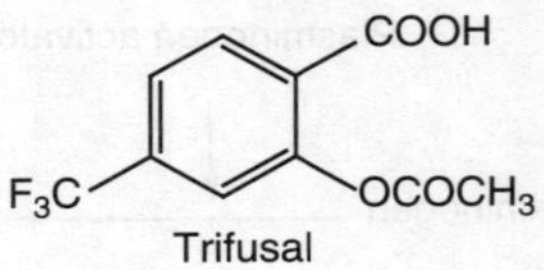

Trifusal

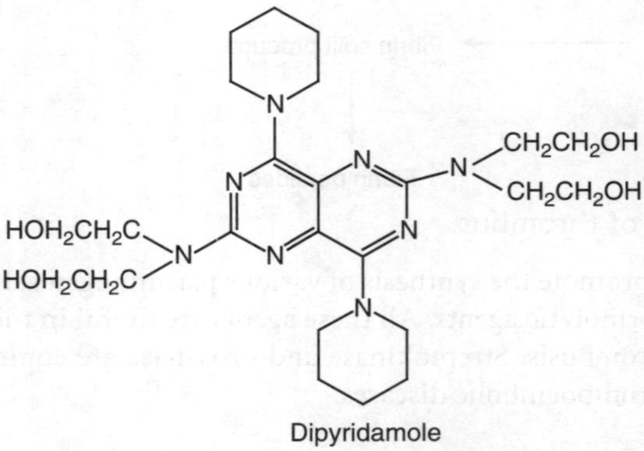

Dipyridamole

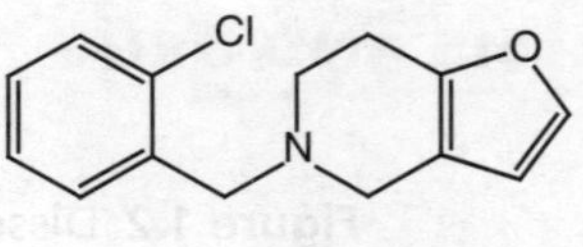

Ticlopidine

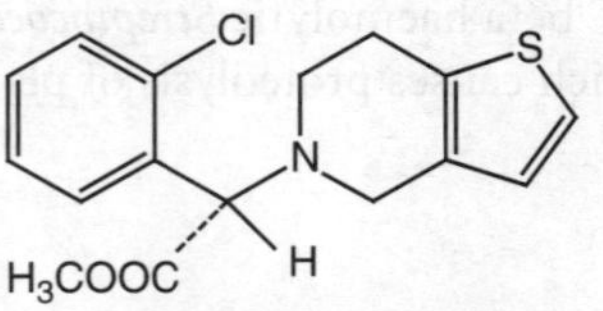

Clopidogrel

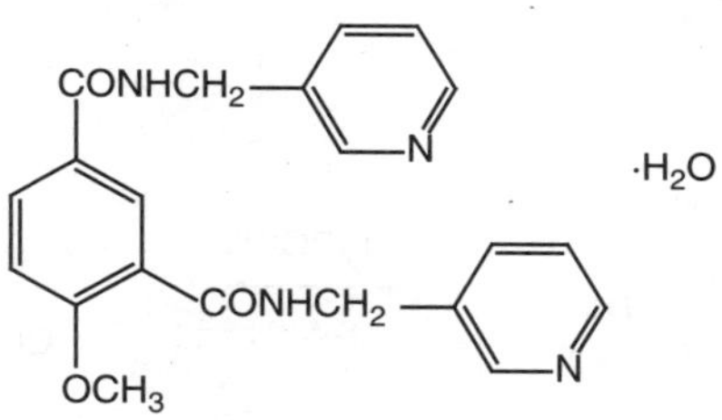

Picotamide monohydrate

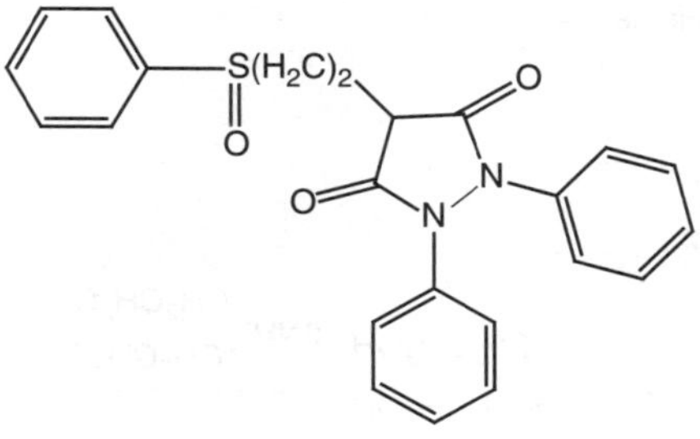

Sulphinapyrazone

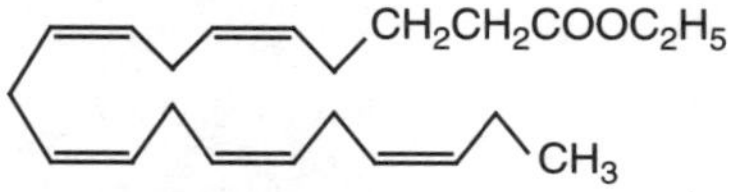

Ethyl icosapentate

SYNTHESIS AND DRUG PROFILE

i. Aspirin

Mode of action: Aspirin inhibits the enzyme cycloxygenase and thromboxane synthetase (TxA_2) by binding irreversibly and interfering with the platelet aggregation.

Synthesis and drug profile of Aspirin is discussed in under sec I, Chapter NSAIDs.

ii. Dipyridamole (Persantine, Cardiwell)

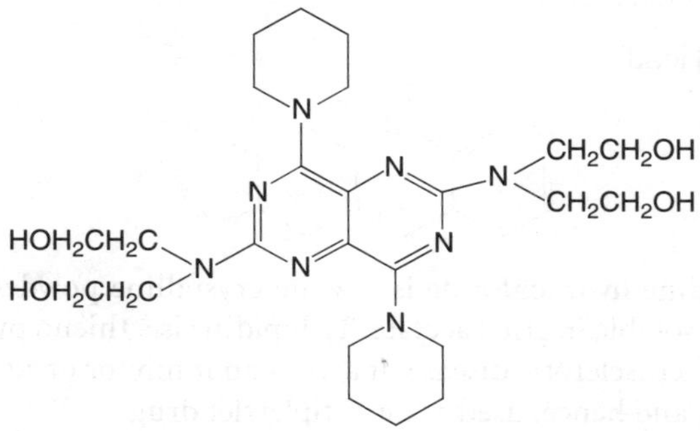

Synthesis

Pyrimido[5,4-d]pyrimidine-2,4,6,8-tetraol → (PCl$_5$/POCl$_3$) → Perchloropyrimido[5,4-d]pyrimidine → (2 piperidine) → intermediate → (2 NH(CH$_2$CH$_2$OH)$_2$) → Dipyridamole

Properties and uses: Dipyridamole is a bright yellow crystalline powder, practically insoluble in water, soluble in acetone, ethanol, and dilute solutions of mineral acids. It is an adenosine reuptake inhibitor, inhibitor of platelet aggregation, and useful in transient ischaemic attacks and secondary prevention of myocardial infarction.

Assay: Dissolve the sample in methanol and titrate against 0.1 M perchloric acid. Determine the end point potentiometrically.

Dose: 50–75 mg 8 hrly in combination with aspirin.

Dosage forms: Dipyridamole tablets B.P.

iii. Ticlopidine HCl (Tyklid, Ticlid)

Properties and uses: Ticlopidine hydrochloride is a white crystalline powder, sparingly soluble in water and ethanol, and very slightly soluble in ethyl acetate. Ticlopidine is a thieno pyridines used for thrombosis prevention in patients with atherosclerotic disease. It acts as an inhibitor of adenosine diphosphate (ADP)-mediated platelet aggregation, and hence, used as an antiplatelet drug.

Synthesis

*[Synthesis scheme for Ticlopidine: Thiophene-2-carbaldehyde → 2-(2-Isocyanatovinyl)thiophene → thieno[3,2-c]pyridinone → 4-chloro thienopyridine → (H) reduction → thienopyridine → NaBH4 → tetrahydrothienopyridine (NH) → acylation with 2-chlorobenzoyl chloride (Cl-COCl) → N-CO-(2-chlorophenyl) intermediate → LiAlH4 → **Ticlopidine**. Alternative route: 2-chlorobenzyl chloride (Cl-CH2Cl) + tetrahydrothienopyridine, Kf/Celite in THF 50°C for 3 hrs.]*

Dosage: The oral dose is 250 mg twice a day.

Assay: Dissolve the sample in anhydrous acetic acid and add acetic anhydride. Titrate against 0.1 M perchloric acid and determine the end point potentiometrically.

iv. Sulphinpyrazone (Anturane)

[Structure of Sulphinpyrazone: a pyrazolidine-3,5-dione with two N-phenyl groups and a 4-(2-(phenylsulfinyl)ethyl) substituent — Ph-S(O)-(CH2)2- attached at C-4 of the pyrazolidinedione ring bearing two N-phenyl groups.]

Properties and uses: Sulphinpyrazone is a white powder, very slightly soluble in water, sparingly soluble in alcohol, but soluble in dilute solutions of alkali hydroxides. It has antiplatelet and potent uricosuric effects, and hence, used in the treatment of gout.

Synthesis

Assay: Dissolve the sample in acetone and titrate against 0.1 M sodium hydroxide using bromothymol blue as indicator until the colour changes from yellow to blue.

Dose: The dose is 300 mg four times a day.

Dosage forms: Sulphinpyrazone tablets B.P.

v. Picotamide Monohydrate

Properties and uses: Picotamide monohydrate is a white crystalline powder, slightly soluble in water, soluble in ethanol, methylene chloride, and dilute mineral acids. It acts as thromboxane synthetase inhibitor and thromboxane receptor antagonist; used as antiplatelet agent.

Assay: Dissolve the sample in a mixture of anhydrous acetic acid and acetic anhydride (1:1) and titrate against 0.1 M perchloric acid. Determine the end point potentiometrically.

PROBABLE QUESTIONS

1. Classify anticoagulants with suitable examples and write the synthesis of any two of them.
2. Enumerate the coumarin derived anticoagulants and write the synthesis of one of them.
3. Write a short note on in vivo anticoagulants.
4. Write a note on indanedione derivatives.
5. Describe in detail about antithrombocytic and fibrinolytic agents.

SUGGESTED READINGS

1. *British Pharmacopoeia*. Medicines and Healthcare products regulatory agency. London, 2008.
2. Bruntan LL, Lazo JS, and Parker KL. *Goodman and Gilman's: The Pharmacological Basis of Therapeutics* (11th edn). New York: McGraw Hill, 2006.
3. Colmon RW, Hirsch J, Marder VJ, and Salzman EW. *Hemostasis and Thrombosis* (2nd edn). Philadelphia: JB Lippincott, 1987.
4. Coller BS. 'Platelets and thrombolytic therapy'. *N Engl J Med* 322: 33, 1990.
5. Gennaro AR. *Remington: The Science and Practice of Pharmacy* (21st edn). New York: Lippincot Williams and Wilkins, 2006.
6. Ito M, Smith A, and Lee M. 'Ticlopidine hydrochloride'. *Clin Pharm* 11: 603–17, 1992.
7. *Indian Pharmacopoeia*. Ministry of Health and Family Welfare. New Delhi, 1996.
8. Jakabowski JA, Smith GF, and Sail DJ. 'Future antithrombatic therapy'. *Ann Rept Med Chem* 27: 99–108, 1992.
9. Reynolds EF (ed). *Martindale the Extra Pharmacopoeia* (31st edn). London: The Pharmaceutical Press, 1997.
10. Simmons ML. 'Thrombolytic therapy in acute mycocardial infarction'. *Ann Rev Med* 40: 181, 1989.
11. Shebuski RJ. 'Emerging drug discovery targets in thrombosis and coagulation'. *Ann Rept Med Chem* 26: 93–101, 1997.

Chapter 2

Plasma Expanders

INTRODUCTION

A haemorrhagic shock may result from the loss of blood during burns, wounds, or surgery. Mild shock results when there is a loss of 15% to 20% in the total blood volume. Further loss of blood, up to 40% of total blood volume may lead to severe shock during which the cardiovascular functioning is severely affected. To restore this functioning, saline should be administered as an initial emergency measure. Plasma expanders can also be used to overcome the initial losses.

There are of two types of plasma expanders: (i) Natural products and (ii) Synthetic products

Natural products: These include transfusion of whole blood or the preparations of plasma proteins. Blood products containing plasma proteins are human albumin (albumisol) and plasma protein fraction (PPF). Both of these preparations are usually given by intravenous infusion.

Synthetic products: Dextran, hetastarch, perfluorochemicals, polyvinylpyrrolidone, and gelatin are some of the synthetic plasma expanders, out of which dextran has been used extensively.

i. Dextran

Dextran could be considered as being almost close to ideal plasma expanders. Dextrans are colloidal glucose polymers that are obtained from sucrose by the action of bacteria, *Leuconostoc mesenteroides*. The dextran molecule consists mainly of 1:6 glucoside linkages with relatively few 1:4 linkages and has an average molecular weight of 40 millions. This form is not clinically suitable. Hence, it is partially hydrolyzed in vitro to give dextran with average molecular weight of 40,000, 70,000, 11,000, and 15,000 daltons. They are known as dextran-40, dextran-70, dextran-110, and dextran-150, respectively. Of these, dextran-40 and dextran-70 are of clinical importance. Solutions of dextran in isotonic sodium chloride is used to increase the circulating blood volume and to maintain the venous pressure, right arterial pressure, stroke volume, and cardiac output. Only dextran solutions are used in the treatment of hypoproteinaemia, nephrosis, and toxaemia of late pregnancy. Dextran does not posses oxygen-carrying capacity.

The dextran solution is pharmacologically inactive and has been reported as having no significant deleterious effect on renal, hepatic, or any other vital functions. Occasionally, sensitization reaction may occur in some patients. The bleeding time, fibrin polymerization on platelet function may be impaired in vivo. Dextrans are contraindicated in patients with anaemia, severe thrombocytopenia, and low plasma fibrinogen level.

ii. Human albumin

It is obtained from pooled human plasma; 100 ml of 20% human albumin solution is the osmotic equivalent of about 400 ml of fresh frozen plasma or 800 ml of whole blood. It can be used without regard to the patient's blood group and does not interfere with coagulation. Unlike whole blood or plasma, it is free of risk of transmitting serum hepatitis because the preparation is heat-treated. There is also no risk of sensitization with repeated infusions. It has been used in acute hypoproteinaemia, acute liver failure, and dialysis.

iii. Degraded gelatin polymer (polygeline)

It is a polypeptide with an average MW 30,000, which exerts osmotic pressure similar to albumin, and is not antigenic and hypersensitivity reactions are rare. It does not interfere with the grouping and cross matching of blood and remains stable for 3 years. It can be used for the priming of heart–lung dialysis machines.

iv. Hydroxyethyl starch (HES, hetastarch)

It is a complex mixture of ethoxylated amylopectin of various molecular sizes, average MW 4.5 lakh (range 10,000–1 million). The colloidal properties of 6% HES approximate those of human albumin. Plasma volume expands slightly in excess of the volume infused. It has been used to improve harvesting of granulocytes because it accelerates erythrocyte sedimentation. Adverse effects are vomiting, mild fever, itching, chills, flu-like symptoms, swelling of salivary glands, urticaria, perorbital oedema, and bronchospasm are the anaphylactoid reactions.

v. Polyvinylpyrrolidone (PVP)

It is a synthetic polymer (average MW 40,000) used as a 3.5% solution. It interferes with the blood grouping and cross matching. It has been found to bind penicillin and insulin in circulation, so that the same is not available for action. It is not frequently used as a plasma expander.

PROBABLE QUESTIONS

1. What are plasma expanders? Write their uses and describe briefly about any two of the products used as plasma expanders.
2. Write a brief note on dextran.

SECTION V

DRUGS ACTING ON ENDOCRINE SYSTEM

1	Oral Hypoglycaemic Drugs	165
2	Steroids	192
3	Antithyroid Drugs	215

Chapter 1

Oral Hypogylcaemic Drugs

INTRODUCTION

Diabetes mellitus is a metabolic disorder characterized by hyperglycaemia, glycosuria, hyperlipidemia, negative nitrogen balance, and ketonaemia. Most patients can be classified, clinically, as having either type I diabetes mellitus (insulin dependent diabetes mellitus (IDDM) or type II noninsulin dependent diabetes mellitus (NIDDM). The incidence of each type of diabetes varies widely throughout the world. In the United States, about 5% to 10% of the diabetic patients have type I diabetes mellitus, with an incidence of 17 per 100,000 found in United Kingdom. The vast majority of diabetic patients have type II diabetes mellitus.

Type I diabetes is also called juvenile onset diabetes mellitus. There is β-cell destruction in the pancreatic islets of langerhans. Majority of the cases are due to autoimmune (type I A) antibodies that destroy β cells, are detectable in blood, but some are idiopathic (type I B) no β (beta) cell antibody is found. In all type I cases, circulating insulin levels are low or very low and ketosis may occur. Genetic predisposition is also a cause for this condition.

Type II diabetes is also called maturity onset diabetes mellitus. There is no loss or moderate reduction in the β cell mass, insulin in circulation levels is low and generally has a late onset of disease after middle age. This may be due to an abnormality in the glucoreceptors of β cells, therefore, they respond at higher glucose concentrations or at relative β cell deficiency. The reduced sensitivity of peripheral tissues to insulin and reduction in the number of insulin receptors are a consequence for producing diabetes. When glucagons exceed a normal amount, it produces hypoglycaemia. The insulin is secreted by the β cells of langerhans, synthesized by a single chain precursor of 110 amino acid preproinsulin. After translocation through the membrane of rough endoplasmic reticulum, the 24 amino acid N-terminal peptide of preproinsulin is rapidly cleared off to form proinsulin. Here, the molecules folds and the disulphide bonds are formed. In the conversion of proinsulin to insulin in the Golgi complex, four basic amino acids and the remaining connector or C peptide are removed by proteolysis. This gives rise to two peptide chains (A and B) of insulin molecules, which contains one intrasubunit and two intersubunits disulphide bonds. The A chain consists of 21 amino acids and B with 30 amino acids and molecular mass is about 5734 daltons.

The regulatory factors of insulin secretion are chemical, hormonal, and neural. Chemical regulation depends upon the glucose entry in to the β cells by glucose transport. Once, after the entry of glucose and its phosphorylation by glucokinase, glucoreceptor activation indirectly inhibits the adenosine triphosphate (ATP) sensitive potassium channels and increases intracellular calcium, which triggers the exocytic release of insulin. Hormonal change in corticosteroids modify the release of insulin. Insulin inhibits glucagon secretion and glucagons increase the insulin secretion.

The neural control is mediated by α_2 and β_2 receptors. Stimulation of α_2 receptor decreases the insulin release and stimulation of β_2 receptors increases insulin release. Cholinergic stimulation increases the insulin secretion.

Hypoglycaemic drugs are agents, which decrease the blood sugar level. Oral hypoglycaemic agents must be distinguished from more hypoglycaemic drugs, such as salicylates, which are too toxic for clinical use in doses that effectively lower the blood sugar. An ideal antidiabetic drug should be nontoxic and correct the basic metabolic defects in diabetics, in addition to lowering the blood sugar.

CLASSIFICATION

I. Sulphonylureas

$$R^1-\text{C}_6\text{H}_4-SO_2-NH-\underset{\underset{O}{\|}}{C}-NH-R$$

a. First-generation drugs

Name	R	R^1
Carbutamide	$-^nC_4H_9$	$-NH_2$
Tolbutamide	$-^nC_4H_9$	$-CH_3$
Chloropropamide	$-^nC_3H_7$	$-Cl$
Tolazamide	(azepane ring, −N<)	$-CH_3$
Acetohexamide	(cyclohexyl)	$-COCH_3$

b. Second-generation drugs

Name	R	R
Glibenclamide (Glyburide)	(cyclohexyl)	(2-methoxy-5-chlorophenyl)−CO−NH(CH$_2$)$_2$
Glipizide	(cyclohexyl)	(5-methylpyrazin-2-yl)−CO−NH(CH$_2$)$_2$

(Continued)

(Continued)

Name	R	R
Gliclazide	(N-bicyclic pyrrolidine group)	–CH$_3$
Glibornuride	(bornyl group with CH$_3$, OH, (H$_3$C)$_2$)	–CH$_3$

II. Biguanides

(General structure: R–N(R$_1$)–C(=NH)–NH–C(=NH)–NH$_2$)

Name	R	R$_1$
Phenformin	C$_6$H$_5$–CH$_2$CH$_2$–	–H
Metformin	–CH$_3$	–CH$_3$
Buformin	–CH$_2$CH$_2$CH$_2$CH$_3$	–H

III. Substituted benzoic acid derivatives (Meglitinides)

i. Meglitinide

(Structure: 5-chloro-2-methoxy-N-[2-(4-carboxyphenyl)ethyl]benzamide)

ii. Repaglinide

iii. Nateglinide

IV. Thiazolidinediones (Glitazones)

Name	R
Pioglitazone	5-ethylpyridin-2-yl-CH$_2$—
Ciglitazone	1-methylcyclohexyl-CH$_2$—
Rosiglitazone	N-methyl-N-(pyrimidin-2-yl)amino-CH$_2$CH$_2$—

V. α-Glucosidase inhibitors

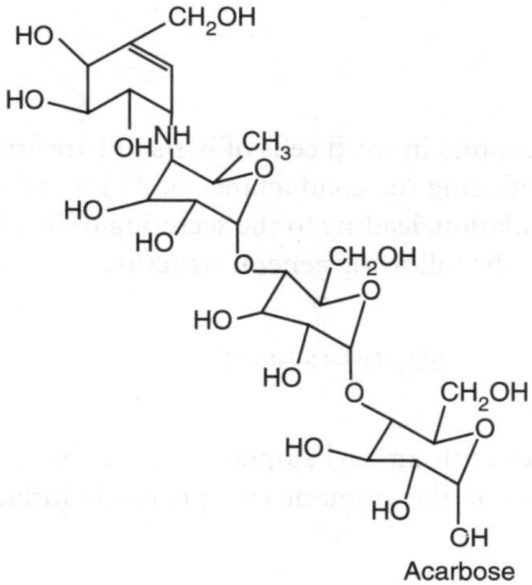

Acarbose

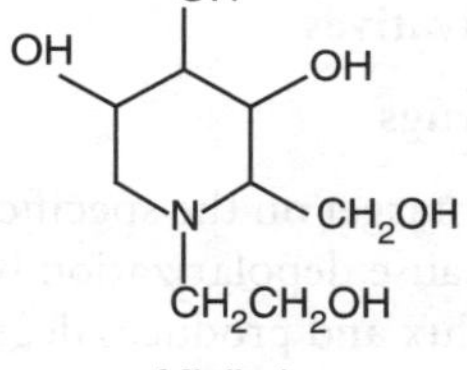

Miglitol

VI. Aldose reductase inhibitors

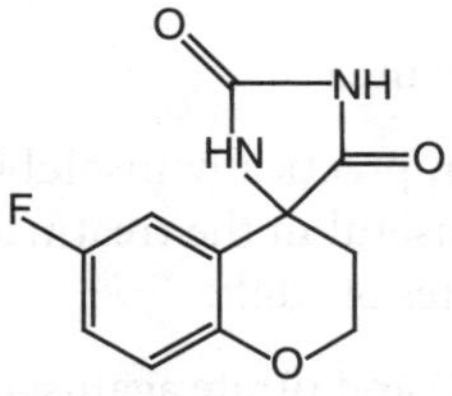

Sorbinil

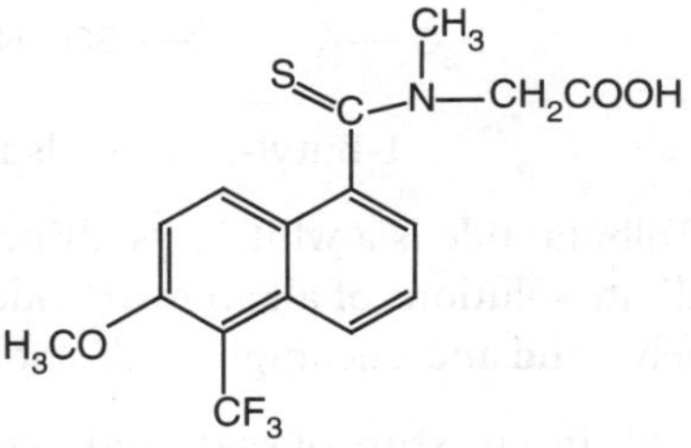

Tolrestat

VII. Miscellaneous

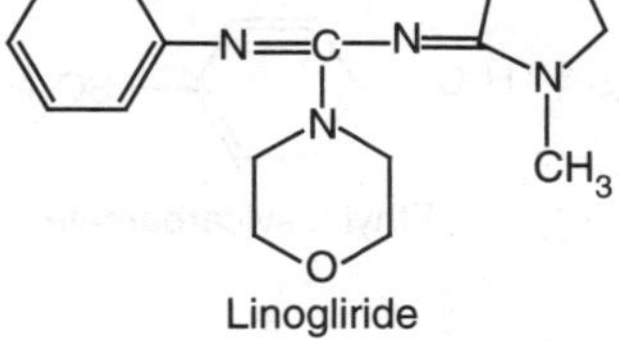

Linogliride

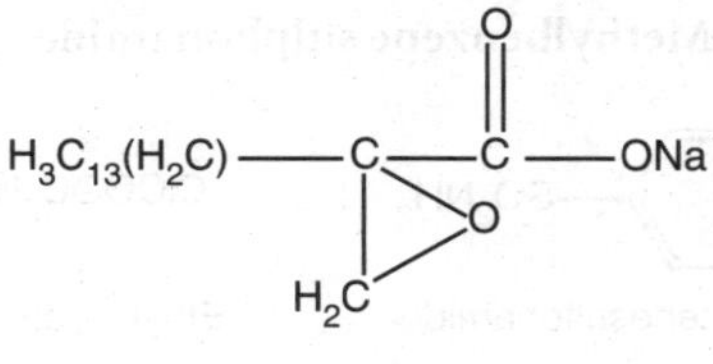

Palmoxirate sodium

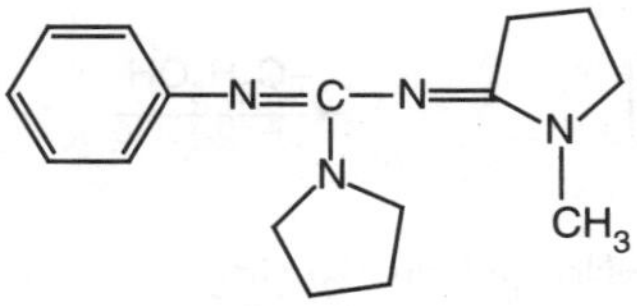

Pirogliride

SYNTHESIS AND DRUG PROFILE

I. Sulphonylurea derivatives

a. First-generation drugs

Mode of action: They target on the specific receptors in the β cells of islets of Langerhans called sulphonylurea receptors, and cause depolarization by reducing the conductance of ATP sensitive K^+ channels. This enhances the Ca^{2+} influx and produces degranulation, leading to the secretion of insulin.

The sulphonylureas may be represented by the following general structure

$$R-\text{C}_6\text{H}_4-SO_2-NH-\overset{O}{\overset{\|}{C}}-NH-R^1$$

All members of this group are urea derivatives with an aryl sulphonyl group in the 1st position and an aliphatic group at the 3rd position. The R group on the aromatic ring primarily influences the duration of action of the compound.

i. Tolbutamide (Orinase)

$$H_3C-\text{C}_6\text{H}_4-SO_2-NH-\overset{O}{\overset{\|}{C}}-NH(CH_2)_3CH_3$$

1-Butyl-3-(*p*-tolylsulphonyl) urea

Properties and uses: Tolbutamide is a white crystalline powder, practically insoluble in water, soluble in acetone, alcohol, and dilute solutions of alkali hydroxides. It is useful in the treatment of selected cases of diabetes mellitus, namely, mild and uncomplicated, stable diabetes of adult.

Assay: Dissolve the sample in a mixture of water and alcohol (1:2) and titrate against 0.1 M sodium hydroxide using phenolphthalein as indicator.

Synthesis

Route I. From: 4-Methylbenzene sulphonamide

$$H_3C-C_6H_4-SO_2NH_2 + ClCOOC_2H_5 \xrightarrow{-HCl} H_3C-C_6H_4-SO_2NHCOOC_2H_5$$

4-Methylbenzenesulfonamide   Ethyl chloro formate   Ethyl tosylcarbamate

$+$ $NH_2-(CH_2)_3CH_3$ (Butylamine)

$$\xrightarrow{-C_2H_5OH} H_3C-C_6H_4-SO_2-NH-\overset{O}{\overset{\|}{C}}-NH(CH_2)_3CH_3$$

Tolbutamide

Route II. From: Toluene

Toluene → (ClSO₃H, −H₂O) → 4-Methylbenzene-1-sulphonyl chloride → (NH₃, −HCl) → 4-Methylbenzenesulfonamide → (ClCOOC₂H₅ Ethyl chloro formate, Pyridine, −HCl) → Ethyl-*N*-*p*-tolyl sulphonyl carbamate → (CH₃(CH₂)₃NH₂, −C₂H₅OH) → Tolbutamide

Dose: The usual dosage is 250 and 500 mg with an initial dose of 500 mg.

Dosage forms: Tolbutamide tablets B.P.

ii. Chloropropamide (Diabenese)

1-[(*p*-Chlorophenyl sulphonyl)]-3-propyl urea

Synthesis

Route I. From: 4-Chlorobenzenesulphonamide

4-Chlorobenzenesulphonamide + Propyl isocyanate → Chloropropamide

Ruote II. From: Chlorobenzene

Chlorobenzene →(ClSO₃H, −H₂O)→ 4-Chlorobenzene-1-sulphonyl chloride (SO₂Cl) →(NH₃, −HCl)→ 4-Chlorobenzene sulphonamide (SO₂NH₂) →(ClCOOC₂H₅ / Pyridine, −HCl)→ Ethyl-N-p-chloro sulphonyl carbamate (SO₂–NH–COOC₂H₅) →(CH₃(CH₂)₃NH₂, −C₂H₅OH)→ Chloropropamide (SO₂–NH–C(O)–NH(CH₂)₂CH₃)

Metabolism: It is metabolized by ω or ω-1 hydroxylation of the propyl group. This reaction is slow and significant amount of the drug is excreted unchanged in urine.

Properties and uses: Chloropropamide is a white crystalline powder, practically insoluble in water, soluble in acetone, methylene chloride, alcohol, and dilute solutions of alkali hydroxides. Used in the treatment of diabetes mellitus.

Assay: Dissolve the sample in alcohol and add water. Titrate against 0.1 M sodium hydroxide using phenolphthalein as indicator until a pink colour is obtained.

Dose: The usual dose is 100–250 mg per day.

iii. Tolazamide (Tolamide, Tolinase)

H₃C–C₆H₄–SO₂NHCONH–N(hexahydroazepine)

1-(Hexahydro-azepine-1-yl)-3-(*p*-tolylsulphonyl)urea

Metabolism of tolbutamide and tolazamide: They undergo a more rapid benzylic oxidation, leading to an inactive benzoic acid derivative. An alternative hydroxylation of the aliphatic ring of tolazamide becomes active and results in a metabolite of prolonged duration of action.

Oral Hypoglycaemic Drugs

Synthesis

Properties and uses: Tolazmide is a white crystalline powder, very slightly soluble in water, soluble in chloroform and acetone, slightly soluble in ethanol. Used as an oral hypoglycaemic agent with action and uses similar to Tolbutamide.

Assay: Dissolve the sample in butan-2-one with the aid of gentle heat. Allow to cool, add 30 ml of ethanol and titrate with 0.1 M sodium hydroxide using phenolphthalein as indicator.

Dose: The dose is 100–250 mg daily.

Dosage forms: Tolazamide tablets B.P.

iv. Acetohexamide

H_3COC—⟨phenyl⟩—$SO_2NHCONH$—⟨cyclohexyl⟩

1-[(4-Acetylphenyl) sulphonyl]-3-cyclohexyl urea

Synthesis

Acetophenone →($ClSO_3H$, $-H_2O$)→ 4-Acetylbenzene-1-sulphonyl chloride (COCH$_3$–Ph–SO$_2$Cl) →(NH_3, $-HCl$)→ 4-Acetylbenzene sulphonamide (COCH$_3$–Ph–SO$_2NH_2$)

→(ClCOOC$_2$H$_5$ Ethyl chloro formate / Pyridine, $-HCl$)→ Ethyl-N-p-acetylsulphonyl carbamate (COCH$_3$–Ph–SO$_2$-NH-COOC$_2$H$_5$)

→(H$_2$N–cyclohexyl, Aminolysis, $-C_2H_5OH$)→ Acetohexamide (COCH$_3$–Ph–SO$_2$NHCONH–cyclohexyl)

Metabolism: The major metabolite of acetohexamide is a reduced product of the keto group, forming an alcohol. The hydroxy metabolite exhibits 2.5 times the hypoglycaemic activity of the parent molecule.

Properties and uses: It is a white, odourless crystalline powder, soluble in alcohol and chloroform, but insoluble in water or ether. It is an orally active hypoglycaemic drug.

b. Second-generation drugs

i. Glibenclamide (Glyburide)

Structure: 5-chloro-2-methoxybenzamide with CONH(CH$_2$)$_2$–phenyl–SO$_2$NHCONH–cyclohexyl

5-Chloro-N-[2-4[[[(cyclohexylamino) carbonylamino] sulphonyl] phenyl] ethyl]-2-methoxy benzamide

Synthesis

Route I. From: 5-Chloro-2-methoxybenzoylchloride

5-Chloro-2-methoxybenzoyl chloride + Phenyl ethylamine $\xrightarrow[-HCl]{\text{Condensation}}$ intermediate $\xrightarrow[-H_2O]{ClSO_3H}$ sulfonyl chloride intermediate $\xrightarrow[-HCl]{NH_3}$ sulfonamide intermediate

+ Isocyanatocyclohexane $\xrightarrow{NaOH}$ Glibenclamide

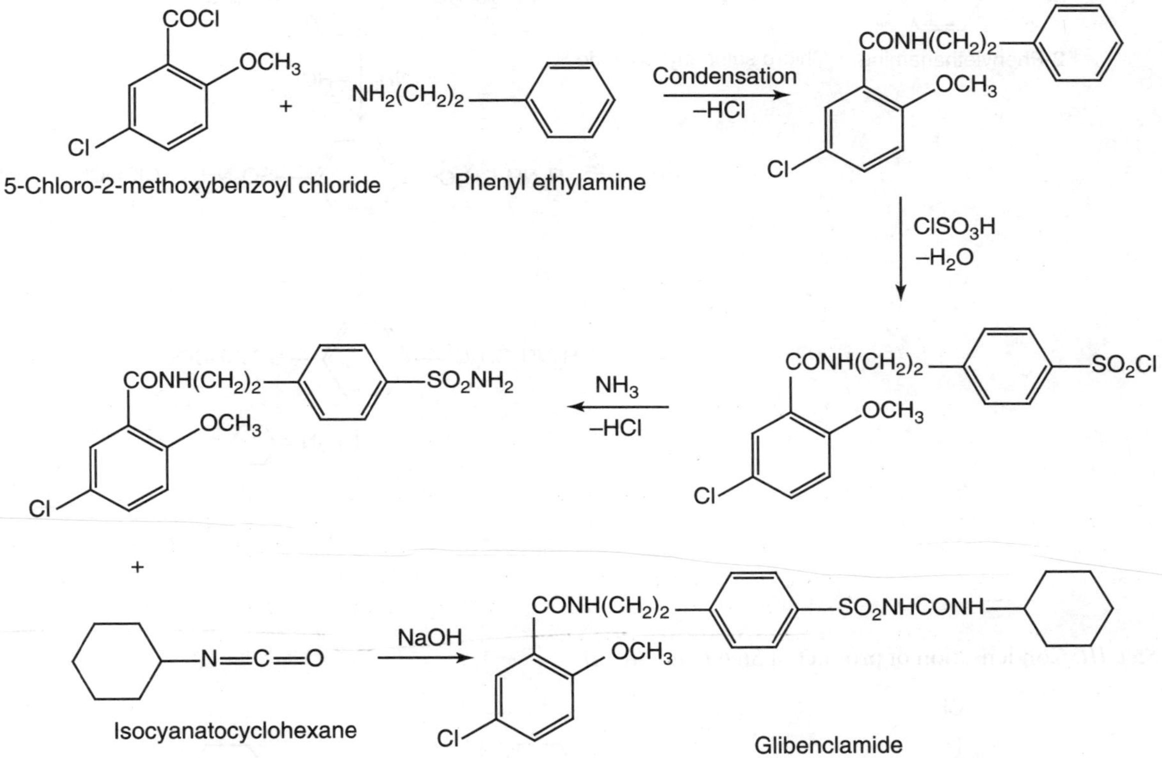

Route II.

Step I: Synthesis of 5-chloro-2-methoxybenzoyl chloride

4-Chlorophenol $\xrightarrow{\text{CO}_2 \text{ under reduced pressure}}$ → $\xrightarrow{\text{Methylation}}$ → $\xrightarrow{SOCl_2}$ 5-Chloro-2-methoxybenzoyl chloride

I

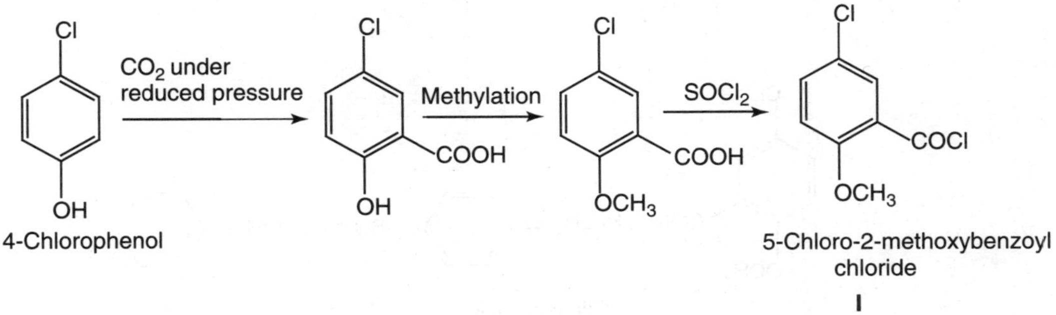

Step II: Synthesis of 4-(Aminoethyl)-1-cyclohexylamino carbonyl benzene sulphonamide

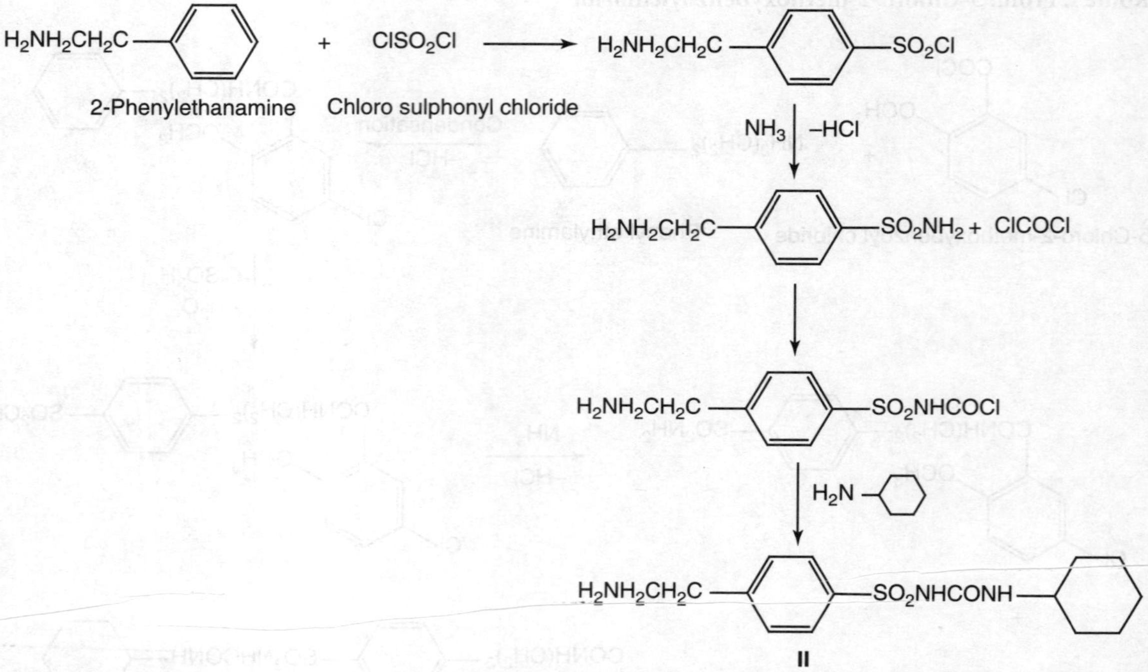

H₂NH₂CH₂C—⟨C₆H₄⟩ + ClSO₂Cl ⟶ H₂NH₂CH₂C—⟨C₆H₄⟩—SO₂Cl

2-Phenylethanamine   Chloro sulphonyl chloride

↓ NH₃ | –HCl

H₂NH₂CH₂C—⟨C₆H₄⟩—SO₂NH₂ + ClCOCl

↓

H₂NH₂CH₂C—⟨C₆H₄⟩—SO₂NHCOCl

↓ H₂N—⟨C₆H₁₁⟩

H₂NH₂CH₂C—⟨C₆H₄⟩—SO₂NHCONH—⟨C₆H₁₁⟩

II

Step III: Condensation of product of *Step I* and *Step II*

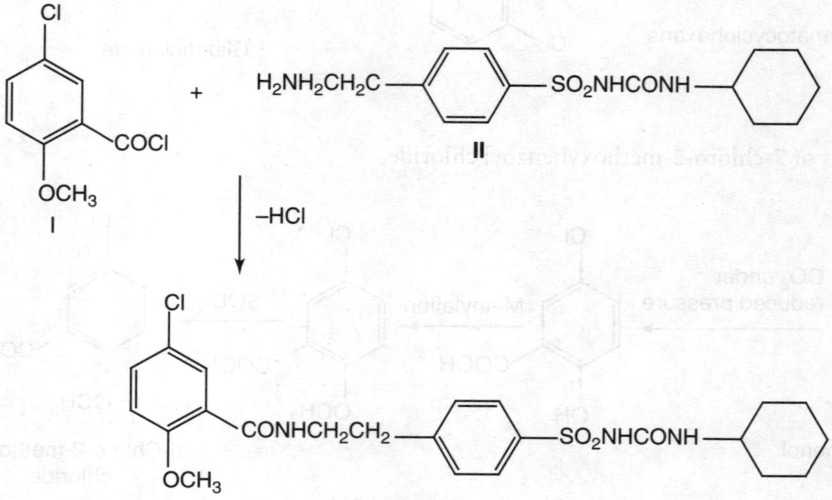

⟨Cl, OCH₃-substituted C₆H₃⟩—COCl + H₂NH₂CH₂C—⟨C₆H₄⟩—SO₂NHCONH—⟨C₆H₁₁⟩

I   **II**

↓ –HCl

⟨Cl, OCH₃-substituted C₆H₃⟩—CONHCH₂CH₂—⟨C₆H₄⟩—SO₂NHCONH—⟨C₆H₁₁⟩

Glibenclamide

Properties and uses: Glibenclamide is a white crystalline powder, practically insoluble in water, sparingly soluble in methylene chloride, slightly soluble in alcohol and methanol. Used in the treatment of mild uncomplicated NIDDM unresponsive to diet alone.

Assay: Dissolve the sample in alcohol by heating and titrate against 0.1 M sodium hydroxide, using phenolphthalein as indicator, until a pink colour is obtained.

Dose: The dose is 2.5–5 mg per day to be taken with breakfast.

Dosage forms: Glibenclamide tablets B.P.

ii. Glipizide (Dibizide, Glucolip, Glynase)

1-Cyclohexyl-3-[[p-[2-(5-methylpyrazine carboxamide) ethyl] phenyl] sulphonyl] urea

Synthesis

Metabolism: It is extensively metabolized to less active or inactive metabolites. Its metabolites are excreted primarily in the urine.

Properties and uses: Glipizide is a white crystalline powder, practically insoluble in water and ethanol, very slightly soluble in methylene chloride and acetone, soluble in dilute solutions of alkali hydroxides. It is an orally active hypoglycaemic drug.

Assay: Dissolve the sample in dimethylformamide and titrate against 0.1 M lithium methoxide add quinaldine red as indicator, until the colour changes from red to colourless.

Dose: The dosage is 25–50 mg once a day or in divided doses.

Dosage forms: Glipizide tablets B.P.

iii. Gliclazide

1-(3-Azabicyclo-oct-3-3-yl)-3-(*p*-tolylsulphonyl)urea

Properties and uses: Gliclazide is a white powder, practically insoluble in water, soluble in methylene chloride, sparingly soluble in acetone, and slightly soluble in alcohol. It is an orally active hypoglycaemic drug.

Assay: Dissolve the sample in anhydrous acetic acid and titrate against 0.1 M perchloric acid. Determine the end point potentiometrically.

Dosage forms: Gliclazide tablets B.P.

SAR of Sulphonylureas

$$R-\text{C}_6\text{H}_4-SO_2-NH-\underset{\underset{O}{\|}}{C}-NH-R_1$$

1. The benzene ring should contain a substitutent preferably in the para position. The substituents, such as methyl, acetyl, amino, chloro, bromo, trifluoro methyl, and dithiomethyl were found to enhance the antihyperglycaemic activity.
2. When the para position of benzene is substituted with aryl carboxamidoalkyl group (second-generation sulphonylureas, such as glibenclamide) the activity was found to be enhanced further.
3. The size of the group attached to the terminal nitrogen is crucial for activity. The group should also impart lipophilicity to the compound N-methyl and ethyl substituents that show no activity, whereas N-propyl and higher homologues were found to be active and the activity is lost when the N-substituent contains 12 or more carbons.

II. Biguanides

Mode of action: Biguanides do not have direct action on increasing or decreasing the glucose level. This reduces glucose levels primarily by decreasing hepatic gluconeogenisis by increasing the insulin action on muscles and fat. It also reduces the absorption of glucose from intestine.

i. Phenformin

$$\text{Ph}-CH_2CH_2NH-\underset{\underset{NH}{\|}}{C}-\underset{\underset{H}{|}}{N}-\underset{\underset{NH}{\|}}{C}-NH_2$$

1-Phenyl ethyl biguanide

Synthesis

Route-I. From: 2-Phenylethylamine

2-Phenylethylamine + Cyano guanidine (NC–NH–C(=NH)–NH$_2$) → Phenformin

Route-II. From: 1-(2-Chloroethyl) benzene

C₆H₅–CH₂CH₂Cl + NH₂–C(=NH)–NH₂ →(–HCl) C₆H₅–CH₂CH₂–NH–C(=NH)–NH₂ + NH₂–C(=NH)–NH₂

1-(2-Chloroethyl)benzene + Guanidine

↓ (–NH₃)

C₆H₅–CH₂CH₂NH–C(=NH)–N(H)–C(=NH)–NH₂

Phenformin

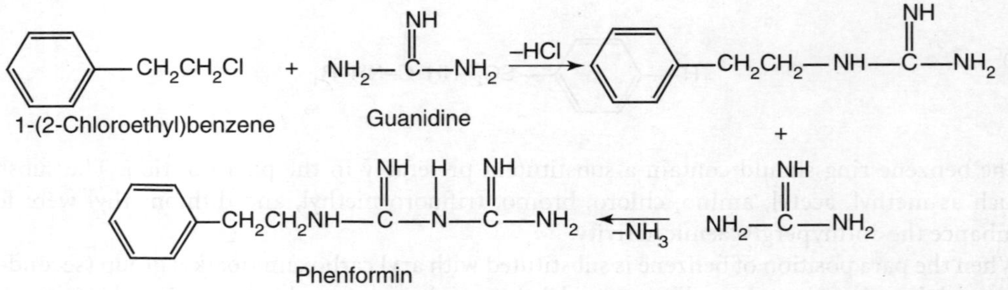

Properties and uses: Used only in stable type II diabetics, it may be used alone or in conjunction with another oral hypoglycaemic agents, such as sulphonylureas or with insulin.

Dose: The normal dose is 25 mg tablets 1–4 times a day, usually 50–150 mg daily with breakfast.

ii. Metformin (Diamet, Diaphage Glyciphage, Glycomet)

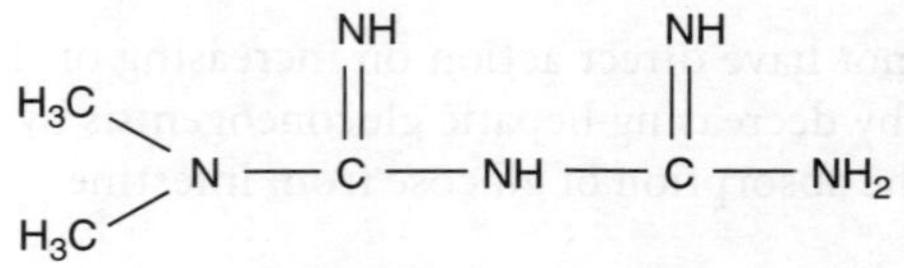

(H₃C)₂N–C(=NH)–NH–C(=NH)–NH₂

1,1-Dimethyl biguanide

Synthesis

Route I. From: Dimethylamine

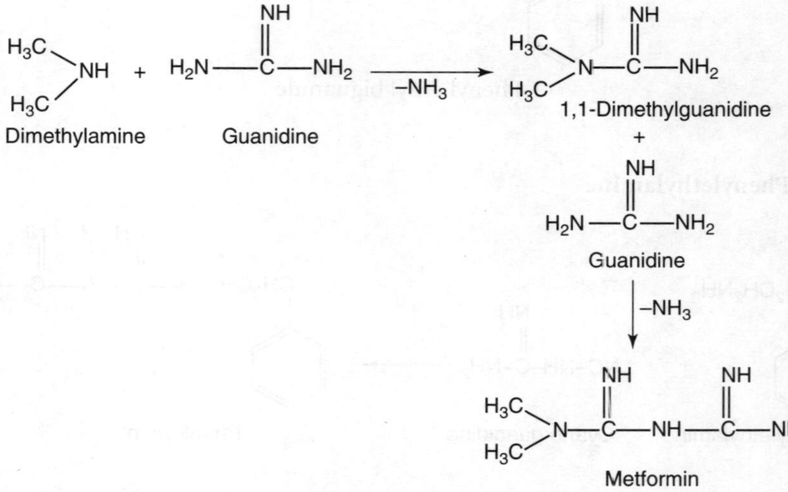

(H₃C)₂NH + H₂N–C(=NH)–NH₂ →(–NH₃) (H₃C)₂N–C(=NH)–NH₂

Dimethylamine + Guanidine → **1,1-Dimethylguanidine**

+

H₂N–C(=NH)–NH₂

Guanidine

↓ –NH₃

(H₃C)₂N–C(=NH)–NH–C(=NH)–NH₂

Metformin

Route II. From: Dimethylamine

Dimethylamine + cyanoguanidine $\xrightarrow{135°C \text{ reflux}}$ Metformin

Properties and uses: Metformin hydrochloride exists as white crystals, freely soluble in water, slightly soluble in alcohol, practically insoluble in acetone and methylene chloride. It is usually given along with sulphonylureas.

Assay: Dissolve the sample in anhydrous formic acid, add acetonitrile, and titrate against 0.1 M perchloric acid. Determine the end point potentiometrically.

Dose: Initial dose is 500 mg thrice daily or 850 mg twice daily with meals.

Dosage forms: Metformin tablets B.P.

III. Meglitinides (Benzoic acid derivatives)

The meglitinides are similar in structure to sulphonylureas. The sulphonylurea and meglitinide classes of oral hypoglycaemic drugs are referred to as endogenous insulin secretagogues because they induce the pancreatic release of endogenous insulin.

Mode of action: Even though, these are not sulphonylureas they act on sulphonylurea receptors as well as the other variant receptors and closes the ATP dependent k⁺ channels, leading to insulin secretion by depolarization.

i. Meglitinide

Synthesis

5-Chloro-2-methoxybenzoic acid + 4-(2-Aminoethyl)benzoic acid $\xrightarrow{SOCl_2}$ Meglitinide

ii. Repaglinide (Repide, Repa, Eurepa)

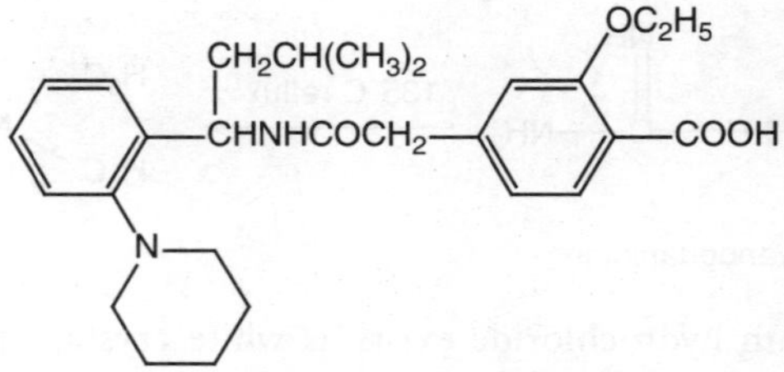

Synthesis

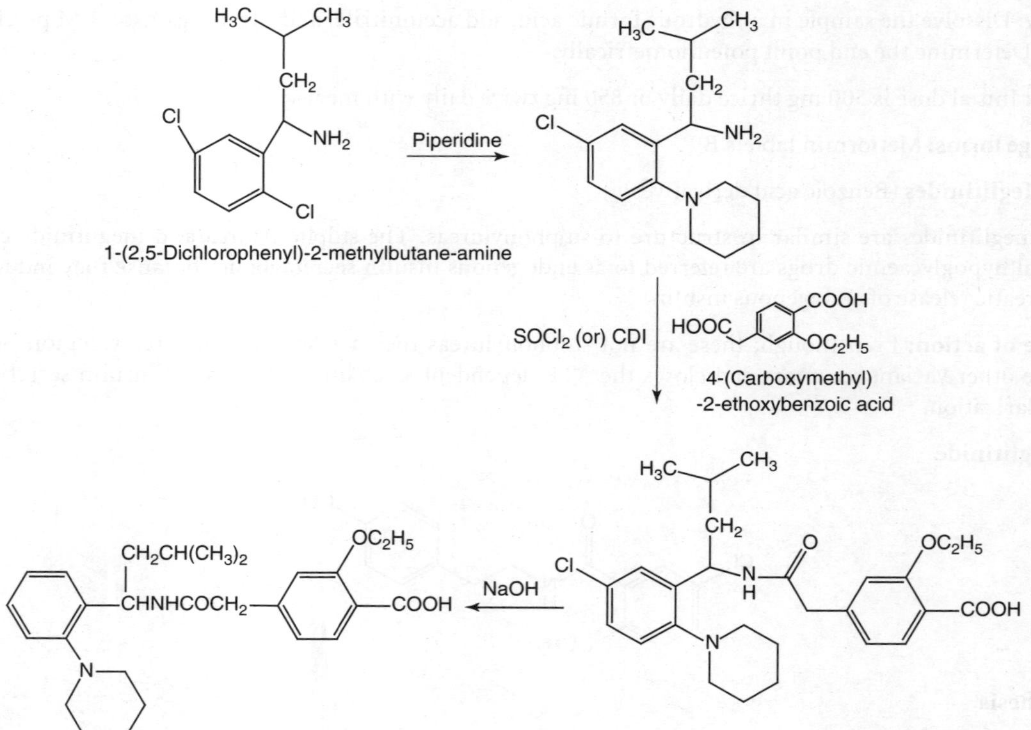

1-(2,5-Dichlorophenyl)-2-methylbutane-amine

4-(Carboxymethyl)-2-ethoxybenzoic acid

Repaglinide

Properties and uses: Repaglinide is a white powder, practically insoluble in water, soluble in methanol, and methylene chloride. It stimulates insulin release and is used in the treatment of diabetes mellitus.

Assay: Dissolve the sample in methanol and add anhydrous acetic acid and titrate against 0.1 M perchloric acid. Determine the end point potentiometrically

Dose: The usual initial dose for adults is 0.5 mg, taken within 30 min of main meals. Initial doses of 1 or 2 mg may be used in patients who have had previous hypoglycaemic treatment. Dose may be adjusted at intervals of 1–2 week up to 4 mg before meals; maximum dose is 16 mg daily.

iii. Nateglinide

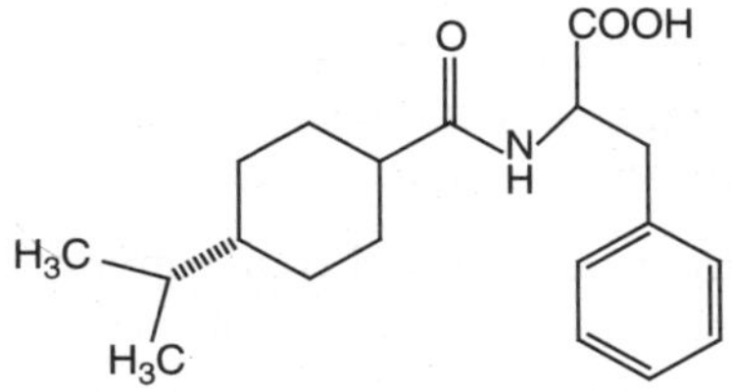

Metabolism: It is metabolized in the liver and 16% is excreted in the urine unchanged. The major metabolites are hydroxyl derivative (CYP2C9 70%, CYP3A4 30%) that are further conjugated to the glucuronide derivative (Fig 1.1).

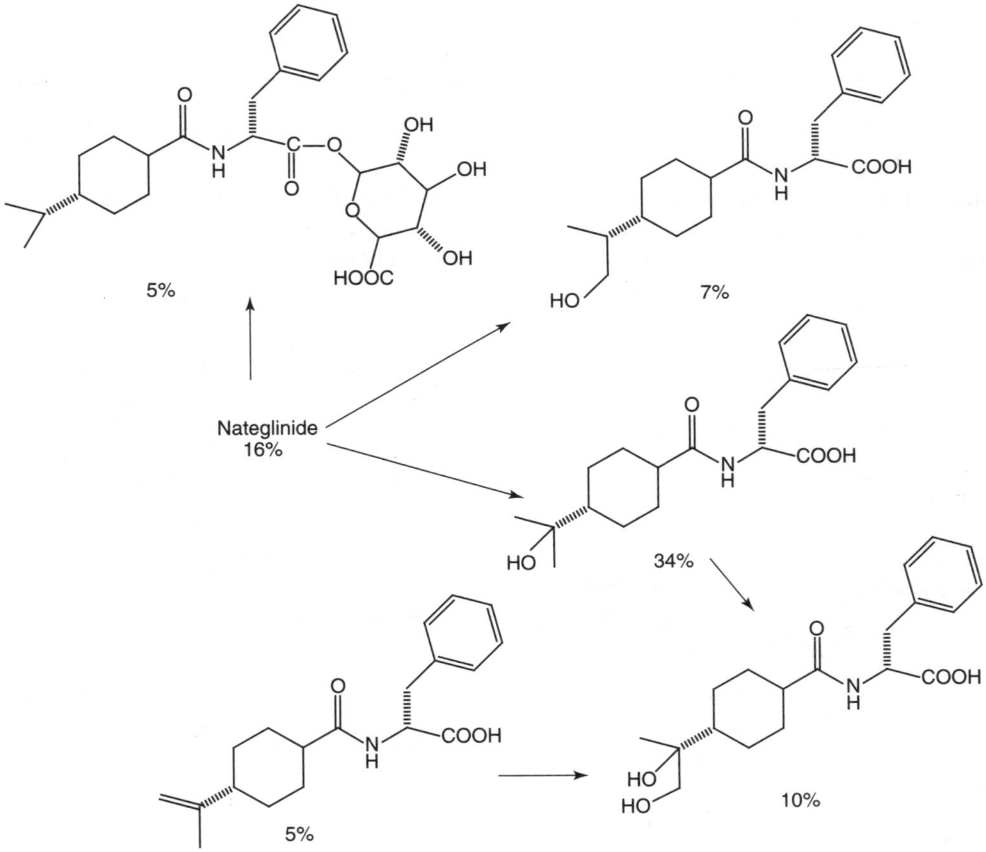

Figure 1.1 Metabolic pathway of nateglinide.

Uses: It is used as an oral hypoglycaemic agent in type II diabetic mellitus.

IV. Thiazolidinediones

Thiazolidinediones are a new class of oral antidiabetic agents (commercially known as glitazones) that enhance insulin sensitivity in peripheral tissues. It is relatively safe in patients with impaired renal function because they are highly metabolized by the liver and excreted in the faeces.

Mode of action: These drugs produce gene-mediated transcription for the release of insulin by forming new proteins. They act on the nuclear peroxisome proliferator activated receptor γ (*ppar γ*) and elicit the genes. It also inhibits the resistance to insulin by activating glucose transporters (Glut and Glut 1) in the plasma membrane.

i. Pioglitazone

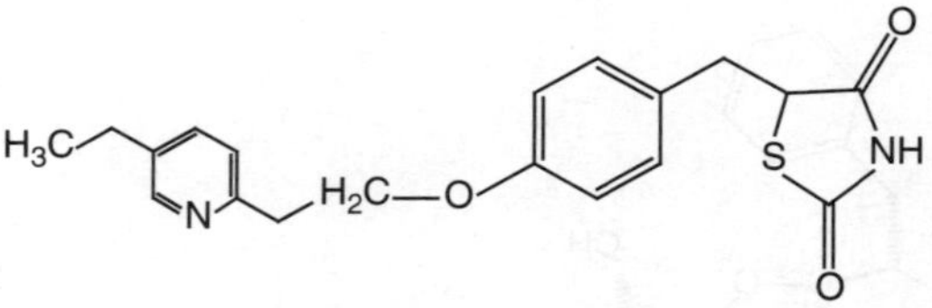

Metabolism: It is metabolized and gives eight metabolic products. These products result from oxidation at either carbon adjacent to the pyridine ring. They are found as various conjugates in the urine and bile. Three metabolites appear to contribute to the biological activity of pioglitazone (Fig 1.2).

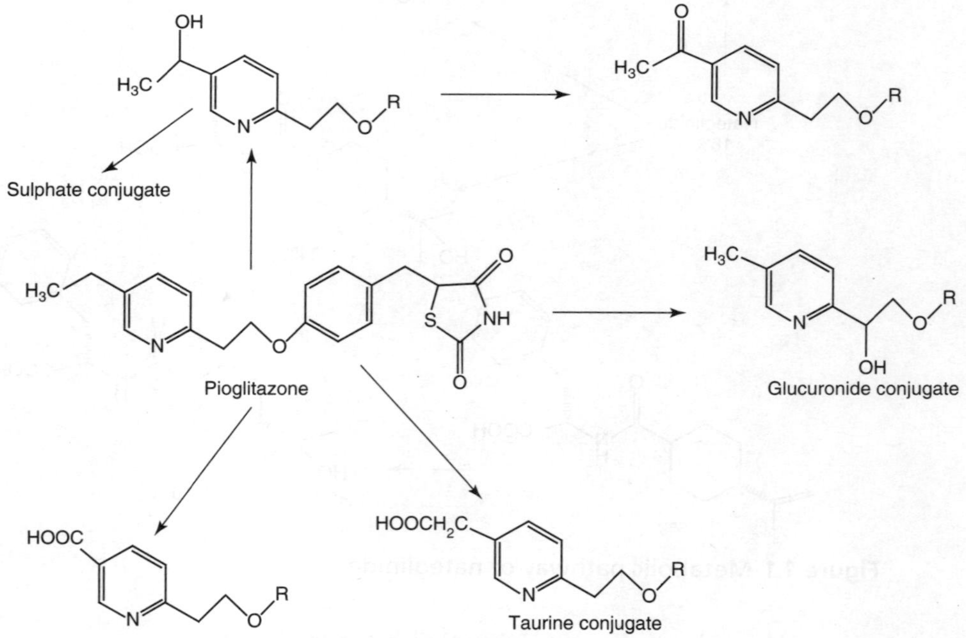

Figure 1.2 Metabolic pathway of pioglitazone.

ii. Ciglitazone

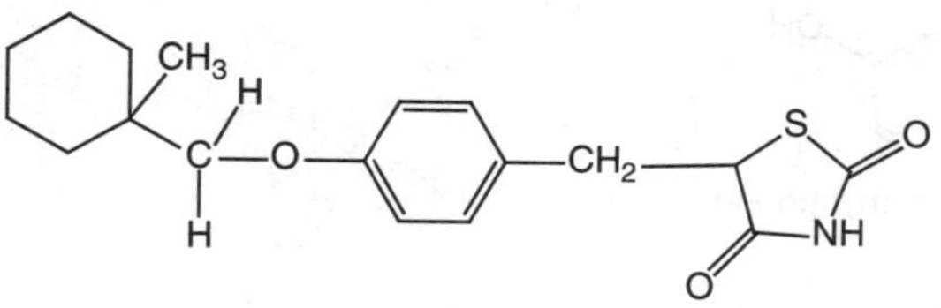

Synthesis

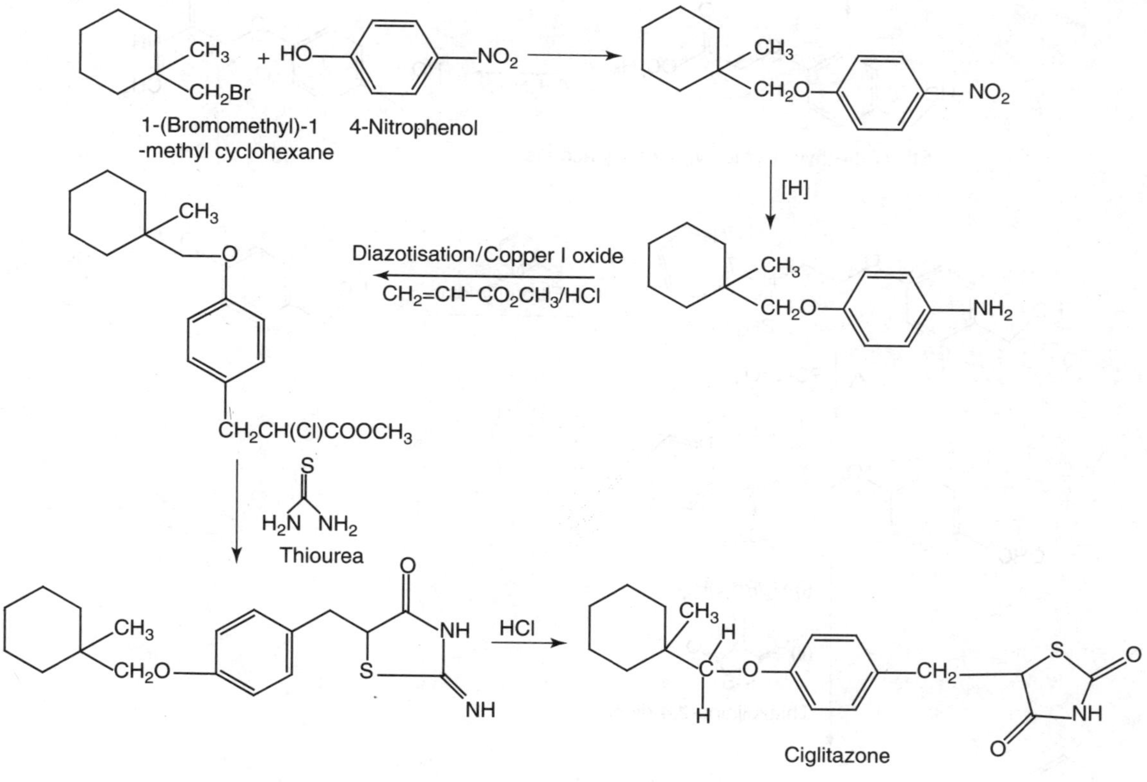

1-(Bromomethyl)-1-methyl cyclohexane + 4-Nitrophenol → [intermediate with NO₂]

[H] → amine intermediate (—NH₂)

Diazotisation/Copper I oxide, $CH_2=CH-CO_2CH_3$/HCl → $CH_2CH(Cl)COOCH_3$ intermediate

Thiourea ($H_2N-CS-NH_2$) → imino-thiazolidinone intermediate

HCl → **Ciglitazone**

Use: It is used in the treatment of NIDDM.

iii. Rosiglitazone (Rosicon, Reglit, Rosinorm)

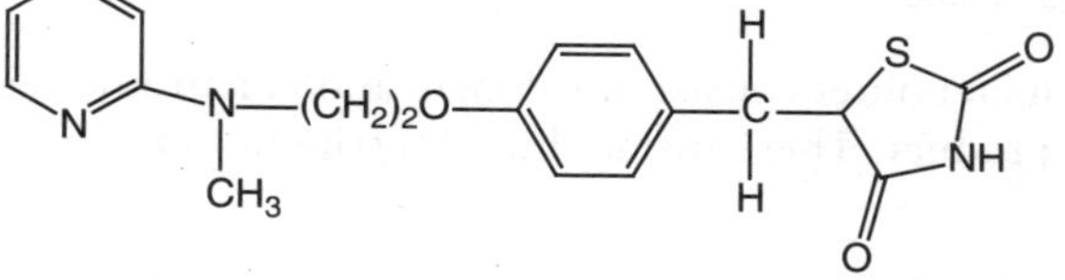

(±)-5-[[4-[2-Methyl-2-pyridinylamino]ethoxy]phenyl methyl]-2,4- thiazolidinedione

Synthesis

[Scheme: Synthesis of Rosiglitazone]

4-(Hydroxymethyl)phenol → (I CH$_2$COOC$_2$H$_5$, K$_2$CO$_3$) → Ethyl 2-(4-(hydroxymethyl)phenoxy)acetate → (CH$_3$NH$_2$) → amide intermediate → (BH$_3$) → secondary amine → (2-Fluoropyridine) → N-pyridyl intermediate → (Δ, PS–CrO$_3$) → aldehyde intermediate → (i) H$_2$/Pd(OH)$_2$; (ii) Thiazolidine-2,4-dione → **Rosiglitazone**

Metabolism: The primary metabolites consist of sulphate and glucuronic acid conjugates of hydroxylation and N-demethylation product. These metabolites contribute to the biological activity of rosiglitazone (Fig 1.3).

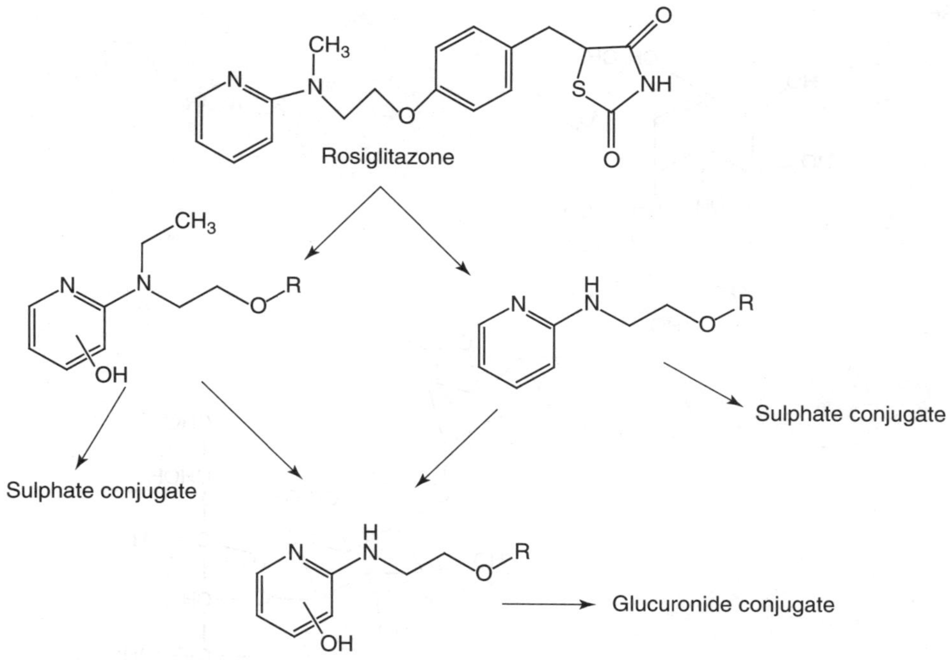

Figure 1.3 Metabolic pathway of rosiglitazone.

Uses: It is used in the treatment of NIDDM.

Dose: The dosage for type 2 diabetes mellitus for adult is 4 mg daily, which may be increased after 8–12 week of therapy, according to response and the maximum dosage is 8 mg daily.

iv. α-Glucosidase inhibitors

α-Glucosidase enzyme is responsible for breaking down the complex polysaccharides and sucrose to monosaccharides, which are then absorbed; α-glucosidase inhibitors decrease the rate of breakdown. They are also called starch blockers.

Mode of action: These acts on the final enzymes in the digestion of carbohydrates present in the brush border of small intestine and transport of polysaccharides and sucrose.

Properties and uses: Acarbose is a white or yellowish amorphous hygroscopic powder, very soluble in water, soluble in methanol, and practically insoluble in methylene chloride. It is an alpha-glucosidase inhibitor and used in the treatment of diabetes mellitus.

Assay: It is assayed by adopting liquid chromatography technique.

i. Acarbose

ii. Miglitol

Properties and uses: It is a crystalline substance, soluble in water. It is a α-glucosidase inhibitor and used as an antidiabetic agent.

V. Aldose reducatse inhibitors

In diabetic complications, high concentrations of glucose is converted into sorbitol by aldose reductase by the polyol pathway (Fig. 1.4). Sorbitol is converted into fructose and these products accumulate in the nerves, kidneys, and retina, etc. Galactone is converted to galacitol, which is not metabolized and causes osmotic swelling. Aldose reductase inhibitors interfere in the polyol pathway of sorbitol and fructose and thereby cause hypoglycaemic effects.

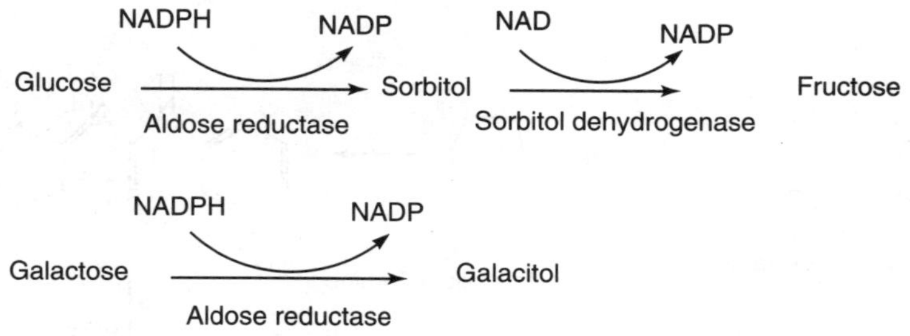

$$\text{Glucose} \xrightarrow[\text{Aldose reductase}]{\text{NADPH} \quad \text{NADP}} \text{Sorbitol} \xrightarrow[\text{Sorbitol dehydrogenase}]{\text{NAD} \quad \text{NADP}} \text{Fructose}$$

$$\text{Galactose} \xrightarrow[\text{Aldose reductase}]{\text{NADPH} \quad \text{NADP}} \text{Galacitol}$$

Figure 1.4 Polyol pathway.

i. Sorbinil

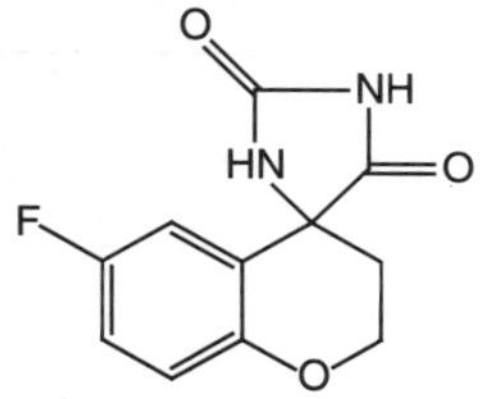

Uses: It is used in the treatment of diabetic neuropathy.

ii. Tolrestat

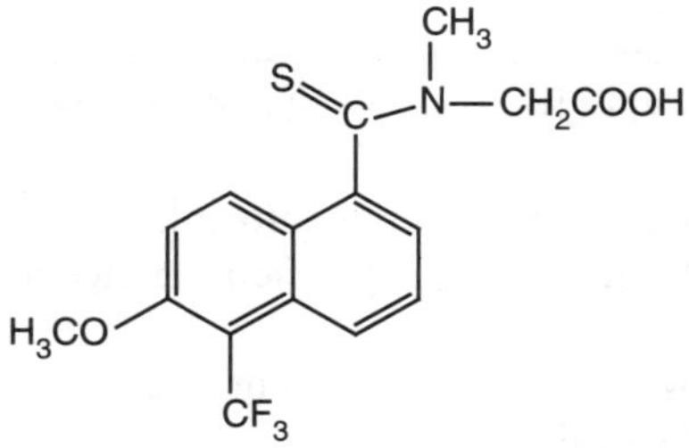

N-[6-Methoxy-5-trifluoromethyl-1- naphthyl(thiocarbonyl)]-N-methylglycine

Uses: It is useful in the prophylaxis of diabetic neuropathy and cataracts.

VI. Miscellaneous

Linogliride

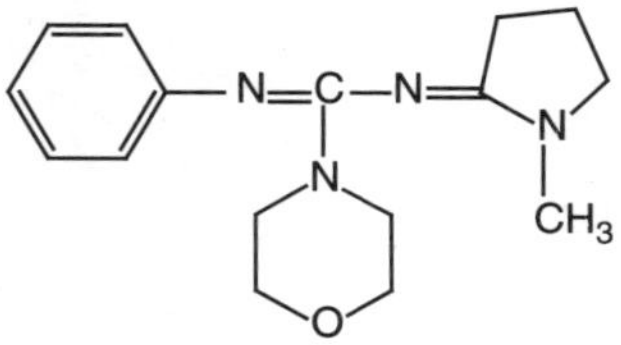

Synthesis

Phenyl isothiocyanate + 1-Methylpyrrolidin-2-imine → (intermediate thiourea) → (CH₃I) → SCH₃ intermediate → (Morpholine) → Linogliride

Uses: Used in the treatment of diabetes mellitus.

PROBABLE QUESTIONS

1. Explain type I and type II diabetes with some typical examples.
2. How do you classify the oral hypoglycaemic agents? Write the structure, chemical names, and uses of at least two compounds.
3. Write the mode of action of Tolbutamide and Phenformin.
4. Write in detail about Thiazolindiones with specific reference to the following drugs Rosiglitazone Troglitazone.
5. Write a short note on the following oral hypoglycaemic agents:
   (a) Biguanides (b) α-Glucosidase inhibitors.
6. Write a brief account of the following with a few examples:
   (a) First-generation sulphonylureas (b) Second-generation sulphonylureas
7. How will you synthesize the following drugs?
   (a) Chloropropamide (b) Tolbutamide (c) Glipizide
8. Explain about the meglitinides' specific mechanism of actions. Write the structure, synthesis, metabolism, and uses of any one of them.

SUGGESTED READINGS

1. Boyd AE. 'Sulfonylurea receptors ion channels, and fruit flies'. *Diabetes* 37: 847–50, 1988.
2. *British Pharmacopoeia*. Medicines and Healthcare Products Regulatory Agency. London, 2008.
3. Bruntan LL, Lazo JS, and Parker KL. *Goodman and Gilman's: The Pharmacological Basis of Therapeutics* (11th edn). New York: McGraw Hill, 2006.
4. Cook NS. *Potassium Channels: Structure, Classification, Function and Therapeutic Potential*. New York: John Wiley, 1990.
5. Datt N. 'Insulin pharmacotherapy'. *J Pharm Pract* 5: 260–70, 1992.
6. Ferner RE. 'Oral hypoglycemic agents'. *Med Clin North Am* 72: 1323–335, 1988.
7. Gennaro AR. *Remington: The Science and practice of Pharmacy* (21st edn). New York: Lippincot Williams and Wilkins, 2006.
8. Gerich JE. 'Oral hypoglycemic agents'. *N Engl J Med* 321: 1231, 1989.
9. *Indian Pharmacopoeia*. Ministry of Health and Family Welfare. New Delhi, 1996.
10. Lednicer D and Mitscher LA. *The Organic Chemistry of Drug Synthesis*. New York: John Wiley, 1995.
11. Lebovitz HE. 'Oral antidiabetic agents'. *Drugs* 44 (Suppl) 3: 21–28, 1992.
12. Miyahera RL. 'Pharmacotherapy of oral hypoglycaemic agents'. *J Pharm Pract* 5: 271–79, 1992.
13. Pandeya SN and Murthi KN. 'Recent developments in antidiabetics'. *Eastern Pharmacist* 35 (416): 69–76, 1992.
14. Pandey SK, Theberge JF, Bernier M, and Srivastava AK. *Biochemistry* 38: 14667–675, 1999.
15. Srivastava V and Pandeya SN. 'Recent trends in hypoglycemic research'. *J Sci Industr Res* 47: 706–21, 1988.

Chapter 2

Steroids

INTRODUCTION

The steroids form a group of structurally related compounds, which are widely distributed in animals and plants. The structures of steroids are based on the 1, 2-cyclopentano phenanthrene skeleton.

1,2-Cyclopentanophenanthrene

Steroids consist of four rings. Perhydrophenanthrene (rings A, B, and C) is a completely saturated derivative of phenanthrene, while D is a five-membered cyclopentane ring.

The major therapeutic classes of steroids are the following:

- Anti-inflammatory agents: Cortisone
- Sex hormones: Estrogen, progesterone, and testosterone
- Oral contraceptives: Norethisterone
- Cardiac steroids: Digitoxigenin
- Diuretics: Spironolactone
- Antibiotics: Fusidic acid
- Neuromuscular blockers: Pancuronium chloride
- Vitamin D precursor: Ergosterol

STEROID NOMENCLATURE AND STRUCTURE

Steroids consist of four fused rings (A, B, C, and D). Chemically, these hydrocarbons are cyclopentano per hydro phenenthrenes. They contain a five-membered cyclopentane (D) ring and the three rings of phenanthrene. A perhydro phenanthrene (ring A, B, and C) is the saturated derivative of phenanthrene.

Steroid template

Phenanthrene

Steroid backbone

Cholestane template

The polycyclic hydrocarbon, known as 5α-cholestane, is used to illustrate the numbering system for a steroid.

- The ring juncture or backbone carbons are shown in the structure of 5α-cholestane with a heavy dark line.
- Solid lines denote groups above the plane of the nucleus (β-configuration) and dotted or broken lines denote groups below the plane (α-configuration). If the configuration of substituent is unknown, its bond to the nucleus is drawn as a wavy line.
- The configuration of the H at C-5 is always indicated in the name.
- Circles were sometimes used to indicate α-hydrogens and dark dots to indicate β-hydrogens.
- Compounds with 5α-cholestane belong to allo-series, while compounds derived from 5 β-cholestane belong to the normal series.
- If the double bond is not between sequentially numbered carbons, in such cases, both carbons are indicated in the same.
- When a methyl group is missing from the side chain, this is indicated by the prefix 'nor' with the number of carbon atom, which has disappeared.

5 β, 19–norandrost-3-one

The symbol Δ is often used to designate a C = C bond in a steroid. If C = C is in between carbons 5 and 4, the compound is referred to as a Δ⁴ steriod, and if the C = C bond is between positions 5 and 10, the compound is designated as Δ $^{5(10)}$ steroid. Example, Estra-1,3,5(10) triene-3,17b-diol.

17β–estradiol
[Estra-Δ1,3,5(10)triene-3,17β–diol]

Since 17 β-estradiol contains 18 carbon atoms, it is considered as a derivative of estrane, a basic nucleus.

5 (α or β)–Estrane (C=18)

Stereochemistry: The absolute stereochemistry of the molecule and any substituent is shown with solid (β) and dashed (α) bonds; a (axial) bond is perpendicular to the plane of the molecule while equatorial bond (e) is horizontal to the plane of the molecule.

5α–Androstane

The aliphatic side chain at position is always assumed to be of β-configuration.

The term *cis* and *trans* are used occasionally to indicate the backbone stereochemistry between rings. For example, 5 α-steroids are A/B *trans* and 5 β-steroids are A/B *cis*. The terms syn and anti are used analogously to *trans* and *cis*.

Conformations: There are six asymmetric carbon atoms in the nucleus 5, 8, 9, 10, 13, and 14. Therefore, there are $2^6 = 64$ optically active forms possible. Cholestane, androstane, and pregnane can exist in two conformations, that is, chair form and boat form.

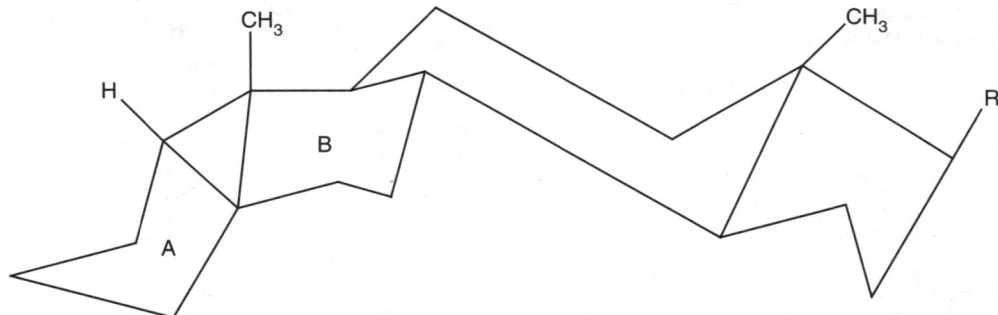

Chair confirmation is more stable than boat confirmation due to less angle strain, and hence, all cyclohexane rings in the steriod nucleus exist in the chair confirmation.

Classification

The adrenal cortex synthesizes two classes of steroids. They are as follows:

Glucocorticoids: These steroids regulate the carbohydrates, proteins, and the fat metabolism and are intimately involved in the operation of the processes that enable the body to resist infections and stress.
   Example—hydrocortisone and cortisone.

Mineralocorticoids: These steroids mainly influence salt and water balance (and hence, the control of blood volume and blood pressure) by maintaining proper electrolyte balance.
   Example—aldosterone, 11-deoxycorticosterone.

i. Cortisone (Cortogen, Cortone)

Synthesis

3α:21-Diacetoxy pregnane-11:20-dione

Reagents in scheme:
- HCN
- (i) POCl$_3$–C$_5$H$_5$N(–H$_2$O)
- (ii) KOH
- (iii) Ac$_2$O
- OsO$_4$
- (i) CrO$_3$
- (ii) Na$_2$SO$_3$
- (i) Ac$_2$O
- (ii) Br$_2$
- (i) –HBr
- (ii) Hydrolysis
- (iii) Ac$_2$O

(i) Cortisone (R=H)
(ii) Cortisone acetate (R=COCH$_3$)

Properties and uses: It is a white, crystalline powder, insoluble in water, and soluble in alcohol. It is used in rheumatoid arthritis, severe shock, allergic conditions, and chronic lymphatic leukaemia.

Dose: The dosage for adults is 20–100 mg per day by oral or IM.

ii. Hydrocortisone (Hydrocortone, Lortef)

Synthesis

Progesterone →(*Rhizopus nigrican* Oxidation)→ 11-α Hydroxyprogesterone →(Oxidation)→ →(Ethyl oxalate)→ →(Br₂)→ →(CH₃COONa, Favorsky reaction)→ →(i) LiAlH₄ (ii) Ac₂O (iii) HCl→ →(i) OsO₄/H₂O₂ (ii) NaOH→

R = Hydrocortisone
R = Ac (Hydrocortisone acetate)

Properties and uses: It exists as white crystalline powder, soluble in water and in alcohol. It is used as an anti-inflammatory agent.

Dose: The dose as injection is 100 mg intramuscular (IM) and as topical cream 1%–2.5% for skin, ear, and eye.

iii. Prednisolone (Prelone, Emsolone)

Synthesis

Hydrocortisone $\xrightarrow[\text{Selective dehydrogenation at 1 and 2 position}]{\text{Corynebacterium simplex}}$ Prednisolone

Properties and uses: It is a white crystalline powder, sparingly soluble in alcohol. It is four times as potent as hydrocortisone.

Dose: The oral dose for adult is 5–60 mg per day. As IM, IV, and intra-articular (IA) injection, the dose is 10–40 mg, and for topical use (skin and eyes), the dose is 0.25%.

iv. Dexamethazone (Dalalone)

Synthesis

Dexamethasone

Properties and use: It exists as white crystalline powder, soluble in alcohol and insoluble in water. Used as an anti-inflammatory and antiallergic drug.

Dose: Oral adult dose is 500 µg to 9 mg daily. The topical dose for conjunctiva is 1 drop of 0.1% suspension.

PROGESTOGENS

The natural progestational hormone or progestogen is progesterone, which is secreted mainly by the corpus luteum in the second part of the menstrual cycle. Small amounts are also secreted by the testis in the male and the adrenal cortex in both sexes, and large amounts are secreted by the placenta.

Classification

Progestogens could be broadly classified into two major classes:

1. Progesterone derivatives

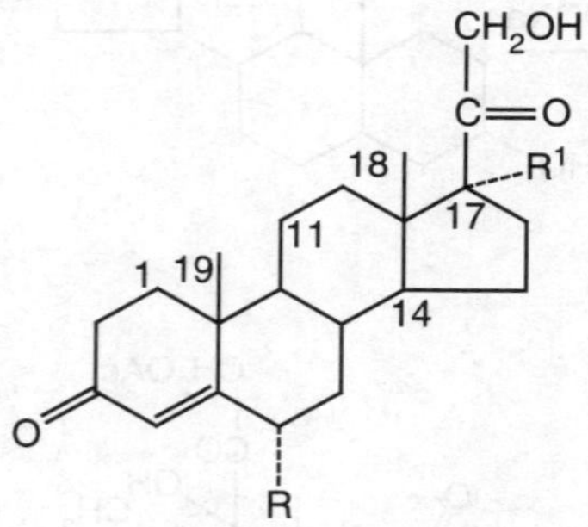

Name	R	R¹
Progesterone	–H	–H
Hydroxy progesterone caproate	–H	–OCO(CH$_2$)$_4$CH$_3$
Methoxy progesterone acetate	–CH$_3$	–OCOCH$_3$

2. 19-Nor testosterone derivatives

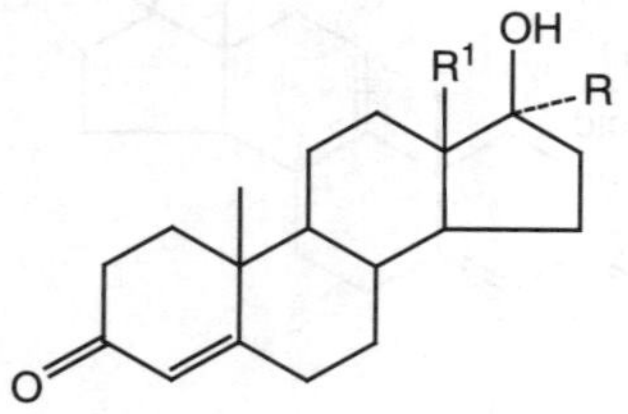

Name	R	R¹
Norethisterone, Norethindrone	–C≡CH	–CH$_3$
Norgestrel	–C≡CH	–C$_2$H$_5$
19-Nortestosterone	–H	–CH$_3$

i. Progesterone (Alza)

Synthesis
Method-I From: Diosgenin

Method-II From: Ergosterol

Properties: It exists as white crystalline powder, insoluble in water and in alcohol.

Dose: The dose for uterine bleeding is 5–10 mg injected per day up to 5–10 days. For habitual abortion, the dosage is 5–20 mg twice or thrice a week by IM injection.

ii. Hydroxyprogesterone caproate

Synthesis

17α-Hydroxyprogesterone caproate

Properties and uses: It exists as white crystalline powder, insoluble in water, it is more potent than progesterone, and has longer duration with short onset of action.

iii. Norethindrone (Norethiesterone, Micronor)

Synthesis

Properties and uses: It exists as white crystalline powder, insoluble in water. It is an important oral contraceptive and has the ability to postpone menstruation and prevent ovulation by suppressing pituitary gonadotropin. It is used in combination with mestranol and ethinestradiol.

Assay: Dissolve the sample in tetrahydrofuran, add silver nitrate, and titrate the solution with 0.1 N NaOH. Determine the end point potentiometrically.

Dose: The oral dose for contraception is 2.5–10 mg daily for 21 days.

iv. Norgestrel (Ovrette, Ovval)

Synthesis

Properties and uses: It exists as white crystalline powder, insoluble in water, slightly soluble in alcohol. Used as an oral contraceptive.

Dose: The oral dose as a single agent is 75 µg per day.

Drugs Acting on Endocrine System

OESTROGENS

The mammalian ovary is a source of steroid hormones that maintain reproductive functions and oestrogen secretion in females.

Classification

Oestrogens could be classified as follows:

i. **Natural steroidal:** Oestradiol, Oesterone
ii. **Synthetic steroidal:** Ethynyl oestradiol, Mestranol
iii. **Nonsteroidal synthetic:** Stilbesterol

i. Oestradiol derivatives

Name	R	R_1	R_2
Oestradiol	–H	–H	–H
Oestradiol valerate	–H	–CO(CH$_2$)$_3$CH$_3$	–H
Oestradiol cypionate	–H	–CO(CH$_2$)$_2$–⬠	–H
Oestradiol dipropionate	–COC$_2$H$_5$	–COC$_2$H$_5$	–H
Oestradiol benzoate	C$_6$H$_5$CO–	–H	–H
Ethynyl oestradiol	–H	–H	–C≡CH
Mestranol	CH$_3$	–H	–C≡CH
Quinestrol	⬠–	–H	–C≡CH

Oestradiol Derivatives

Properties: It exists as a creamy white crystalline powder hygroscopic, insoluble in water and soluble in alcohol.

ii. Diethylstilbestrol (Stilbetin, Stilphstrol)

Properties: It is a white crystalline powder, insoluble in water and soluble in alcohol.

Dose: The dose for menopausal symptoms orally is 0.1–2 mg. For secondary amenorrhoea, the dose is 0.2–0.5 mg and for carcinoma, of the prostate the intake is 3 mg per day.

Synthesis

Method-I From: Anisaldehyde (Dodds method)

Method-II From: Anethole

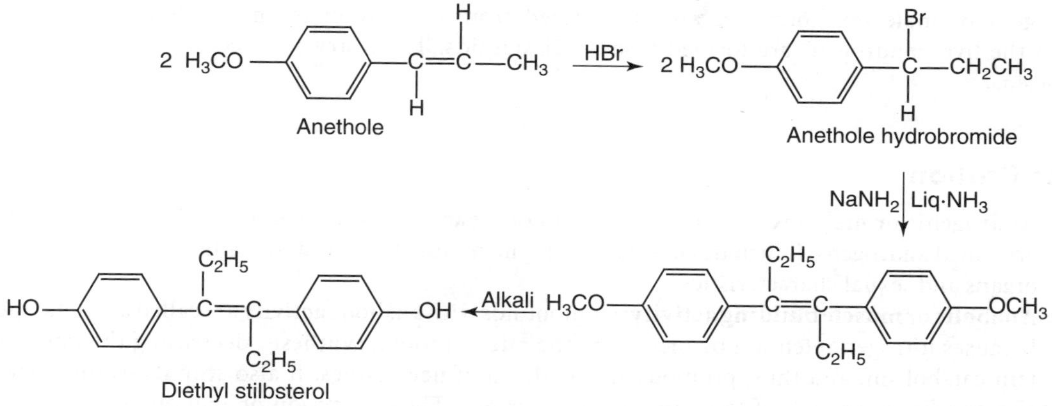

2 H₃CO—C₆H₄—CH=CH—CH₃ (Anethole) →[HBr] 2 H₃CO—C₆H₄—CHBr—CH₂CH₃ (Anethole hydrobromide)

↓ NaNH₂ / Liq·NH₃

H₃CO—C₆H₄—C(C₂H₅)=C(C₂H₅)—C₆H₄—OCH₃

→[Alkali]

HO—C₆H₄—C(C₂H₅)=C(C₂H₅)—C₆H₄—OH
Diethyl stilbsterol

iii. Dienestrol (Estragard)

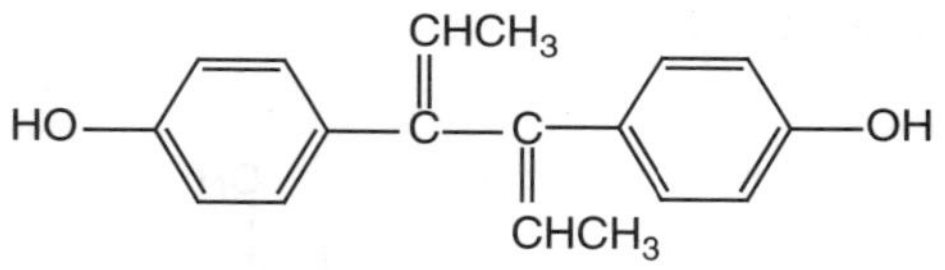

HO—C₆H₄—C(=CHCH₃)—C(=CHCH₃)—C₆H₄—OH

Synthesis

Diethyl stilbsterol →[CH₃COCl] Diethyl stilbsteroldiacetate

↓ Br₂

H₃COC—O—C₆H₄—C(C₂H₅)(Br)—C(Br)(C₂H₅)—C₆H₄—O—COCH₃

↓ Pyridine, Heat, −H₂O

H₃COC—O—C₆H₄—C(=CHCH₃)—C(=CHCH₃)—C₆H₄—O—COCH₃ →[NaOH] HO—C₆H₄—C(=CHCH₃)—C(=CHCH₃)—C₆H₄—OH
Dienestrol

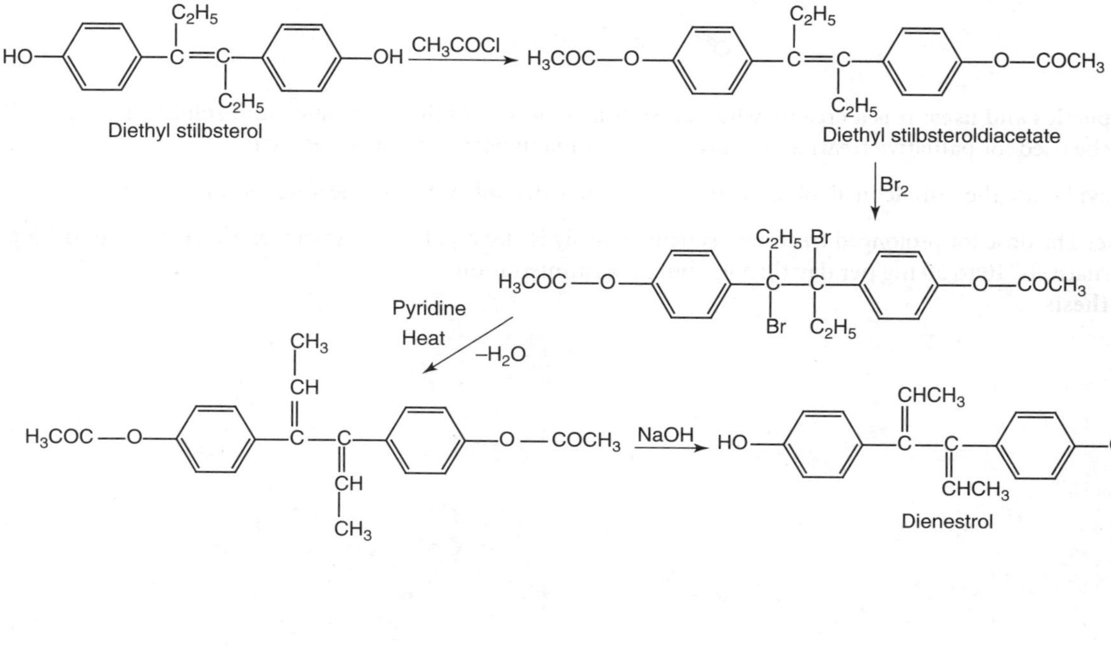

ANDROGENS AND ANABOLIC AGENTS

Androgens or male sex hormones are synthesized from cholesterol in the testes and adrenal cortex. In the liver, androgens are formed from C-21 steroids. The ovary also secretes small amounts of androgens.

Classification

1. **Androgenic or male sex characteristics promoting activity:** Compounds with androgenic activity are called androgens. It includes normal development, functioning, and maintenance of the male sex organs and sexual characteristics.
2. **Anabolic or muscle building activity:** Compounds with anabolic activity are called anabolic agents. It causes nitrogen retention by increasing the rate of protein synthesis, decreasing the rate of protein catabolism, and thus, promotes laying down of new tissues. It also stimulates the thickness rise and linear growth of the bones to some extent. The distinction of anabolic therapy of such wasting conditions such as cancer, trauma, osteoporosis, and also effects of immobilizations are also treated by the anabolic agents.

i. Testosterone (Nuvir, Andriol, Testoviron)

Properties and uses: It is a creamy white crystalline powder, insoluble in water, and soluble in alcohol. It may be used for palliative treatment of breast carcinoma in postmenopausal women.

Assay: Dilute the sample in alcohol to 50 ml with ethyl alcohol. Measure the absorption at 241 nm.

Dose: The dose for prolonged treatment subcutaneously is 600 mg. For breast cancer, the dose is up to 1.5 g; alternatively, 10 to 30 mg per day through buccal administration.
Synthesis

Steroids

Synthesis scheme from Cholesterol to Testosterone and its esters:

Cholesterol → (i) Ac$_2$O (ii) Br$_2$ → **Cholesteryl acetate dibromide** → CrO$_3^-$ / CH$_3$COOH → (5,6-dibromo-3-acetoxy-17-keto intermediate) → (i) Zn–CH$_3$COOH (ii) Hydrolysis → **Dehydroepiandrosterone**

From Dehydroepiandrosterone:

- (i) Ac$_2$O, (ii) Na–C$_2$H$_5$OH → 3-acetoxy-17-hydroxy intermediate → (i) C$_6$H$_5$COCl, (ii) Mild hydrolysis, (iii) CH$_3$OH–NaOH → 17-benzoate-3-hydroxy intermediate → Oppeanuer oxidation → 17-OCOC$_6$H$_5$-3-keto-Δ5 intermediate → Hydrolysis KOH → **Testosterone**

- Oxidizing agent O$_2$ → **Androst-4-ene-3:17-dione** → **Testosterone**

Testosterone transformations:

- + ⟨cyclopentyl⟩–CH$_2$CH$_2$COCl, Pyridine → **Testosterone cypionate**
- + CH$_3$(CH$_2$)$_5$COCl → **Testosterone enanthate**
- + (CH$_3$CH$_2$CO)$_2$O → **Testosterone propionate** (OCOC$_2$H$_5$)

ii. Methyl testosterone

Synthesis

Dehydroepiandrosterone —CH₃MgI→ (intermediate) —Oppneauer oxidation→ Methyl testosterone

iii. Fluoxymesterone (Halotestin)

Properties: It exists as a white crystalline powder and insoluble in water. It is used in the treatment of postmenopausal osteoporosis in combination with an estrogen.

Dose: The dose orally for adults in the replacement therapy is 1–3 mg twice a day.

Synthesis

17-Methyl testosteronre →(Aspergillus)→ [11-hydroxy intermediate] →(i) *p*-Toluene sulphonic acid (ii) OH⁻→ [diene intermediate] →(H₂O | CH₃CONHBr)→ [bromohydrin] →(C₂H₅ONa)→ [epoxide] →(HF)→ **Fluoxymesterone**

PROBABLE QUESTIONS

1. What are steroids? Provide the nomenclature and stereochemistry of steroids.
2. Classify steroids with suitable examples and mention their therapeutic uses.
3. Write a brief account of the androgens. How will you synthesize testosterone from the following:
   (a) Cholesterol (b) Dehydroepiandrosterone
4. Describe the synthesis of cortisone and hydrocortisone
5. Name the steroids used as contraceptives, draw their chemical structure, and write the synthesis of anyone of them.
6. Write a brief note on progesterone derivatives
7. Give the names and official status of at least five derivatives of the following, which are used in medicine.
   (a) Testosterone (b) Estradiol

SUGGESTED READINGS

1. Abraham DJ (ed). *Burger's Medicinal Chemistry and Drug Discovery* (6th edn). New Jersey: John Wiley, 2007.
2. Bhatnagar A, Brodie, AMH et al (eds.) Fourth International Anrnatase Conference. *J Steroid Bio Chem Mol Biol* 61: 107–426, 1997.

3. *British Pharmacopoeia*. Medicines and Healthcare Products Regulatory Agency. London, 2008
4. Bruntan LL, Lazo JS, and Parker KL. *Goodman and Gilman's: The Pharmacological Basis of Therapeutics* (11th edn). New York: McGraw Hill, 2006.
5. Gennaro AR. *Remington: The Science and Practice of Pharmacy* (21st edn). New York: Lippincot Williams and Wilkins, 2006.
6. *Indian Pharmacopoeia*. Ministry of Health and Family Welfare. New Delhi, 1996.
7. Lednicer D and Mitscher LA. *The Organic Chemistry of Drug Synthesis*. New York: John Wiley, 1995.
8. Lemke TL and William DA. *Foye's Principle of Medicinal Chemistry* (6th edn). New York: Lippincott Williams and Wilkins, 2008.
9. Reynolds EF (ed). *Martindale the Extra Pharmacopoeia* (31st edn). London: The Pharmaceutical Press, 1997.
10. Zeelen FJ. *Medicinal Chemistry of Steroids*. Elsevier: Amsterdam, 1990.

Chapter 3

Antithyroid Drugs

INTRODUCTION

Antithyroid drugs are compounds that act within the thyroid gland to inhibit the biosynthesis of the thyroid hormones. Excessive amount of thyroid hormones in the circulation are associated with a number of diseased states, including Grave's disease, toxic adenoma, goitre, and thyroidities among others.

CLASSIFICATION

Antithyroid drugs are classified as follows:
I. Thioureylenes
i. Thiouracil derivatives

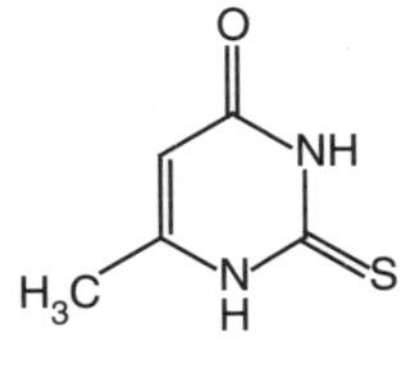

Methylthiouracil

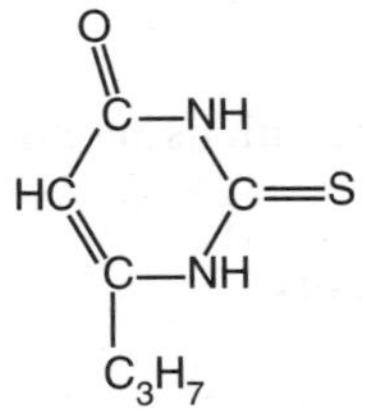

Propylthiouracil

ii. Imidazoles

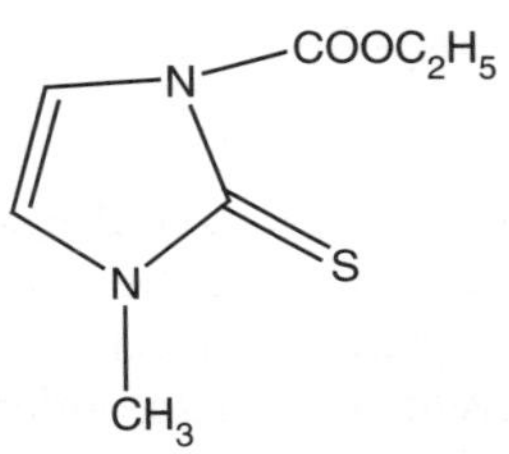

Carbimazole

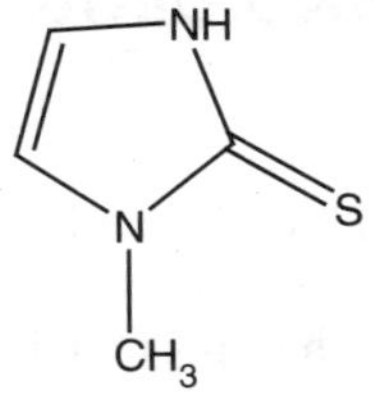

Methimazole

iii. Aniline derivatives

Sulphanilamide: 4-aminobenzenesulfonamide (H_2N-C$_6$H$_4$-SO_2NH_2)

Sulphaguanidine: 4-aminobenzenesulfonyl guanidine

p-Aminosalicylic acid: 4-amino-2-hydroxybenzoic acid

Carbutamide: H_2N-C$_6$H$_4$-$SO_2NHC(O)NHC_4H_9$

Mode of action: These agents interfere with some of the process catalyzed by thyroid peroxidase, such as iodide oxidation, organification, and coupling of iodotyrosines.

II. Polyhydric phenols
i. Resorcinol

Resorcinol (benzene-1,3-diol)

Mode of action: The only clinical agent from this category is resorcinol. It possesses same mechanism of action similar to that of thioamides.

III. Ionic inhibitors

(a) Potassium perchlorate
(b) Thiocynate

Mode of action: These anions resemble iodide ions and affect the power of thyroid gland to accumulate iodine.

IV. Miscellaneous agents

(a) Lithium carbonate and
(b) Adrenergic blockers

SYNTHESIS AND DRUG PROFILE

I. Thioureylenes

Mode of action: Thiourea and thiouracil derivatives are among the primary drugs to treat thyroid hyperactivity. Methyl and propylthiouracil derivatives are effective drugs in the treatment of thyroid-related problems. They prevent iodine incorporation into the organic form perhaps by antagonizing the iodide oxidation by peroxidase. They are also found to prevent coupling of iodotyrosines to form iodothyronines.

The 2-thiouracil derivatives, that is, 4-keto-2-thio pyrimidines, are undoubtedly tautomeric compounds and can be represented as follows:

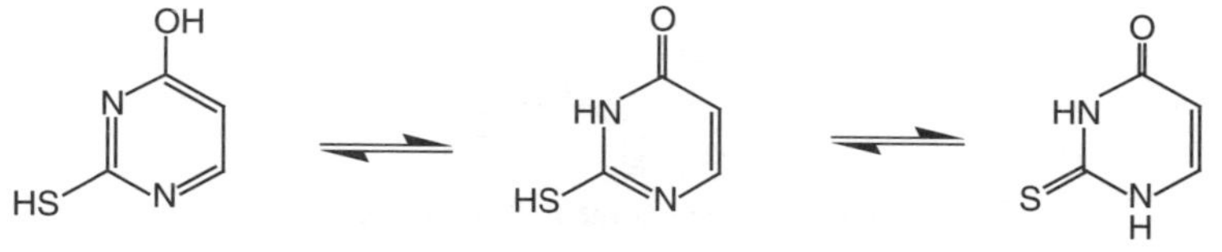

Some 300-related structures have been evaluated for antithyroid activity, but, of these, only the 6-allyl-2-thio uracil and closely related structure possess useful clinical activity. The most serious adverse effect of thiouracil therapy is agranulocytosis.

i. Propylthiouracil (Tietil)

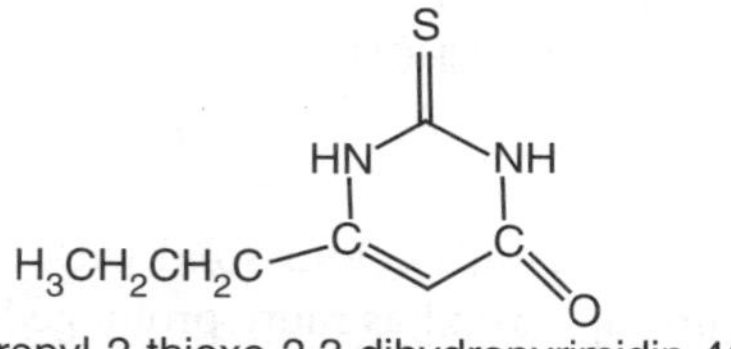

6-Propyl-2-thioxo-2,3-dihydropyrimidin-4(1H)-one

Synthesis

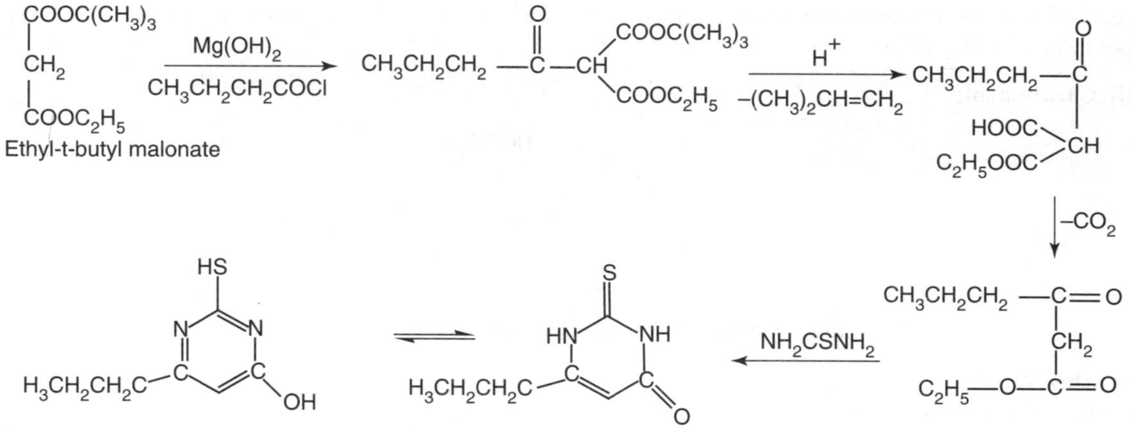

Propylthiouracil

Properties and uses: It is a white powdery crystalline substance with bitter taste, soluble in water, alcohol, chloroform, and ether. Used in the management of hyperthyroidism.

Dose: For hyperthyroidism, the dose for adults initially is 200–300 mg per day in divided doses. When the patient attains normal basal metabolic rate (euthyroidism), the dose is usually reduced to a maintenance dose of 50–75 mg per day in two to three divided doses. In children, over 10 years old, initial dose is 150–300 mg per day in four divided doses until the child becomes euthyroid, then, usually, 100 mg daily is given in two divided doses, for maintenance.

ii. Methimazole (Tapazele)

3-Methyl-1H-imidazole-2(3H)-thione

Synthesis

2,2-Dimethoxyethanamine → (CH₃NCS) → intermediate → (H⁺) → Methimazole

Properties and uses: It exists as white to pale-buff colour solid with characteristic odour and soluble in water. The drug is more potent, more prompt, and has more prolonged action than propylthiouracil. It is indicated in the treatment of hyperthyroidism.

Dose: Usual initial dose is 5–20 mg every 8 h. When condition is stabilized (1–2 months), the dose is reduced to a maintenance dose of 5–15 mg per day. For children, the initial dose is 400 µg/kg body weight per day in divided doses.

iii. Carbimazole

Ethy-l-methyl-2-thioxo-1,2-dihydroimidazole-3-carboxylate

Synthesis
Route I: From: Methimazole

Methimazole → (ClCOOC₂H₅) → Carbimazole

Route II. From: *N*-methylamino acetal

N-Methylamino cetal + HNCS → 1-Methyl-2-mercapto imidazole →[ClCOOC$_2$H$_5$] Carbimazole

PROBABLE QUESTIONS

1. Define and classify antithyroid agents and write the synthesis and uses of any two of them.
2. Write the synthesis and uses of methylthiouracil and propylthiouracil.

SECTION VI

CHEMOTHERAPY

1	History and Development of Chemotherapy	223
2	Antibacterial Sulphonamides	229
3	Quinoline Antibacterials	254
4	Antibiotics	265
5	Antitubercular Agents	331
6	Antifungal Agents	344
7	Antiviral Agents	364

8	Antiamoebic Agents	401
9	Antimalarials	409
10	Anthelmintics	435
11	Antineoplastic Agents	455
12	Antileprotic Drugs	511

Chapter 1

History and Development of Chemotherapy

INTRODUCTION

Chemotherapy is the treatment of systemic disease or infection with appropriate drugs, which are capable to produce retardation in multiplication of microorganism or to suppress their growth without affecting the host system. The word chemotherapy is applicable for the treatment of infection due to viral, bacterial, fungal, and protozoal infections. Antibiotics are substances produced by microorganisms, which selectively suppress the growth and proliferation or kill other microorganisms at very low concentration. As the analogues of the antibiotic products are produced semisynthetically they are also called as chemotherapeutic agents.

HISTORICAL BACKGROUND

There are three phases to explain the history of chemotherapy, such as empirical period, Ehrlich's phase, and the modern phase. In early empirical period of 16th century, Paracelsus used mercury for the treatment of syphilis and during 17th century cinchona bark was used for pyrexia. In 500 to 600 BC, molded curd of soybean was used in Chinese folk medicine for infection and wounds. In early period, during these phases, Hindus used chaulmoogra oil for the treatment of leprosy. In Ehrlich's phase, it was revealed that certain dyes produced toxicity and killed some microorganisms. So neoarsphenamine was developed by Ehrlich for the treatment of syphilis. The word antibiosis was coined after the killing of anthrax bacilli when grown in culture media with other bacteria during the 18th century. The modern phases demonstrated the therapeutic effect of prontosil (a sulphonamide) in pyrogenic infections in 19th century.

In 1929, Sir Alexander Fleming accidentally discovered the antibacterial properties of penicillin by destroying the *staphylococcus* in culture plate; this is broadly cited in modern antibiotic era. Chain and Florey followed up this observation in 1939 and later penicillin was clinically used during 1941. In 1942, Waksman proposed the search of *actinomycetes* and discovered streptomycin in 1944. Later, the advance in medicinal chemistry produced synthetic and semisynthetic agents.

SPECTRUM OF ACTIVITY OF CHEMOTHERAPEUTIC AGENTS

The ability of drug with all ranges (gram positive and gram negative) of antibiotic action, chloramphenicol, and tetracycline, to antagonize numerous pathogens have resulted mention as broad-spectrum antibiotics. Many of the broad-spectrum antibiotics are active only at high concentration. Some drugs are primarily static and they may exert cidal action at high concentration (e.g. sulphonamides, erythromycin, nitrofurantoin, etc). The bacteriostatic agents are those that interfere with the growth or replication of microorganisms, but does not kill it. The bactericidal drugs are those that kills the microorganisms. Concentration of drugs at the site of infection is an important factor for the therapeutic effect in case of antimicrobials. The classes of antibiotics and their spectrum of activity is detailed in Table 1.1.

Table 1.1 Classes of antibiotics and their spectrum of activity.

Class of Antibiotics	Name of the Drug	Susceptible Organism
Natural penicillins	Penicillin G and V	Gram positive bacteria—*streptococci* except *viridians*. Gram positive *Bacilli*, i.e. *B. anthracis*, *Corynebacterium diphtheriae*, and all *Clostridia*
Semisynthetic penicillins	Oxacillin	Penicillinase-resistant
	Ampicillin	Broad spectrum. It is active against all organisms, which are sensitive to penicillin G and many gram-negative organisms, i.e. *Haemophilus influenzae, Escherichia coli, Proteus, Solmonella,* and *Shigella*
	Amoxycillin	Broad spectrum antibacterial action with penicillinase inhibitor. It is less active against *Shigella* and *H. influenzae*
	Aztreonam	*Pseudomonas* and gram-negative organism
Cephalosporins	Cefazolin	It is active against all organisms and sensitive to penicillin, i.e. *Streptococci, Gonococci, Meningococci, C. diphtheriae, H. influenzae, Clostridia,* and *Actinomycetes*. Highly active against *Klebsiella* and *E. coli*
	Cephalothin	Similar in spectrum to Cefazolin, but less active against penicillinase producing *Staphylococci* and *H. influenzae*. Parentral administration produces broad spectrum action

(Continued)

Table 1.1 (Continued)

Class of Antibiotics	Name of the Drug	Susceptible Organism
	Cefotaxime	Potent action against aerobic gram negative and some gram positive, not active against anaerobes; *Staphylococcus aureus* and *Pseudomonas aeruginosa*
Glycopeptide antibiotics	Bacitracin	Gram-positive organisms of both *cocci* and *bacilli*
	Vancomycin	Gram-positive bacteria. It is useful in case of methicillin resistant *Staphylococcus aureus, Streptococcus viridans,* and *Enterococcus*
	Polymyxin	Gram negative, including *Pseudomonas* species
Antimycobacterial antibiotics	Isoniazid, Ethambutol	*Mycobacterium* species
Inhibitors of protein synthesis	Chloramphenicol	Broad spectrum
Aminoglycosides	Streptomycin	Broad spectrum, including *Mycobacterium* species. Primarily active against aerobic gram-negative bacilli.
	Neomycin	Broad spectrum activity
	Gentamycin	Broad spectrum, including *Pseudomonas* species. Ineffective against *Mycobacterium tuberculosis, Streptococcus pyogens,* and Pneumoniae
Tetracyclines	Tetracycline, oxytetracycline, doxycycline, minocycline, and clortetracyclin	All types of pathogens except virus and fungi. Broad spectrum including chlamydia, spirochetes, and rickettsia. *Mycoplasma* and *Actinomyces* are moderately sensitive.
Macrolides	Erythromycin	Gram-positive bacteria, highly active against *Str. pyogens, Neisseria gonorrhoeae, Clostridia, C. diphtheriae*, and *Listera*

(Continued)

Table 1.1 (*Continued*)

Class of Antibiotics	Name of the Drug	Susceptible Organism
	Clarithromycin	Similar to erythromycin, in addition *M. avium* complex. More active against gram-positive cocci, *Moraxella, Legionella, Mycoplasma pneumonea*, and *H. pylori*
	Azithromycin	Less effective in gram-positive cocci. Highly active against respiratory pathogens, i.e. *Mycoplasma, Chlamydia, Moraxella, Pneumoniae,* and *Legionella*
Streptogramins	Quinupristin and dalfopristin	Vancomycin resistant, methicillin resistant gram-positive bacteria
Oxazolidindione	Linezolid	It is active against methicillin resistant *Staphylococcus aureus*. Cidal to *Streptococci, Pnemococci,* and *Bacteriodes fragilis*
Quinolones and fluoroquinolones	Nalidixic acid, gatifloxacin, pefloxacin, norfloxacin, ciprofloxacin, etc	Most susceptible are gram negative *bacilli*. At high concentration gram positive bacteria highly susceptible bacteria are *E. coli, Klebsiella pnemoniae, Enterobacter, Solmonella typhi, Shigella proteus, Camphylobacter jejuni, Vibrio cholerae, Pseudomonas auruginosa, Brucella, Listeria,* and *B. anthracis* are little susceptible
Sulphonamides	Cotrimoxazole and other sulpha drugs	Broad spectrum. Primarily bacteriostatic
Nucleoside and nonneucleoside analogues	Acyclovir, Ganciclovir, ribavirin, lamivudine	Herpes virus
	Cidofovir	Cytomegalo virus
Tricyclic amines	Amantidine, Rimantidine	Influenza virus
8-Hydroxy quinolones	Quinidochlor	Malarial parasites

(*Continued*)

Table 1.1 (Continued)

Class of Antibiotics	Susceptible Organism	Susceptible Organism
Nitrimidazoles	Metronidazole and tinidazole	Broad spectrum action against protozoa, trichomoniasis, and Giardiasis infections
Benzimidazole	Albendazole, mebendazole	*Enterobias, Trichuris* infestations
Polyenes	Amphotericin B	Systemic fungal infection, active against wide range of yeasts and fungi, i.e. *Candida albicans, Histoplasma capsulatum, Blastomyces dermatitidis, Cryptococcus neoformans, Aspergillus, sporothrix,* and *Torulopsis*
Azole derivatives	Ketaconazole, clotrimaxazole, miconazole	Systemic fungal infection, Topical infection. Imidazole and triazole has broad spectrum antifungal action covering dermatophytes, *Candida, nocardia,* some gram positive and anerobic bacteria, i.e. *Staphylococcus aureus, Bacillus fragilis,* and *leishmania*
Allylamines	Terbinafine, Naftidine	Resistant organisms for azoles
Heterocyclic benzofuran	Griseofulvin	Most dermatophytes of skin fungal infection but not against *Candida*

Bacterial Resistance to Antimicrobial Agents

The bacterial resistance development depends on three factors. They are as follows:

- The necessary dose or concentration not reached to target.
- The chemotherapeutic agent is not active.
- The target is altered.

The outer membrane of the gram-negative bacteria is a permeability barrier that excludes large polar molecules, including antibiotic, through a protein called porins. Loss of porin channel may prevent the entry of antibiotics and reduces the concentration in target site. If there is an active transport mechanism for the entry of drug into the cell, mutational changes will occur in the transport to produce resistant. For example, passage of gentamycin across the microbial cell membrane by concentration gradient by involving the respiratory electron transport and oxidative phosphorylation. Mutation in this enzyme pathway decreases the concentration to the target.

Inactivation of drugs are seen in case of aminoglycoside and β-lactums. In aminoglycosides, the acquisition of cell membrane bound inactivating enzymes which phosphorylates/adenylates or acetylates the drug molecule and produces conjugated aminoglycosides. These conjugated amino glycosides do not bind to target ribosome and so are incapable of enhancing active transport. Nosocomial microbes have rich plasmids producing multidrug resistance and cross resistance.

In fluroquinolone, the resistance is occurred by alteration of target. The resistance is noted due to chromosomal mutations producing a DNA gyrase or topoisomerase IV with reduced affinity to the fluroquinolone or due to reduced permeability of the drug.

Selection of Antimicrobial Agents

The selection is based on thorough knowledge of pharmacological and microbiological factors. Antibiotics are used in three general ways such as empirical therapy, definitive therapy, and prophylactic therapy. When used in empirical, the drug intended should cover all the microorganisms, if the pathogen is exactly not known. In the *combination therapy*, treatment with a broad spectrum antibiotic is necessary. After the identification of infecting microorganism, selective drug can be used.

Combination Therapy

It is the combined use of drugs intended to achieve better action; in chemotherapy it is used for the synergistic action (e.g. a sulphonamide used with trimethoprim to produce additive action). Other examples are in the combination of β-lactamase inhibition by clavulanic acid or sulbactum with amoxycillin or ampicillin for β-lacamase producing *H. influenza, Neisseria gonorrhoeae*, and other organisms.. Combination of bactericidal with a bacteriostatic drug produces synergistic action. The combination therapy of antimicrobials are also used in the treatment of mixed infection and initial treatment of severe infections.

Chapter 2

Antibacterial Sulphonamides

INTRODUCTION

The term sulphonamides are employed as a generic name for the derivatives of para amino benzene sulphonamide (sulphanilamide). The sulphonamide drugs were the first effective chemotherapeutic agents to be employed systemically for the prevention and treatment of bacterial infections in humans. The sulphonamides are bacteriostatic antibiotics with a wide spectrum action against most gram-positive bacteria and many gram-negative organisms. Actually it was found to be the metabolic product of Prontosil, which is responsible for antibacterial activity, and this has given the initiation to develop sulphonamides as antibacterial agents.

$$H_2N-\text{C}_6H_3(NH_2)-N=N-\text{C}_6H_4-SO_2NH_2$$
Prontosil

$$\downarrow$$

$$H_2N-\text{C}_6H_4-SO_2NH_2$$
Sulphanilamide

Sulphonamides are total synthetic substances that are produced by relatively simple chemical synthesis. The advent of penicillin and, subsequently of other antibiotics has diminished the usefulness of sulphonamides. Antimicrobial compounds contain sulphonamide (SO_2NH_2) group. This group (SO_2NH_2) is also present in other compounds, such as antidiabetic agents (e.g. Tolubutamide), diuretics (e.g. chlorthiazide and its congeners, furosemide, and acetazolamide), and anticonvulsants such as sulthiame. The sulphonamides exists as white powder, mildly acidic in character, and they form water-soluble salts with bases. The pH of sodium salts with some exception, for example, sodium sulphacetamide, is very high when given intramuscular (IM), the marked alkalinity causes damage to the tissues.

Microorganisms that may be susceptible in vitro to sulphonamides include *Streptococcus pyogens*, *Streptococcus pneumoniae*, *Haemophilus influenzae*, *H. ducreyi*, *Nocardia*, *Actinomyces*, *Calymmatobacterium granulomatis*, and *Chlamydia trachomatis*. The minimal inhibitory concentration ranges from 0.1 µg/ml for *C. trachomatis* to 4–64 µg/ml for *E. coli*. Sulphonamides are selective drugs used to treat urinary tract infections, bacterial respiratory infections, and gastrointestinal (GI) infections.

Mode of action: Sulphonamides are structure analogues and competitive antagonists of para-amino benzoic acid (PABA). They inhibit dihydropteroate synthetase, the bacterial enzyme responsible for the incorporation of PABA into dihydropteric acid, and it is the intermediate precursor of folic acid. Synergistic effect is obtained by a combination of trimethoprim. The compound trimethoprim is a potent and selective inhibitor of microbial dihydrofolate reductase, the enzyme that reduces dihydrofolate to tetrahydrofolate. The simultaneous administration of sulphonamide and trimethoprim blocks the pathway of cell-wall synthesis sequentially.

SAR of Sulphonamides

The major features of SAR of sulphonamides include the following:

- Sulphanilamide skeleton is the minimum structural requirement for antibacterial activity.
- The amino- and sulphonyl-groups on the benzene ring are essential and should be in 1 and 4 position.
- The N-4 amino group could be modified to be prodrugs, which are converted to free amino function in vivo.

- Sulphur atom should be directly linked to the benzene ring.
- Replacement of benzene ring by other ring systems or the introduction of additional substituents on it decreases or abolishes its activity.
- Exchange of the –SO$_2$NH group by –CONH reduces the activity.

- On N-1-substituted sulphonamides, activity varies with the nature of the substituent at the amino group. With substituents imparting electron-rich characters to SO_2 group, bacteriostatic activity increases.
- Heterocyclic substituents lead to highly potent derivatives, while sulphonamides, which contain a single benzene ring at N-1 position, are considerably more toxic than heterocyclic ring analogues.
- The free aromatic amino groups should reside *para* to the sulphonamide group. Its replacement at *ortho* or *meta* position results in compounds devoid of antibacterial activity.
- The active form of sulphonamide is the ionized, maximum activity that is observed between the pKa values 6.6–7.4.
- Substitutions in the benzene ring of sulphonamides produced inactive compounds.
- Substitution of free sulphonic acid ($-SO_3H$) group for sulphonamido function destroys the activity, but replacement by a sulphinic acid group ($-SO_2H$) and acetylation of N-4 position retains back the activity.
- *m*. Sulphonamides bind to the basic centres of arginine, histidine, and lysine sites of proteins. The binding groups are alkyl, alkoxy, and halides. The binding affects the activity of sulphonamides; protein binding appears to modulate the availability of the drug and its half-life.
- The lipid solubility influences the pharmacokinetic and antibacterial activity, and so increases the half-life and antibacterial activity in vitro.

CLASSIFICATION

Sulphonamides can be classified in various ways:

On the basis of the site of action

- Sulphonamides for general infection: Sulphanilamide, Sulphapyridine, Sulphadiazine, Sulphamethoxacine, Sulphamethoxazole.
- Sulphonamides for urinary tract infections: Sulphaisoxazole, Sulphathiazole.
- Sulphonamides for intestinal infections: Phthalylsulphathiazole, Succinyl sulphathiazole, Sulphasalazine.
- Sulphonamides for local infections: Sulpahacetamide, Mafenamide, Silver sulphadiazine.
- Sulphonamides for dermatitis: Dapsone, Solapsone.
- Sulphonamides in combination: Trimethoprim with Sulphamethoxazole.

On the basis of the pharmacokinetic properties

- Poorly absorbed sulphonamides (locally acting sulphonamides)—Sulphasalazine, Phthalylsulphathiazole, Sulphaguanidine, Salicylazo sulphapyridine, Succinyl sulpha thiazole.
- Rapidly absorbed and rapidly excreted (systemic sulphanamides): Sulphamethoxazole, Sulphaisoxazole, Sulphadiazine, Sulphadimidine, Sulphafurazole, Sulphasomidine, Sulphamethiazole, Sulphacetamide Sulphachlorpyridazine.
- Topically used sulphonamides: Sulphacetamide, Mafenide, Sulphathiazole, Silver sulphadiazine.

On the basis of the pharamacological activity

- Antibacterial agents: Sulphadiazine, Sulfisoxazole.
- Drugs used in dermatitis: Dapsone.

On the basis of the duration of action

- Extra long-acting sulphonamides (half-life greater than 50 h): Sulphasalazine, Sulphaclomide, Sulphalene.
- Long-acting sulphonamides (half-life greater than 24 h):Sulphadoxine, Sulphadimethoxine, Sulphamethoxy pyridazine, Sulphamethoxydiazine, Sulphaphenazole, Sulphamethoxine.
- Intermediate-acting sulphonamides (half-life between 10–24 h): Sulphasomizole, Sulphamethoxazole.
- Short-acting sulphonamides (half-life less than 20 h): Sulphamethiazole, sulphaisoxazole.
- Injectables (soluble sulpha drugs): Sulphafurazole, Sulphadiazine, Sulphamethoxine.

On the basis of the chemical structure

- N-substituted sulphonamide:Sulphadiazine, Sulphacetamide, Sulphadimidine.
- N-4 substituted sulphonamides (prodrugs): Prontosil.
- Both N-1 and N-4 substituted sulphonamides: Succinyl sulphathiazole, Phthalylsulphathiazole.
- Miscellaneous: Mefenide sodium.

$$RHN-\underset{3\ \ 2}{\overset{5\ \ 6}{\text{C}_6\text{H}_4}}-SO_2NHR'$$

I. N-1 Substituted sulphonamides

Name	R	R^1
Sulphanilamide	–H	–H
Sulphapyridine	–H	2-pyridyl
Sulphathiazole	–H	2-thiazolyl
Sulphacetamide	–H	–COCH$_3$
Sulphadiazine	–H	2-pyrimidinyl
Sulphadimidine	–H	4,6-dimethyl-2-pyrimidinyl

a. Short-acting sulpha drugs

Name	R	R¹
Sulphamethizole	–H	2-methyl-1,3,4-thiadiazol-5-yl (N–N, S, CH₃)
Sulphasomidine	–H	2,6-dimethylpyrimidin-4-yl
Sulphaisoxazole	–H	3,4-dimethylisoxazol-5-yl

b. Intermediate-acting sulphonamides

Name	R	R¹
Sulphasomizole	–H	3-methyl-5-methylisothiazol-4-yl
Sulphamethoxazole	–H	5-methylisoxazol-3-yl

c. Long-acting sulphonamides

Name	R	R¹
Sulphamethoxy pyridazine	–H	6-methoxypyridazin-3-yl (–OCH₃)
Sulphamethoxy diazine	–H	5-methoxy-1,3-diazin-2-yl (–OCH₃)

(Continued)

(Continued)

Name	R	R₁
Sulpha dimethoxine	–H	pyrimidine with two –OCH₃ groups
Sulphaphenazole	–H	pyrazole with N–C₆H₅

d. **Extra long-acting sulphonamides**

Name	R	R₁
Sulphalene	–H	pyrazine with H₃CO substituent
Sulphormethoxine	–H	pyrimidine with two OCH₃ groups

II. N-4 substituted suphonamides

Prontosil

H_2N–(benzene with NH_2)–N=N–(benzene)–SO_2NH_2

III. Both N-1 and N-4 substituted suphonamides

Name	R	R₁
Succinyl sulphathiazole	–CO–CH₂–CH₂–COOH	thiazole (methyl-substituted)
Phthalylsulphathiazole	–CO–(benzene)–COOH	thiazole

IV. Miscellaneous

a. Topically used sulphonamides

Mafenide

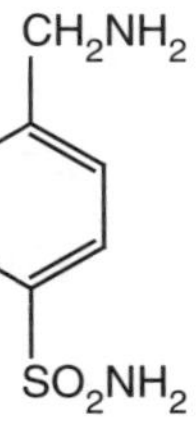

Silver sulphadiazine

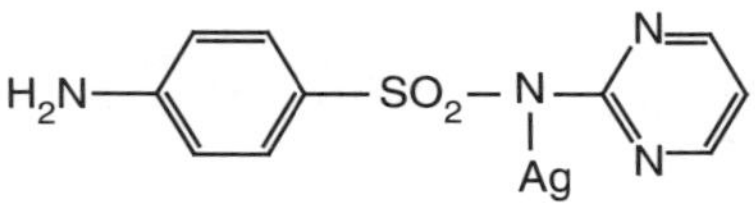

Solapsone

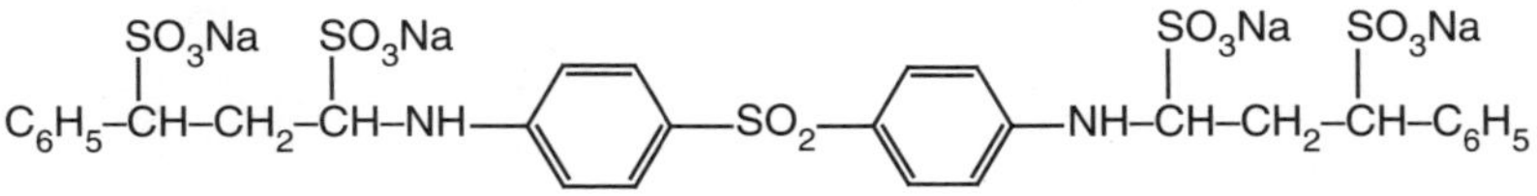

b. Drugs used in combination with sulphonamides

Trimethoprim

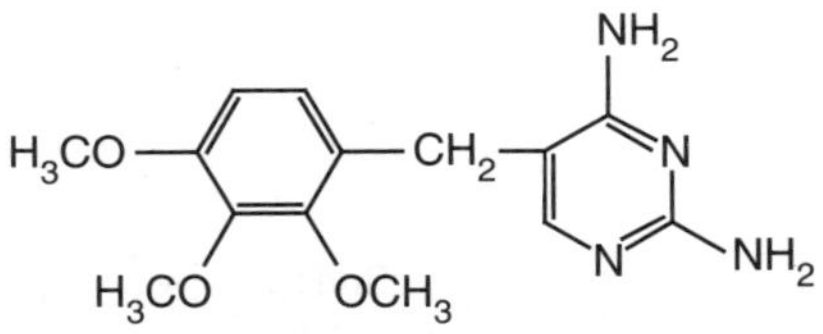

Pyrimethamine

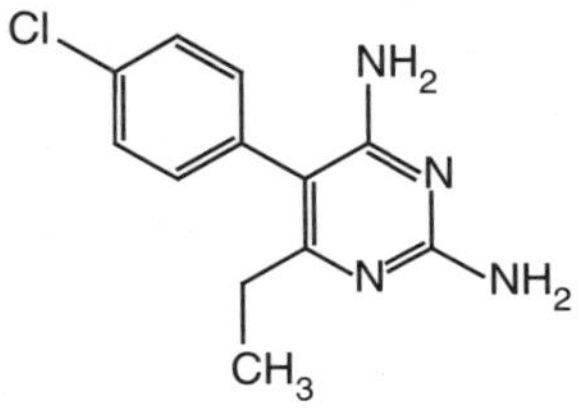

Chemotherapy

SYNTHESIS AND DRUG PROFILE

I. N-1 Substituted sulphonamides

i. Sulphanilamide

$H_2N-C_6H_4-SO_2NH_2$
4-Aminobenzene sulphonamide

Synthesis
Route-I. From: Benzene

Benzene $\xrightarrow{HNO_3/H_2SO_4}$ Nitrobenzene $\xrightarrow{H_2SO_4, \Delta}$ 4-Nitrobenzenesulphonic acid ($NO_2-C_6H_4-SO_3H$) $\xrightarrow{PCl_5}$ 4-Nitrobenzenesulphonyl chloride ($NO_2-C_6H_4-SO_2Cl$) $\xrightarrow{[H] \; Sn/HCl}$ 4-Aminobenzenesulphonyl chloride ($NH_2-C_6H_4-SO_2Cl$) $\xrightarrow{Con. NH_4OH, -HCl}$ Sulphanilamide ($H_2N-C_6H_4-SO_2NH_2$)

Route-II. From: Nitrobenzene

Nitrobenzene $\xrightarrow{ClSO_2OH}$ $NO_2-C_6H_4-SO_2Cl$ $\xrightarrow{Sn/HCl, [H]}$ $NH_2-C_6H_4-SO_2Cl$ $\xrightarrow{NH_4OH}$ $H_2N-C_6H_4-SO_2NH_2$
Sulphanilamide

Route-III. From: Aniline

Aniline → (CH$_3$CO)$_2$O → Acetamido benzene → H$_2$SO$_4$ → 4-acetamidobenzenesulfonic acid (HOO$_2$S-C$_6$H$_4$-NHCOCH$_3$)

NH$_4$OH | PCl$_5$ (−POCl$_3$, −HCl)

→ H$_3$COCHN-C$_6$H$_4$-SO$_2$NH$_2$ → HCl → H$_2$N-C$_6$H$_4$-SO$_2$NH$_2$ (Sulphanilamide)

Uses: It is used in veterinary medicine as an antibacterial agent.

ii. Sulphacetamide (Albucid)

H$_2$N-C$_6$H$_4$-SO$_2$NH-CO-CH$_3$

N-Sulphanilyl acetamide

Synthesis

H$_2$N-C$_6$H$_4$-SO$_2$NH$_2$ (4-Aminobenzenesulphonamide or Sulphanilamide) → (CH$_3$CO)$_2$O, −H$_2$O → CH$_3$CONH-C$_6$H$_4$-SO$_2$NHCOCH$_3$

−CH$_3$COOH | Partial hydrolysis

→ H$_2$N-C$_6$H$_4$-SO$_2$NHCOCH$_3$ (Sulphacetamide)

Properties and uses: It exists as white crystalline powder, bitter in taste. Used in the treatment of bacterial infections of urinary tract.

Assay: Dissolve the sample in water and hydrochloric acid. Titrate with sodium nitrite and determine the end point potentiometrically.

Dose: Dose for eyes, as drops 10%, 15%, 20%, and 30%; in ointments 2.5% and 6% of Sulphacetamide.

iii. Sulphasalazine

HO-C$_6$H$_3$(COOH)-N=N-C$_6$H$_4$-SO$_2$NH-(2-pyridyl)

Synthesis

Metabolism: It undergoes reductive metabolism by gut bacteria, converting the drug into sulfapyridine and 5-amino salicylic acid, which are active components.

Properties and uses: Sulphasalazine is a bright yellow or brownish-yellow fine powder, very slightly soluble in alcohol, practically insoluble in methylene chloride. It dissolves in dilute solutions of alkali hydroxides. It is used in the treatment of ulcerative colitis.

Assay: Dissolve and dilute the sample in 0.1 M sodium hydroxide and add 0.1 M acetic acid and measure the absorbance at the maxima of 359 nm using ultraviolet spectrophotometer.

Dosage forms: Sulphasalazine tablets B.P.

iv. Sulphadiazine

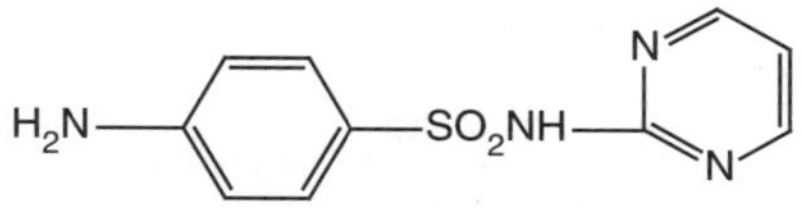

$H_2N-\text{C}_6H_4-SO_2NH-\text{(pyrimidin-2-yl)}$

N'-2 Pyrimidinyl sulphanilamide

Synthesis

Step-I. Preparation of formyl acetic acid

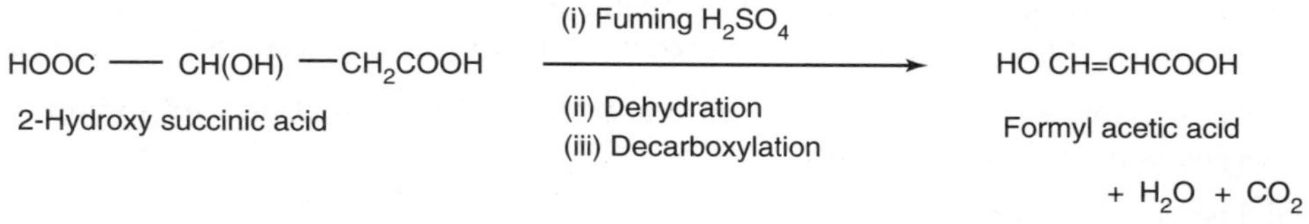

HOOC — CH(OH) — CH$_2$COOH → HO CH=CHCOOH + H$_2$O + CO$_2$

2-Hydroxy succinic acid

(i) Fuming H$_2$SO$_4$
(ii) Dehydration
(iii) Decarboxylation

Formyl acetic acid

Step II. Synthesis of 2-Aminopyrimidine

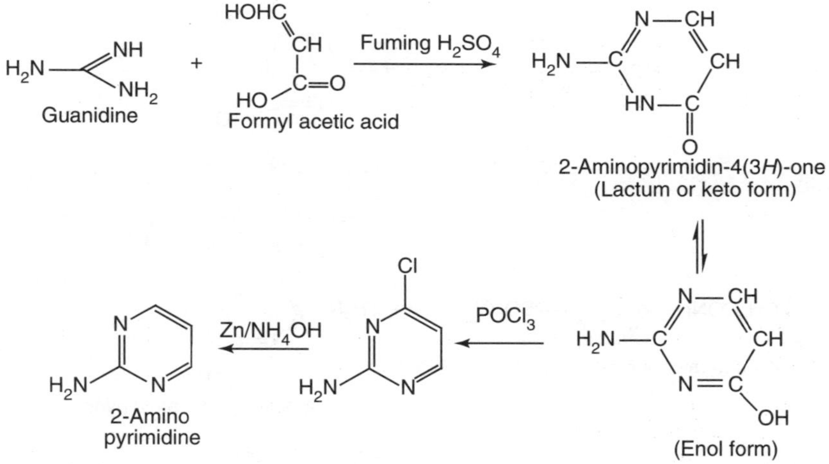

Guanidine + Formyl acetic acid $\xrightarrow{\text{Fuming } H_2SO_4}$ 2-Aminopyrimidin-4(3H)-one (Lactum or keto form) ⇌ (Enol form) $\xrightarrow{POCl_3}$ 4-chloro-2-aminopyrimidine $\xrightarrow{Zn/NH_4OH}$ 2-Amino pyrimidine

Step III. Synthesis of *p*-acetamido benzene sulphonyl chloride (PABS)

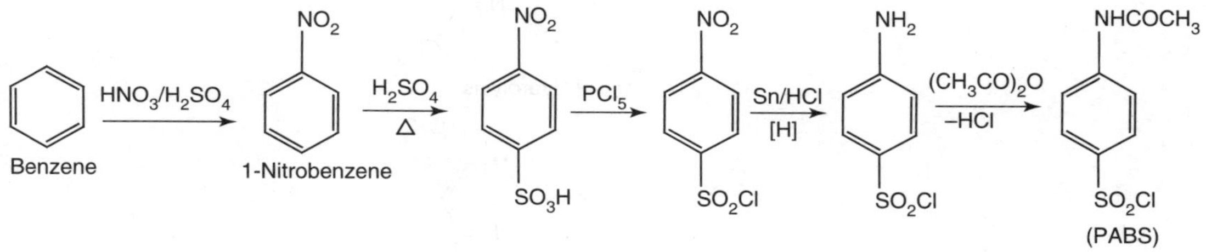

Benzene $\xrightarrow{HNO_3/H_2SO_4}$ 1-Nitrobenzene $\xrightarrow[\Delta]{H_2SO_4}$ (NO$_2$-C$_6$H$_4$-SO$_3$H) $\xrightarrow{PCl_5}$ (NO$_2$-C$_6$H$_4$-SO$_2$Cl) $\xrightarrow[{[H]}]{Sn/HCl}$ (NH$_2$-C$_6$H$_4$-SO$_2$Cl) $\xrightarrow[-HCl]{(CH_3CO)_2O}$ (NHCOCH$_3$-C$_6$H$_4$-SO$_2$Cl) (PABS)

Step IV. Condensation of *p*-acetamido benzene sulphonyl chloride with 2-aminopyrimidine

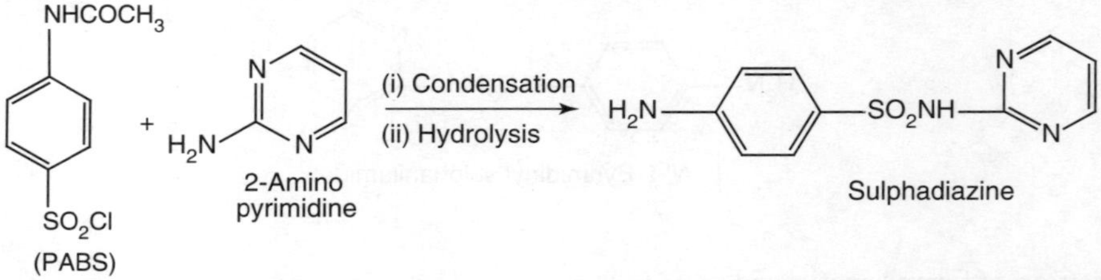

Properties and uses: Sulphadiazine is a white or yellowish-white or pinkish-white crystalline powder or crystals, insoluble in water, slightly soluble in acetone, very slightly soluble in alcohol, and soluble in solutions of alkali hydroxides and in dilute mineral acids. It is used in the treatment of canceroids and rheumatic fever.

Assay: Dissolve the sample in water and hydrochloric acid. Titrate the mixture with sodium nitrite and determine the end point potentiometrically.

Dose: Usual dose is 2–8 g per day

Dosage forms: Sulphadiazine tablets I.P., Sulphadiazine injection B.P.

v. **Sulphadimidine**

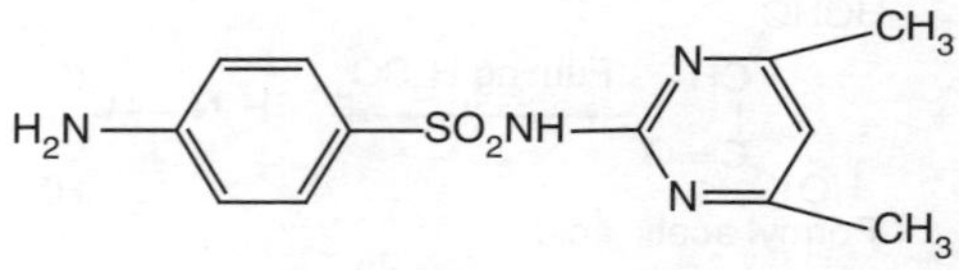

N' (4, 6- Dimethyl -2- pyrimidinyl) Sulphanilamide

Synthesis

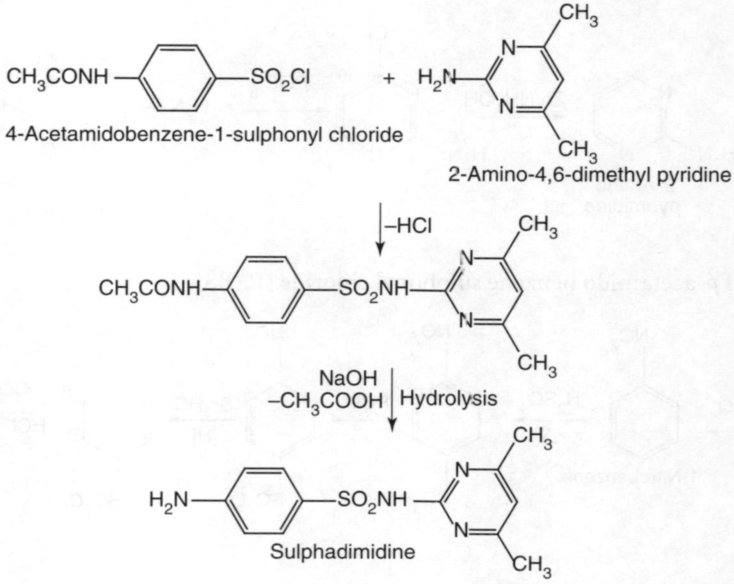

Properties and uses: It exists as white crystalline powder with a bitter taste, insoluble in water, and sparingly soluble in alcohol. It is less effective in meningeal infection because of its poor penetration into the cerebrospinal fluid.

Dose: Dose is 3 g initially and subsequent doses up to 6 g per day in divided doses.

vi. Sulphamerazine (Solumedine)

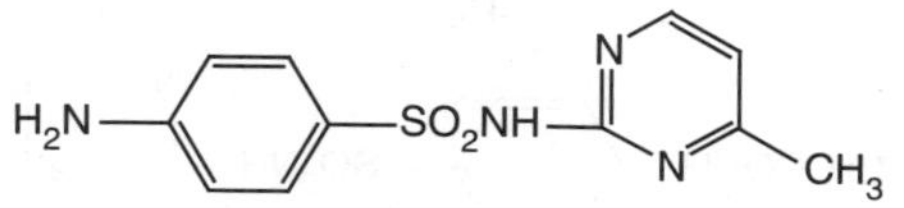

$H_2N-C_6H_4-SO_2NH-$(4-methyl-2-pyrimidinyl)

N'- (4-methyl - 2 - pyrimidinyl) Sulphanilamide

Synthesis

Step I. Preparation of PABS

Synthesized as mentioned under Sulphadiazine

Step II. Preparation of 2-amino-4-methyl pyrimidine

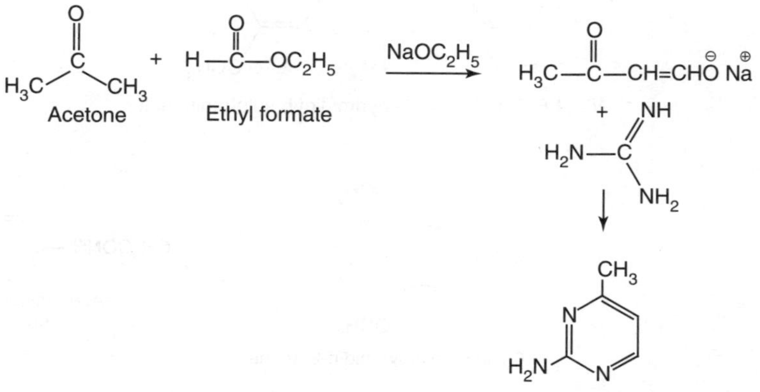

$$H_3C-CO-CH_3 + H-CO-OC_2H_5 \xrightarrow{NaOC_2H_5} H_3C-CO-CH=CHO^{\ominus} Na^{\oplus}$$

$$+ \; H_2N-C(=NH)-NH_2$$

$$\downarrow$$

2-Amino-4-methyl pyrimidine

Step III. Condensation of products of *Step I* and *II*

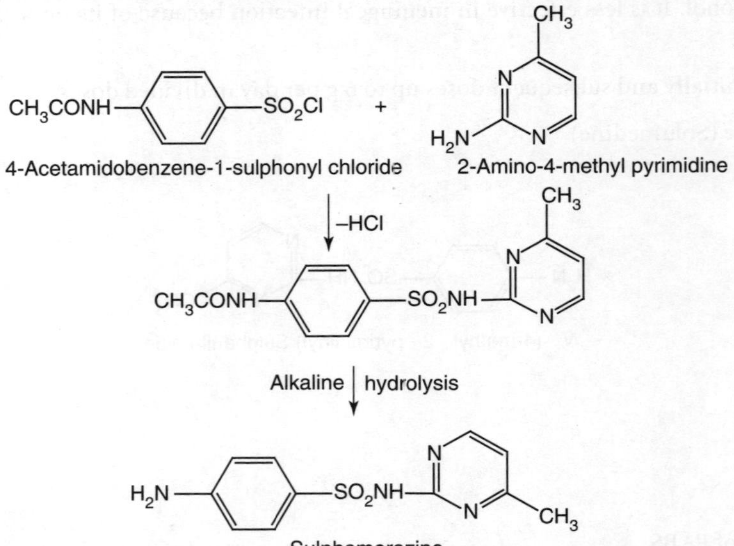

4-Acetamidobenzene-1-sulphonyl chloride + 2-Amino-4-methyl pyrimidine

↓ −HCl

CH₃CONH—C₆H₄—SO₂NH—(4-methylpyrimidin-2-yl)

Alkaline hydrolysis ↓

Sulphamerazine

Uses: Used as an antibacterial agent.
Dose: Dose is 4 g initially, and subsequent dose is 1 g every 6 h

vii. Sulphadimethoxine

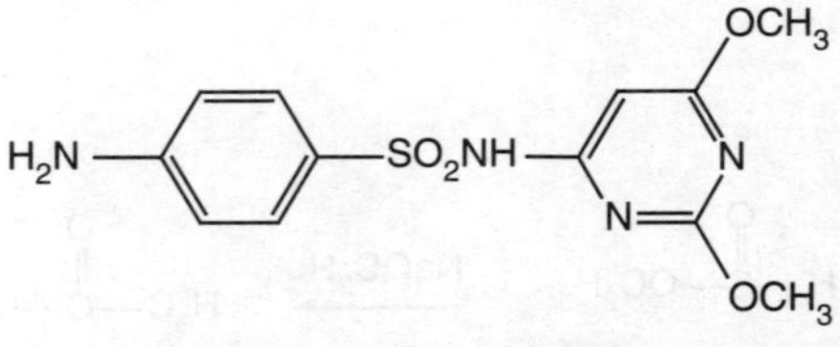

N'- (4,6-Dimethoxy -2- pyrimidinyl) sulphanilamide

Synthesis

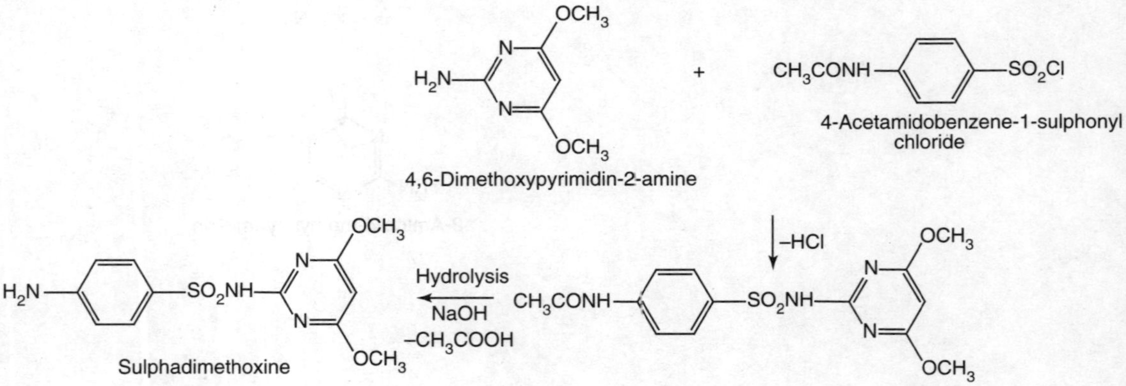

4,6-Dimethoxypyrimidin-2-amine + 4-Acetamidobenzene-1-sulphonyl chloride

↓ −HCl

CH₃CONH—C₆H₄—SO₂NH—(4,6-dimethoxypyrimidin-2-yl)

Hydrolysis
NaOH
−CH₃COOH

Sulphadimethoxine

viii. Sulpha methoxy pyridazine

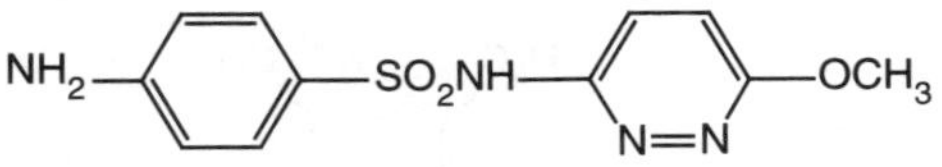

3-(4-Amino benzene sulphonamido)-6-methoxy pyridazine

Synthesis

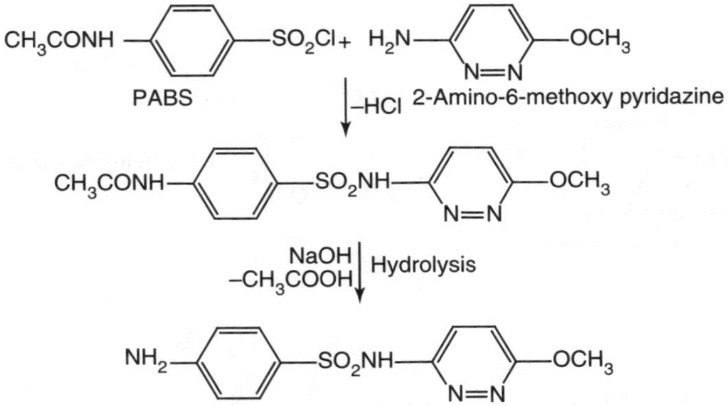

PABS + 2-Amino-6-methoxy pyridazine $\xrightarrow{-HCl}$

$CH_3CONH-C_6H_4-SO_2NH-$(6-methoxy pyridazin-3-yl)

$\xrightarrow[-CH_3COOH]{NaOH \text{ Hydrolysis}}$

Sulphamethoxy pyridazine

ix. Sulphaphenazole

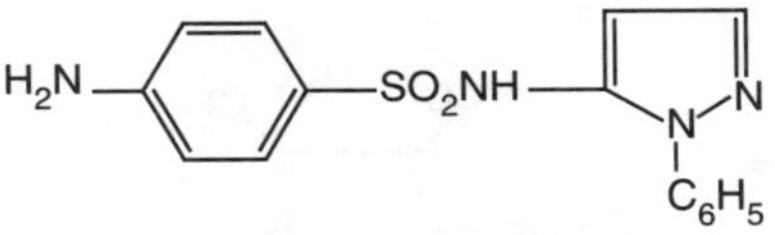

5-(4-Amino benzene sulphamido)N-Phenyl pyrazole

Synthesis

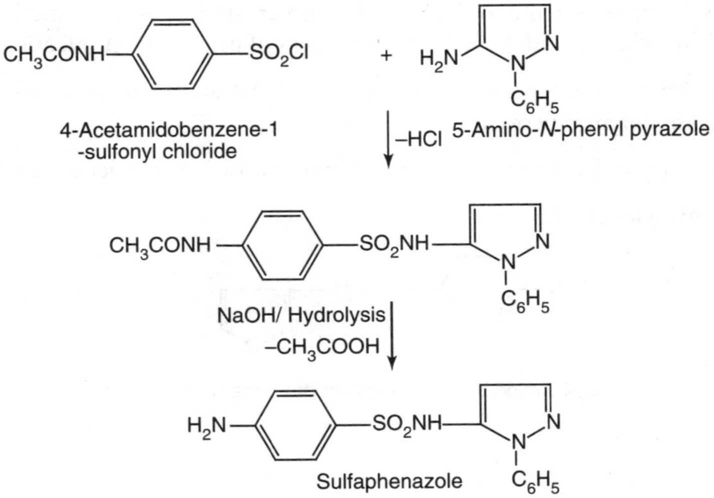

4-Acetamidobenzene-1-sulfonyl chloride + 5-Amino-N-phenyl pyrazole $\xrightarrow{-HCl}$

$CH_3CONH-C_6H_4-SO_2NH-$(1-phenyl pyrazol-5-yl)

$\xrightarrow[-CH_3COOH]{NaOH/ \text{ Hydrolysis}}$

Sulfaphenazole

x. Sulpha Isoxazole (Lipo Gantrisin, Gantrisin)

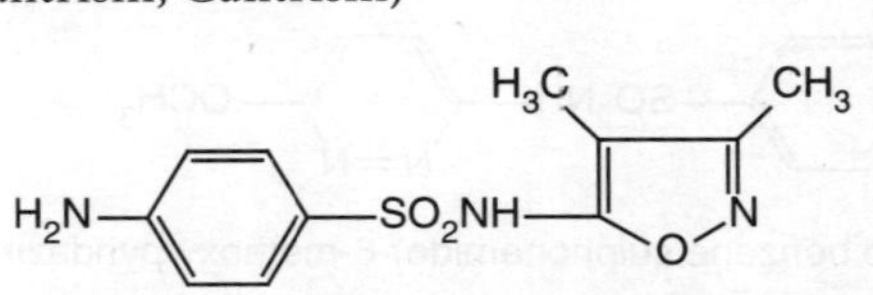

5-(4-Aminobenzene sulphonamido)-3,4-dimethyl isoxazole

Synthesis

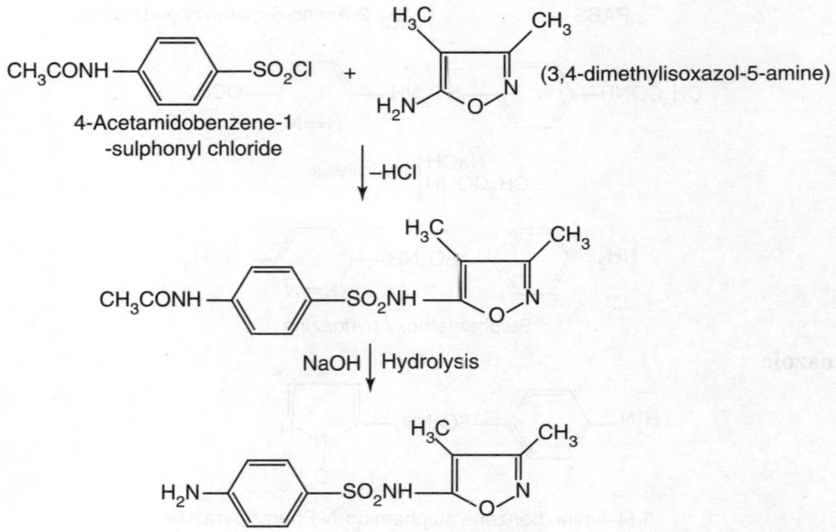

4-Acetamidobenzene-1-sulphonyl chloride + (3,4-dimethylisoxazol-5-amine)

↓ −HCl

↓ NaOH | Hydrolysis

Sulpha isoxazole

Properties and uses: It exists as white to slightly yellowish crystalline powder and is odourless, soluble in water and in dilute hydrochloric acid. Used in the treatment of urinary tract infections.

Assay: Dissolve the sample in water and hydrochloric acid. Titrate the mixture with sodium nitrite and determine the end point potentiometrically.

Dose: Initial dose is 2–4 g orally for adults and maintenance dose is 4–8 g per day in divided doses.

xi. Sulphamethoxazole (Gantanol)

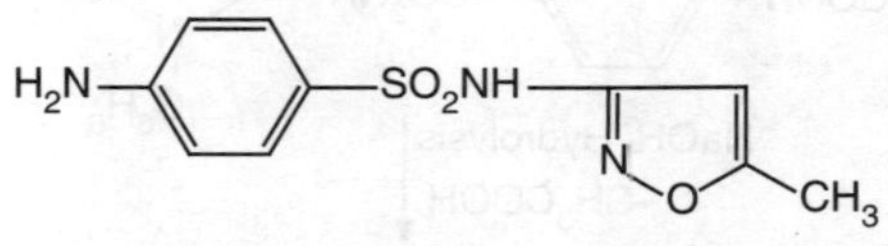

3-(4-Amino benzene sulphamido)-5-methyl isoxazole

Synthesis

N-(5-Methylisoxazol-3-yl)carbamic acid

↓ −CO_2

5-methylisoxazol-3-amine + PABS

↓ −HCl

Sulphamethoxazole

Properties and uses: Sulphamethoxazole is a white or almost white crystalline powder, practically insoluble in water, soluble in acetone, sparingly soluble in ethanol, dissolves in dilute solutions of sodium hydroxide and in dilute acids. Used in the treatment of bacterial infections.

Assay: Dissolve the sample in dilute hydrochloric acid and add potassium bromide. Cool in ice and titrate against 0.1N Sodium nitrate. Determine the end point electrometrically.

Dose: Orally 2 g followed by 1 g every 8 h.

Dosage forms: Co-trimoxazole intravenous infusion B.P., Co-trimoxazole oral suspension B.P., Paediatric co-trimoxazole oral suspension B.P., Co-trimoxazole tablets B.P., Dispersible co-trimoxazole tablets B.P., Paediatric co-trimoxazole tablets B.P.

xii. Sulphaguanidine

N' -(Diamino methylene)sulphanilamide

Properties and uses: Sulphaguanidine is a white, fine crystalline powder, soluble in dilute mineral acids, very slightly soluble in water and ethanol, slightly soluble in acetone, but insoluble in methylene chloride. Used in the treatment of local intestinal infections, specifically, bacillary dysentery.

Assay: Dissolve the sample in dilute hydrochloric acid and add potassium bromide. Cool in ice and titrate against 0.1N sodium nitrate. Determine the end point electrometrically.

Synthesis

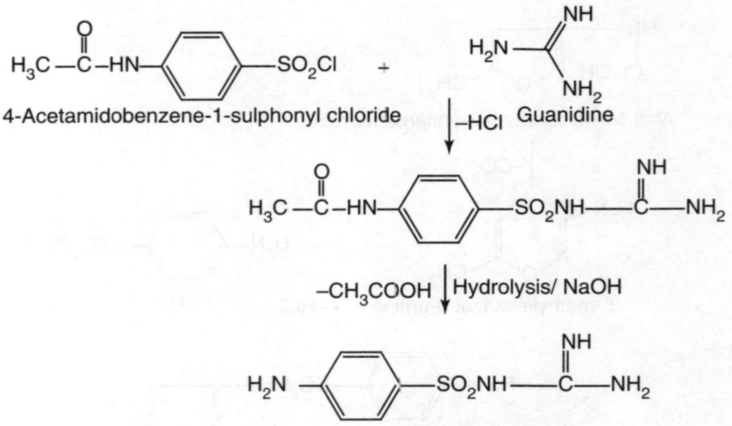

[Structure: 4-Acetamidobenzene-1-sulphonyl chloride + Guanidine → (−HCl) → acetamido sulphonyl guanidine intermediate → (−CH₃COOH, Hydrolysis/NaOH) → Sulphaguanidine]

4-Acetamidobenzene-1-sulphonyl chloride + Guanidine

Sulphaguanidine

III. Both N-1 and N-4 substituted sulphonamides

i. Succinyl sulphathiazole

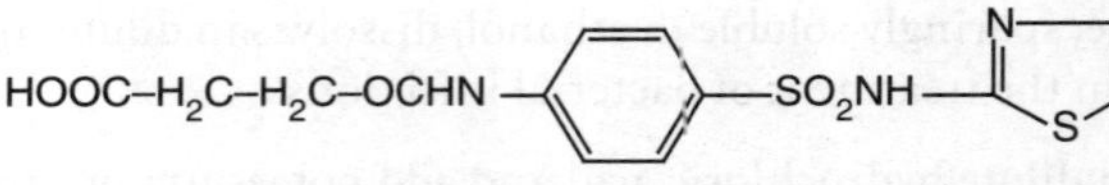

2-[(4-Succinylaminobenzene) sulphonamido] thiazole

Synthesis

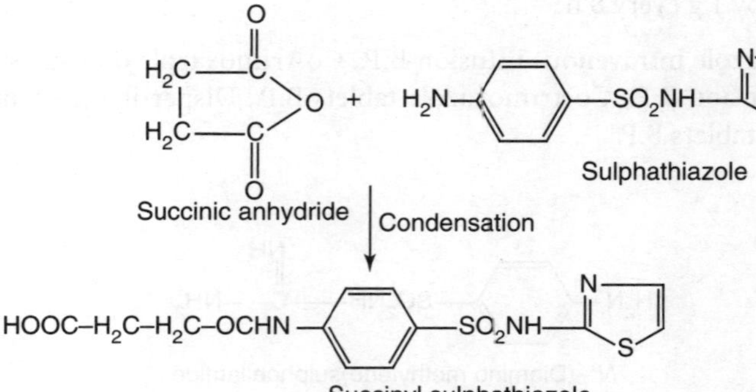

Succinic anhydride + Sulphathiazole → (Condensation) → Succinyl sulphathiazole

Uses: Used in bacillary dysentery and cholera.

Dose: Dose is 10–20 g per day in divided doses.

ii. Phthalyl Sulphathiazole (Thalazole)

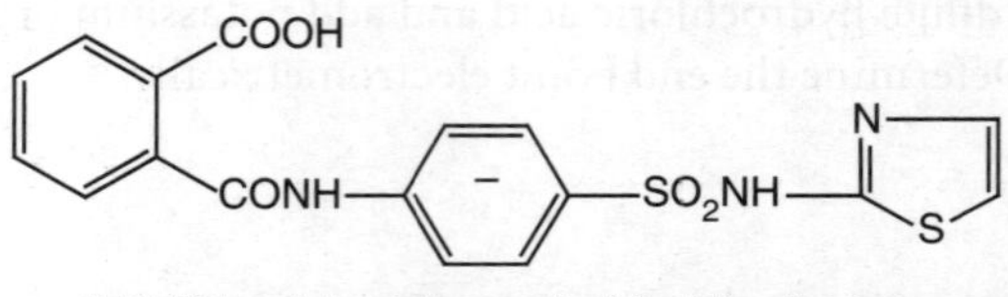

4'-(2-Thiazolyl sulphamoyl) phthalylamino benzene

Synthesis

Phthalic anhydride + Sulphathiazole (H₂N–C₆H₄–SO₂NH–thiazole)

$$\xrightarrow[-H_2O]{\text{Condensation}}$$

Phthalyl sulphathiazole (2-COOH-C₆H₄-CONH–C₆H₄–SO₂NH–thiazole)

Properties and uses: Slightly soluble in alcohol and ether, but insoluble in water. It is used in the treatment of acute bacillary dysentery, bowel irregularities, and ulcerative colitis.

Dose: Dose is 5–10 g per day in divided doses.

IV. Miscellaneous

a. Topically used sulphonamides

i. Mafenide (Sulfamylon)

4-(Aminomethyl)benzene sulphonamide — structure: benzene ring with CH_2NH_2 and SO_2NH_2 para substituents.

Uses: It is used in the treatment and cure of gas gangrene. It is also effective against *Clostridium welchii* on topical application.

Dose: Dose is 5% solution of mafenide hydrochloride or mafenide propionate for topical use.

Synthesis

Benzylamine $\xrightarrow{(CH_3CO)_2O}$ (acetanilide intermediate) $\xrightarrow[-H_2O]{ClSO_2OH}$ (sulfonyl chloride intermediate) $\xrightarrow[-HCl]{NH_3}$ (sulfonamide intermediate) $\xrightarrow[\text{Hydrolysis } -CH_3COOH]{NaOH}$ **Mafenide**

ii. Silver Sulphadiazine

4-Amino-N-(2-pyrimidinyl)mono silver salt of benzene sulphonamide

Uses: It is an effective topical antimicrobial agent, especially, against *Pseudomonas* species; it finds extensive use in burn therapy.

iii. Dapsone (Avcosulfon)

p,p'-Diamino diphenyl sulphone (DDS)

Action and use: Dapsone is a white or slightly yellowish-white crystalline powder, very slightly soluble in water, soluble in acetone and dilute mineral acids, sparingly soluble in alcohol. Used as folic acid synthesis inhibitor in the treatment of leprosy and nocardiosis.

Assay: Dissolve the sample in dilute hydrochloric acid, add potassium bromide, cool in ice, and titrate against 0.1N sodium nitrate. Determine the end point electrometrically.

Dose: The dose as a leprostatic is 25 mg twice a week initially for 1 month followed by 25 mg per day each month. As suppressant for dermatitis herpetiformis the dose is 100–200 mg per day.

Dosage forms: Dapsone tablets B.P.

Synthesis

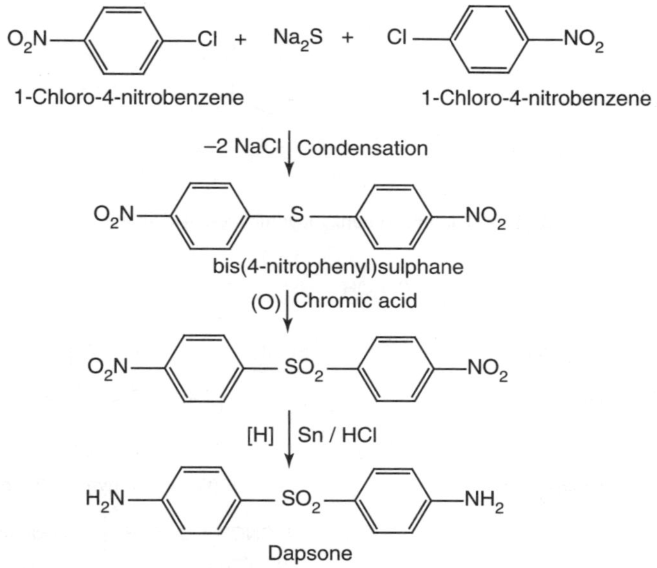

O_2N—⟨C₆H₄⟩—Cl + Na_2S + Cl—⟨C₆H₄⟩—NO_2
1-Chloro-4-nitrobenzene   1-Chloro-4-nitrobenzene

↓ −2 NaCl | Condensation

O_2N—⟨C₆H₄⟩—S—⟨C₆H₄⟩—NO_2
bis(4-nitrophenyl)sulphane

↓ (O) | Chromic acid

O_2N—⟨C₆H₄⟩—SO_2—⟨C₆H₄⟩—NO_2

↓ [H] | Sn / HCl

H_2N—⟨C₆H₄⟩—SO_2—⟨C₆H₄⟩—NH_2
Dapsone

iv. Solapsone

C_6H_5–CH(SO₃Na)–CH_2–CH(SO₃Na)–NH—⟨C₆H₄⟩—SO_2—⟨C₆H₄⟩—NH–CH(SO₃Na)–CH_2–CH(SO₃Na)–C_6H_5

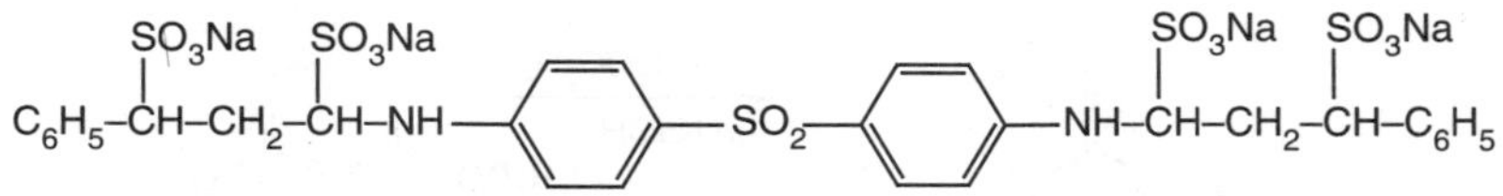

1,1′-[Sulphonyl bis (4,4′-phenyleneimino)] *bis* [3-phenyl-1, 3-propane disulphonic acid] tetra sodium.

Synthesis

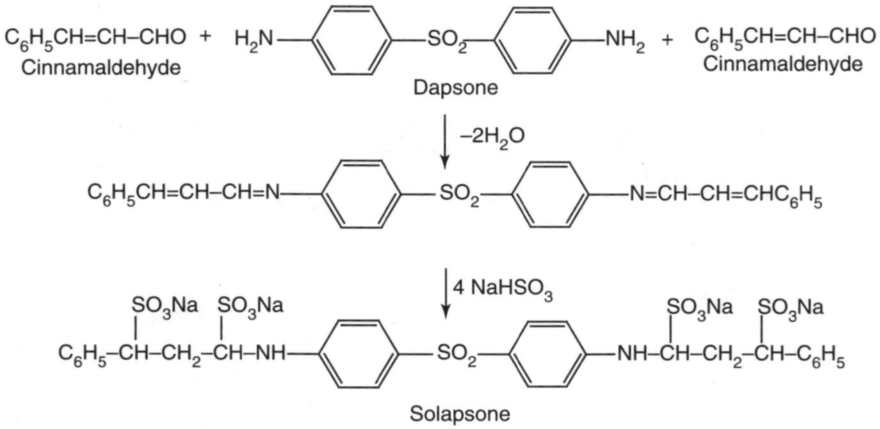

$C_6H_5CH=CH–CHO$ + H_2N—⟨C₆H₄⟩—SO_2—⟨C₆H₄⟩—NH_2 + $C_6H_5CH=CH–CHO$
Cinnamaldehyde   Dapsone   Cinnamaldehyde

↓ −2H_2O

$C_6H_5CH=CH–CH=N$—⟨C₆H₄⟩—SO_2—⟨C₆H₄⟩—$N=CH–CH=CHC_6H_5$

↓ 4 $NaHSO_3$

C_6H_5–CH(SO₃Na)–CH_2–CH(SO₃Na)–NH—⟨C₆H₄⟩—SO_2—⟨C₆H₄⟩—NH–CH(SO₃Na)–CH_2–CH(SO₃Na)–C_6H_5
Solapsone

Uses: It is used in the treatment of leprosy.

V. Drugs used in combination with sulphonamides

i. Trimethoprim

5-(2,3,4-Trimethoxybenzyl)pyrimidine-2,4-diamine

Synthesis

3,4,5-Trimethoxy benzaldehyde → (Zn/HCl, [H]) → benzyl alcohol → (SOCl$_2$) → 5-(Chloromethyl)-1,2,3-trimethoxybenzene

(i) CNCH$_2$COOC$_2$H$_5$ Ethylcyano acetate
(ii) Hydrolysis
(iii) −CO$_2$

→ CH$_2$CH$_2$COOC$_2$H$_5$ intermediate

(i) HCOOC$_2$H$_5$
(ii) NaOH

→ CH$_2$–C(COOC$_2$H$_5$)=CH·OH intermediate

H$_2$N–C(=NH)–NH$_2$, Cyclization, −C$_2$H$_5$OH

→ 2-amino-4-hydroxy pyrimidine intermediate

POCl$_3$ → 4-chloro-2-amino pyrimidine intermediate

−HCl, NH$_3$ → **Trimethoprim**

Properties and uses: Trimethoprim is a white or yellowish-white powder, very slightly soluble in water and slightly soluble in ethanol. It is used as dihydrofolate reductase inhibitor, effective against chloroquine and pyrimethamine resistant strains of *Plasmodium falsiparum*.

Assay: Dissolve the sample in anhydrous acetic acid and titrate with 0.1 M perchloric acid. Determine the end-point potentiometrically.

Dosage forms: Co-trimoxazole intravenous infusion B.P., Co-trimoxazole oral suspension B.P., Paediatric co-trimoxazole oral suspension B.P., Co-trimoxazole tablets B.P., Dispersible co-trimoxazole tablets B.P., Paediatric co-trimoxazole B.P., Tablets trimethoprim oral suspension B.P., Trimethoprim tablets B.P.

ii. Pyrimethamine

5-(4-Chlorophenyl)-6-ethylpyrimidine-2,4-diamine

Synthesis

Properties and uses: Pyrimethamine is a white crystalline powder or colourless crystals, practically insoluble in water, and slightly soluble in alcohol. It is used in combination with sulphadoxine for the treatment of malaria.

Assay: Dissolve the sample in anhydrous acetic acid by heating gently. Cool and titrate with 0.1 M perchloric acid. Determine the end point potentiometrically.

Dosage forms: Pyrimethamine tablets I.P., pyrime thamine tablets B.P.

PROBABLE QUESTIONS

1. What are sulphonamides? Write its mode of action and SAR.
2. Explain how an 'azo-dye' breaks down in vivo to yield sulphanilamide? N1-Substitution in sulphanilamide is more effective and useful than N4-substitution. Explain.
3. What are the different ways to classify sulphonamides and explain with suitable examples about the chemical classification.
4. Write the synthesis, metabolism, and uses of sulphasalazine and sulphaguanidine.
5. Name the sulphonamides used topically, write the synthesis, and uses of sulphacetamide.
6. How will you synthesize sulphanilamide from the following:
   (a) Nitrobenzene (b) Benzene (c) Aniline
7. Write the structure, synthesis, brand name, assay, dosage forms, and uses of the following:
   (a) Phthalyl sulphathiazole (b) Sulphadiazine (c) Sulphamethoxazole
8. Name the poorly absorbed sulphonamides and write the synthesis and uses of any one of them.
9. How will you synthesize the following drugs, employed for urinary tract infections:
   a. Sulphacetamide from sulphanilamide
   b. Sulphafurazole from *p*-acetamidobenzene sulphonyl chloride
10. Write the structure, chemical name, synthesis, dose, dosage forms, and uses of the following sulphonamides:
    (a) Sulphaisoxazole (b) Sulphaphenazole
11. Mention the sulphonamides used in the following and write the synthesis of any one among them
    (a) Intestinal infections (b) Second-and third-degree burns.

SUGGESTED READINGS

1. Abraham DJ (ed). *Burger's Medicinal Chemistry and Drug Discovery* (6th edn). New Jersey: John Wiley, 2007.
2. *British Pharmacopoeia*. Medicines and Healthcare Products Regulatory Agency. London, 2008.
3. Bruntan LL, Lazo JS, and Parker KL. *Goodman and Gilman's: The Pharmacological Basis of Therapeutics* (11th edn). New York: McGraw Hill, 2006.
4. Busch H and Lane M. *Chemotherapy*. Chicago: Yearbook Medical, 1967.

5. Goldstein A. 'Antibacterial chemotherapy'. *New England J Med.* 240: 258–61, 1949.
6. Hawking F and Lawrence JS. *The Sulfonamides.* New York: Grune and Stratton, 1961.
7. *Indian Pharmacopoeia.* Ministry of Health and Family Welfare. New Delhi, 1996.
8. Lemke TL and William DA. *Foye's Principle of Medicinal Chemistry* (6th edn.). New York: Lippincott Williams and Wilkins, 2008.
9. Lednicer D and Mitscher LA. *The Organic Chemistry of Drug Synthesis.* New York: Wiley, 1995.
10. Northey EN. 'The sulfonamides and allied compounds'. In *American Chemical Society Monograph Series*, WA Hamor (ed), pp. 46–47. New York: Reinhold Publishing, *1948.*
11. Gennaro AR. *Remington: The Science and Practice of Pharmacy* (21st edn). New York: Lippincot Williams and Wilkins, 2006.
12. Reynolds EF. (ed). *Martindale the Extra Pharmacopoeia* (31st edn). London: The Pharmaceutical Press, 1997.
13. Seydel JK. Molecular basis for the action of chemotherapeutic drugs, structure-activity studies of sulfonamides *Proc. III International Pharmacology Congress.* New York: Pergamon, 1966.
14. Schuler FW (ed). *Molecular Modification in Drug Design: Advances in Chemistry* Series No. 45, Washington, DC: American Chemical Society, 1964.

Chapter 3

Quinolone Antibacterials

INTRODUCTION

Quinolones constitute a large class of synthetic antimicrobial agents that are highly effective in the treatment of many types of infectious diseases, particularly those caused by bacteria. Quinolones are potent, broad-spectrum antibacterial agents. The early congeners (nonfluorinated at C-6 position, such as nalidixic acid) were limited to certain gram-negative infections, such as urinary tract infections. However, the modern generation of fluoroquinolones, containing C-6 fluoro substituent and a cyclic basic amine moiety at C-7 position, surpass their predecessors in terms of spectrum of activity and potency. This has allowed for their use against a variety of gram-negative as well as some gram-positive pathogens.

Quinolone

Many analogues have piperazino groups on C-7 because of which they broaden the spectrum, especially to gram-negative organisms, such as *Pseudomonas aeruginosa*, however, they also increase the affinity of the compound for the gamma-aminobutyric acid (GABA) receptor, which contributes to central nervous system (CNS) side effects. Quinolones are easily prepared and administered via parenteral and oral routes, and are well tolerated.

Mode of action: Quinolones inhibit the action of bacterial DNA gyrase enzyme. This enzyme is responsible for supercoiling and compacting bacterial DNA molecules into the bacterial cell during replication. This action is accomplished by modifying the topology of DNA via supercoiling and twisting of these macromolecules to permit DNA replication or transcription.

EFFECTIVE ANTIBACTERIAL QUINOLONE DERIVATIVES

Name	X	R_6	R_1	R_7
Nalidixic acid	–N	–H	–CH$_2$CH$_3$	–CH$_3$
Enoxacin	–N	–F	–CH$_2$CH$_3$	H–N⌒N– (piperazinyl)
Pipemidic acid	–N	–H	–CH$_2$CH$_3$	H–N⌒N– (piperazinyl)
Norfloxacin	–CH	–F	–CH$_2$CH$_3$	H–N⌒N– (piperazinyl)
Pefloxacin	–CH	–F	–CH$_2$CH$_3$	H$_3$C–N⌒N– (4-methylpiperazinyl)
Ciprofloxacin	–CH	–F	cyclopropyl	H–N⌒N– (piperazinyl)
Amifloxacin	–CH	–F	–NHCH$_3$	H$_3$C–N⌒N– (4-methylpiperazinyl)
Sparfloxacin	–CF	–F	cyclopropyl	3,5-dimethylpiperazinyl
Lomefloxacin	–CF	–F	–C$_2$H$_5$	3-methylpiperazinyl

(Continued)

(Continued)

Name	X	R_6	R_1	R_7
Fleroxacin	–CF	–F	–CH$_2$CH$_2$F	–N(piperazinyl)N–CH$_3$
Tefloxacin	–CH	–F	cyclopropyl	–N(piperazinyl)N–CH$_3$
Gatifloxacin	–COCH$_3$	–F	cyclopropyl	3-methylpiperazinyl
Clinafloxacin	–CCl	–F	cyclopropyl	3-aminopyrrolidinyl
Sitafloxacin	–CCl	–F	fluorocyclopropyl	7-amino-5-azaspiro[2.4]heptyl

SYNTHESIS AND DRUG PROFILE

i. **Nalidixic acid**

1-Ethyl-1,4-dihydro-7-methyl-4-oxo 1,8-naphthyridine-3-carboxylic acid

Properties and uses: Nalidixic acid is a white or pale yellow crystalline powder, practically insoluble in water, soluble in methylene chloride, slightly soluble in acetone, alcohol, and dilute solutions of alkali hydroxides. It is particularly effective against gram-negative bacteria that cause urinary tract infection. Nalidixic acid is biotransformed into hydroxy methyl derivative at the 7-methyl group, which is also active. A low incidence of adverse effects observed includes gastrointestinal (GI) disturbances, rashes, drowsiness, headache, and visual disturbances.

Assay: Dissolve the sample in methylene chloride and add 2-propanol and carbon dioxide-free water and pass nitrogen through the solution throughout the titration by maintaining a temperature between 15°C and 20°C and titrate against 0.1 M ethanolic sodium hydroxide. Determine the end point potentiometrically.

Dosage forms: Nalidixic acid oral suspension B.P., Nalidixic acid tablets B.P.

Synthesis

ii. Fluoroquinolones

Synthesis

iii. Ciprofloxacin

1-Cyclopropyl-6-fluro-1,4-dihydro-4-oxo-7-piperazine

Synthesis

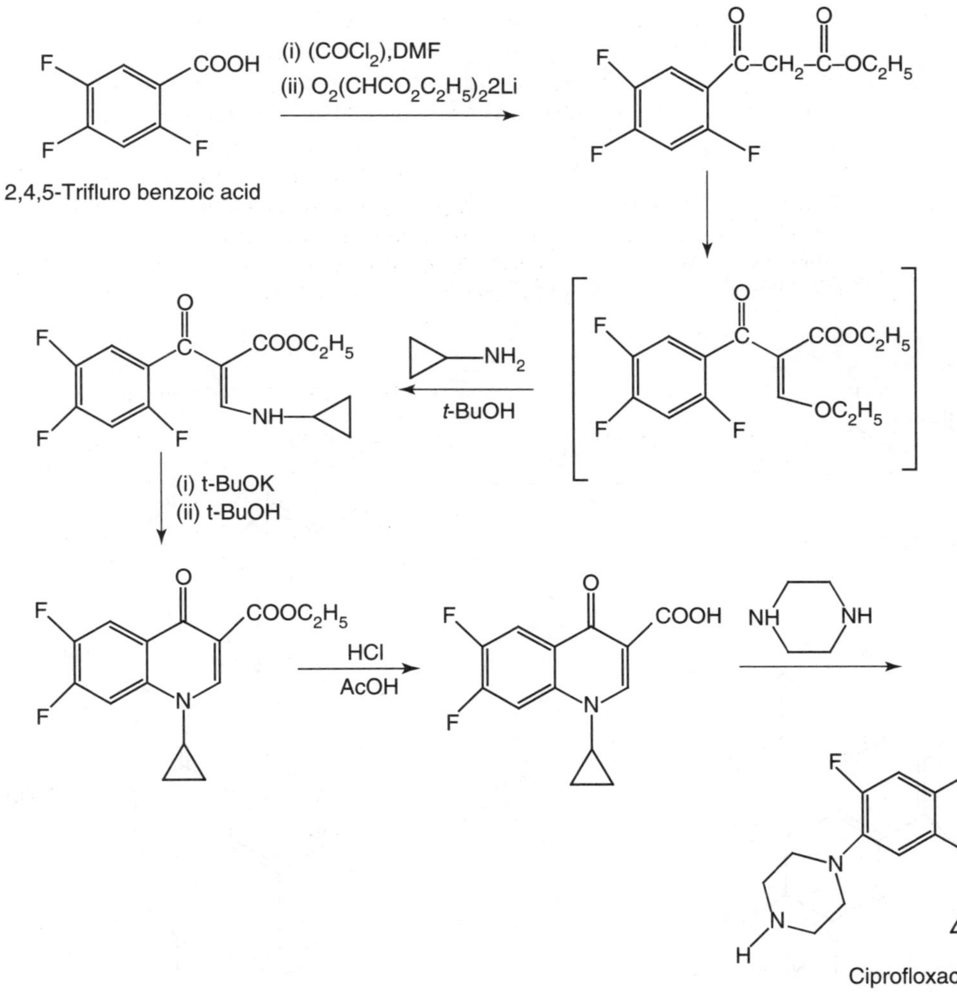
COOH
F
F
F
2,4,5-Trifluro benzoic acid
(i) (COCl2),DMF
(ii) O2(CHCO2C2H5)22Li
C–CH2–C–OC2H5
COOC2H5
OC2H5
NH2
t-BuOH
NH
(i) t-BuOK
(ii) t-BuOH
HCl
AcOH
N
NH
H
Ciprofloxacin

Properties and uses: Ciprofloxacin hydrochloride is pale yellow, crystalline in nature, slightly hygroscopic powder, soluble in water, slightly soluble in methanol, very slightly soluble in ethanol, but insoluble in acetone, ethyl acetate, and methylene chloride. It is very effective for the treatment of urinary tract infection, prostatitis, and for acute diarrhoeal disease caused by *Escherichia coli, Shigella, Salmonella,* and *Campylobacter.*

Assay: It is assayed by adopting liquid chromatography technique.

Dosage forms: Ciprofloxacin tablets B.P.

iv. Ofloxacin

9-Fluoro-3-methyl-10-(4-methylpiperazin-1-yl)-7-oxo-3,7-dihydro-2H-[1,4]oxazino[2,3,4-ij]quinoline-6-carboxylic acid

Synthesis

Properties and uses: Ofloxacin is a pale yellow or bright yellow crystalline powder, slightly soluble in water and methanol, and soluble in glacial acetic acid and methylene chloride. It is one of the most promising newer members of the fluoroquionolone family. In this product, *N*-ethyl moiety has been made rigid by incorporation into a heterocyclic ring. It is useful in the treatment of genitourinary, respiratory, gastrointestinal, skin, soft tissue infections, peridonitis, and gonorrhoea.

Assay: Dissolve the sample in anhydrous acetic acid and titrate against 0.1 M perchloric acid. Determine the end point potentiometrically.

v. Pefloxacin

1-Ethyl-6-fluoro-7-(4-methylpiperazin-1-yl)-4-oxo-1,4-dihydroquinoline-3-carboxyli cacid

Synthesis

Properties and uses: Pefloxacin mesilate is a white powder, soluble in water, slightly soluble in alcohol, and very slightly soluble in methylene chloride, used as an antibacterial agent.

Assay: Dissolve the sample in anhydrous acetic acid, add acetic anhydride, and titrate against 0.1 M perchloric acid. Determine the end point potentiometrically.

SAR of Quinolones

1. **Substituent at N-1 position:** The optimum substituents at position 1 appear to be ethyl, butyl, cyclopropyl, and difluorophenyl, and these substituents have resulted in potent compounds. Addition of a fluorine atom into the N-1 cyclopropyl group or the 1-butyl substituent resulted in compounds with overall improved activity against gram-positive bacteria.
2. The simple replacement of C-2 hydrogen has been generally disadvantageous (e.g. C-2 methyl or hydroxy groups); however, some derivatives containing a suitable C-1, C-2 ring have shown to possess notable activity.

Prulifloxacin

3. **The carboxy functions at position:** Modification of C-3 carboxylic acid group leads to decrease in antibacterial activity. However, replacement of C-3 carboxylic group with isothiazolo group afforded most active isothiazolo quinolone, which has been 4–10 times greater in *in vitro* antibacterial activity than ciprofloxacin. The isothiazolo system possesses aromatic character and the nitrogen proton is very acidic and can be considered as an carboxylic acid mimic, whereas other groups, such as sulphonic acid, phosphonic acid, tetrazole as well as derivatization, as an ester lead to loss of antibacterial activity.

4. The C-4-oxo group of the quinolone nucleus appears to be essential for antibacterial activity. Replacement with 4-thioxo or sulphonyl group leads to a loss of activity.
5. The incorporation of a group at the C-5 position has proven beneficial in terms of antibacterial activity. The order of activity is NH_2: CH_3>F, H>OH, or SH, SR.
6. The incorporation of a fluorine atom at the C-6 position of the quinolone is monumental. The order of activity is F>Cl, Br, CH_3>CN.
7. The introduction of a piperazine moiety at the C-7 position is essential. Other aminopyrrolidines also are compatible for activity.

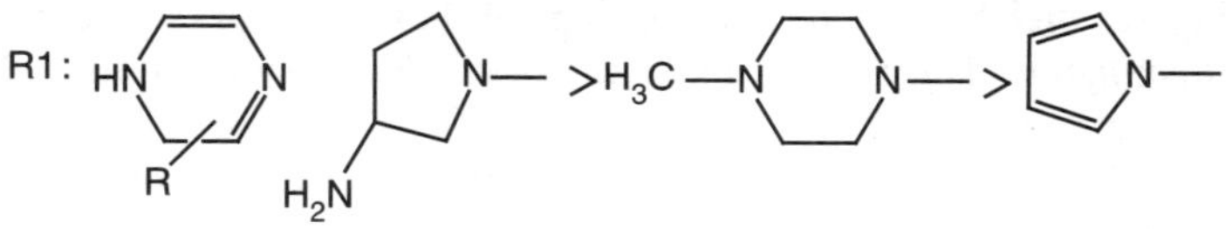

R1: [structures shown: HN-substituted ring with R, aminopyrrolidine with H_2N, > H_3C-N piperazine N-, > pyrrole N-]

8. In general, a C-8 fluoro substituent offers good potency against gram-negative pathogens, while a C-8 methoxy moiety is active against gram-positive bacteria. The order of activity is F, Cl, OCH_3>H, CF_3>methyl, vinyl, propargyl.
9. A halogen (F or Cl) at the C-8 position improves oral absorption.
10. Linking of N-1 group to the C-8 position with oxazine ring leads to active oflaxacin.

Uses: Fluoroquinolones are used to treat upper and lower respiratory infections, gonorrhoea, bacterial gastroenteritis, skin soft tissue infections, urinary tract infections, bone and joint infections, and against tuberculosis.

Adverse Effects

The most common adverse reactions are nausea, headache, and dizziness. Some CNS problems, such as hallucination, insomnia, and visual disturbances can occur. Some side effects of the quinolones are class effects and cannot be modulated by molecular variation. Most of the fluoroquionolones produce photosensitivity reactions and cause convulsions particularly in concurrent administration of NSAID fenopofen. Increasing steric bulk through alkylation ameliorates these effects. Phototoxicity is determined by the nature of the 8-position substituent with halogen causing the greatest photoreaction while hydrogen and methoxy show little light produced toxicity. These drugs are not recommended for use in pretubertal children or pregnant women.

PROBABLE QUESTIONS

1. Draw the structure and number the quinolone nucleus. Mention the position of substituents introduced in quinolone antibacterials. Write the SAR of quinolone antibacterials.
2. Enumerate the quinolone antibacterials with their chemical structures and write the synthesis and uses of ciprofloxacin.

SUGGESTED READINGS

1. Abraham DJ (ed). *Burger's Medicinal Chemistry and Drug Discovery* (6th edn). New Jersey: John Wiley, 2007.
2. Bruntan LL, Lazo JS, and Parker KL. *Goodman and Gilman's: The Pharmacological Basis of Therapeutics* (11th edn). New York: McGraw Hill, 2006.
3. *British Pharmacopoeia*. Medicines and Healthcare Products Regulatory Agency. London, 2008.
4. Chu DTW and Fernandes PB. 'Recent developments in the field of quinolone antibacterial agents', in *Advances in Drug Research* Vol. 21, Testa B (ed), pp. 39–144. New York: Academic Press, 1991.
5. Gennaro AR. *Remington: The Science and Practice of Pharmacy* (21st edn). New York: Lippincot Williams and Wilkins, 2006.
6. Hooper DC and Wolfson JS. 'Mode of action of the quinolone antimicrobial agents: Review of recent information'. *Rev Infect Dis* 11 (Suppl 5): S902, 1989.
7. *Indian Pharmacopoeia*. Ministry of Health and Family Welfare. New Delhi, 1996.
8. Lednicer D and Mitscher LA. *The Organic Chemistry of Drug Synthesis*. New York: John Wiley, 1995.
9. Lemke TL and William DA. *Foye's Principle of Medicinal Chemistry* (6th edn). New York: Lippincott Williams and Wilkins, 2008.
10. Siporin C, Hefetz CL, and Domagala JM (eds). *The New Generation of Quinolones*. New York: Marcel Dekker, 1990.
11. Suto MJ, Domagala JM, and Miller PF. 'Antibacterial agents, targets and approaches', In *Annual Reports in Medicinal Chemistry*, Vol. 27, JA Bristol (ed), p. 119. San Diego, CA: Academic Press, 1992.
12. Rosen T. 'The fluoroquinolone antibacterial agents'. *Progress in Med Chem* 27: 235–95, 1990.

Chapter 4

Antibiotics

INTRODUCTION

The term antibiotic has its origin in the word antibiosis (i.e. against life). Antibiotics are chemical substances obtained from various species of microorganisms (bacteria, fungi, actinomycetes) that suppress the growth of other microorganisms and eventually may destroy them. The probable points of difference amongst the antibiotics may be physical, chemical, pharmacological properties, antibacterial spectra, and mechanism of action. They have made it possible to cure diseases caused by bacteria, such as pneumonia, tuberculosis, and meningitis, and they save the lives of millions of people around the world.

CLASSIFICATION

Antibiotics are classified on the basis of their mechanism of action and by its chemical nature.

Classification Based on Mechanism of Action

1. *Agents that inhibit the synthesis of bacterial cell wall*: These include the penicillins and cephalosporins that are structurally similar and dissimilar agents, such as cycloserine, vancomycin, bacitracin and the imidazole antifungal agents.
2. *Agents that act directly on the cell membrane of the microorganisms, affecting permeability, and leading to leakage of intracellular compounds*: These include polymyxin, polyene antifungal agents, nystatin, and amphotericin B that bind to cell wall sterols.
3. *Agents that affect the function of 30s and 50s ribosomal subunits to cause reversible inhibition of protein synthesis*: These include tetracyclines, erythromycins, chloramphenicol, and clindamycin.
4. *Agents that bind to the 30s ribosomal subunit and alter protein synthesis*: These include aminoglycosides that leads to cell deaths eventually.
5. *Agents that affect nucleic acid metabolism:* Such as rifamycins, which inhibit DNA dependent RNA polymerase.

Classification Based on Chemical Structure

1. β-lactam antibiotics
2. Aminoglycoside antibiotics
3. Tetracycline antibiotics
4. Polypeptide antibiotics
5. Macrolide antibiotics
6. Lincomycins
7. Other antibiotics

1. β-lactam antibiotics

These consists of two major class of agents, that is penicillins and cephalosporins.

a. Penicillins

Penicillin, the most important antibiotic, was first extracted from the mould *Penicillium notatum*. Subsequently, a mutant of a related mould, *P. chrysogenum*, was found to give the highest yield of penicillin and is employed for the commercial production of this antibiotic. Penicillin belongs to a group of antibiotics called β-lactam antibiotics. The basic structure of the penicillins consists of a thiazolidine ring fused with a β-lactam ring, which is essential for antibacterial activity. These two rings constitute the fundamental nucleus of all the penicillins, namely, 6-amino penicillanic-acid (6-APA) A variety of semisynthetic penicillins are produced by altering the composition of the side chain attached to 6-APA nucleus. Both the 6-APA nucleus and side chain are essential for the antibacterial activity.

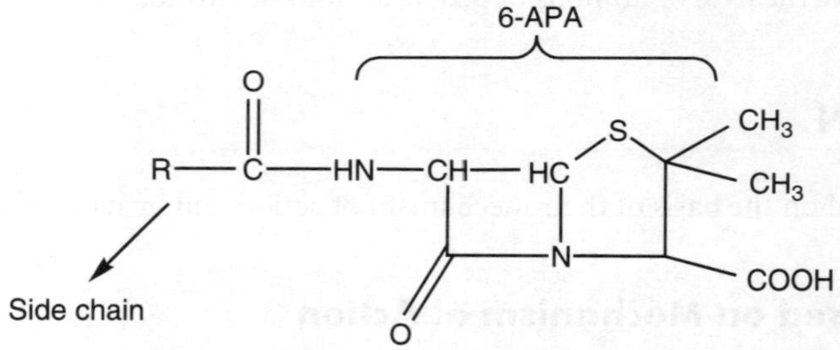

Basic structure of penicillin

Nomenclature

Penicillins are named in the following ways:

a. Chemical abstract

1. The penicillins are described as 4-thia-1-azabicyclo (3.2.0) heptanes.
2. Benzylpenicillin is 6-(2-phenylacetamido)-3, 3-dimethyl-7-oxo-4-thia-1-azabiclo(3.2.0)heptane-2-carboxylic acid.

b. Penam

In order to simplify the unsubstituted bicylic ring system of penicillin, it is given the name penam. Accordingly, the penicillins are 6-acylamino-2, 2-dimethyl penam-3-carboxylates.

c. Pencillanic acid derivatives

— Pencillanic acid

CLASSIFICATION

Name	Nature of Substituent (R)
Penicillin G (Benzyl penicillin)	C₆H₅–CH₂– (benzyl)
Penicillin V (Phenoxy methyl penicillin)	C₆H₅–O–CH₂–
Phenethicillin	C₆H₅–O–CH(CH₃)–

I. Penicillinase-susceptible penicillins

The general impact on antibacterial activity is as follows:

- Good gram-positive potency against susceptible *Staphylococci* and *Streptococci*
- Useful against some gram-positive *cocci*
- Not effective against gram-negative bacilli

Name	R
(i) Methicillin	2,6-dimethoxyphenyl (H_3CO groups at ortho positions)
(ii) Oxacillin ($R_1=R_2=H$)	3-phenyl-5-methylisoxazol-4-yl
(iii) Cloxacillin ($R_1=H, R_2=Cl$)	3-(2-chlorophenyl)-5-methylisoxazol-4-yl
(iv) Dicloxacillin ($R_1=R_2=Cl$)	3-(2,6-dichlorophenyl)-5-methylisoxazol-4-yl
(v) Floxacillin ($R_1=F, R_2=Cl$)	3-(2-chloro-6-fluorophenyl)-5-methylisoxazol-4-yl

(Continued)

(Continued)

Name	R
(vi) Nafcillin	[structure: 2-ethoxy-1-methylnaphthalene group]

II. Penicillinase-resistant penicillins

General impact on antibacterial activity is as follows:

- Decreased susceptibility to many penicillinase.
- Active against microrganisms, resistant to early penicillin.
- Oxacillins offer good oral activity.

III. Aminopenicillins

Name	R
Ampicillin	[structure: phenyl-CH(NH$_2$)–]
Amoxicillin	[structure: 4-HO-phenyl-CH(NH$_2$)–]
Talampicilin	[full penicillin structure with phenyl-CH(NH$_2$)-C(=O)-NH- side chain and COOR$_1$ ester; R$_1$ = 3-phthalidyl group]

General impact on antibacterial activity is as follows:
- Extended spectrum of activity against some gram-negative bacteria and retention of gram-positive potency
- Ineffective against *Pseudomonas aeruginosa*

IV. Antipseudomonal penicillins (Carboxy Penicillins)

Name	R
Carbenicillin (R_1=H)	Ph-CH(COOR$_1$)-
Indanyl carbenicillin (R_1=5-indanol)	Ph-CH(COOR$_1$)-
Ticarcillin (R_1 = H)	(thiophene)-CH(COOR$_1$)-

V. Ureidopenicillins

Name	R
Aziocillin	Ph-CH(CH$_3$)-NH-C(=O)-N(imidazolidinone)
Piperacillin	Ph-CH(CH$_3$)-NH-C(=O)-N(piperazine-2,3-dione-N'-C$_2$H$_5$)

General impact on antibacterial activity is as follows:

- Enhanced spectrum of activity against *P. aeruginosa* and expanded activity against *Klebsiella*.
- Good potency against gram-positive bacteria, but generally not effective against penicillinase producers.
- Good pharmacokinetic profile.
- Good activity against *Escherichia coli, Klebsiella, Shigella, Salmonella,* and many other resistant species.

VI. Miscellaneous penicillins

Name	R
Quinicillin	quinoxaline-2-carboxylic acid group
Amidinopencillins (Mecillinam)	N-C=N- (hexahydroazepine amidine)
Azidocillin	phenyl-CH(N$_3$)-C(=O)-NH-
Bacampicillin	phenyl-CH(NH$_2$)-C(=O)-NH- [penicillin nucleus with COOR$_1$]; $R_1 = -CH(CH_3)-O-C(=O)-O-C_2H_5$

The chemical degradation of penicillins is depicted in Figure 4.1

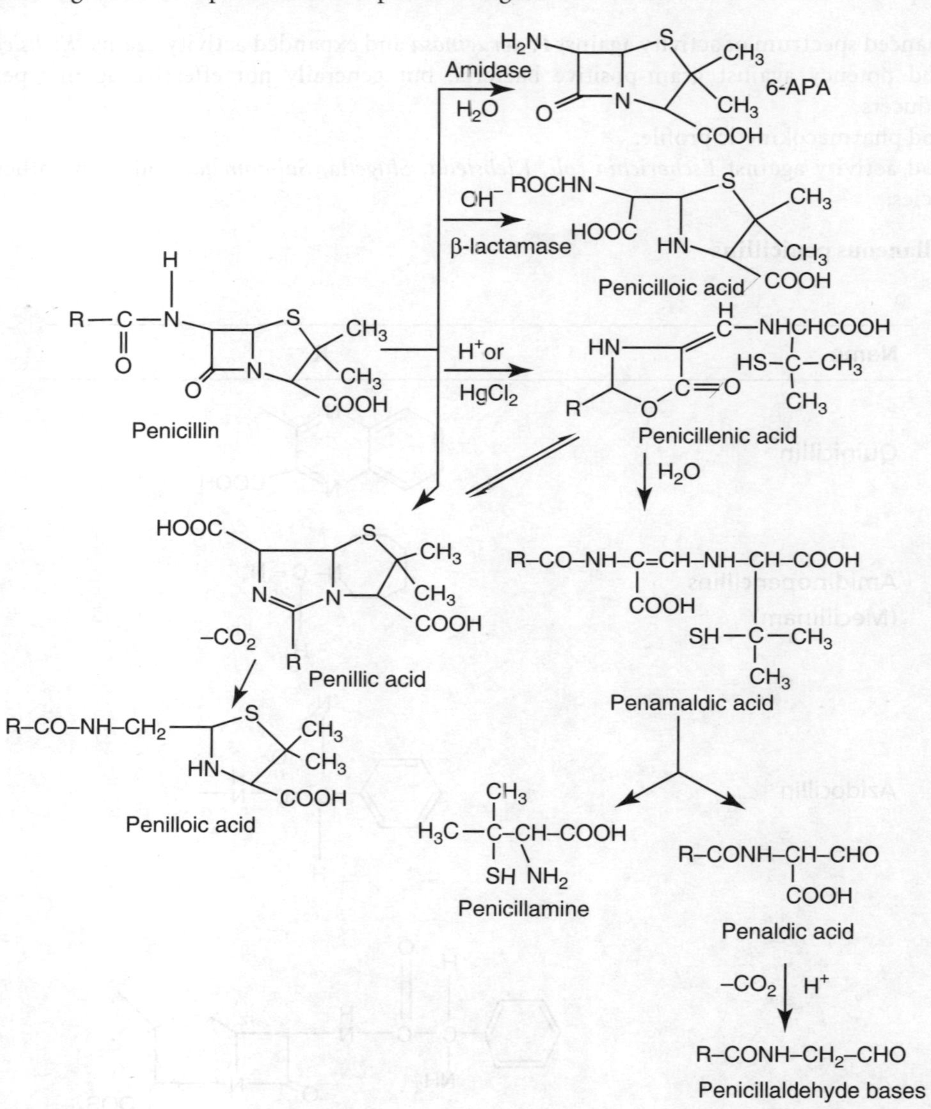

Figure 4.1 Chemical degradation of penicillins.

Inactivation of penicillins by acids, bases, and β-lactamases is as follows:
- The penicillins are very reactive due to the strained amide bond in the fused β-lactum of the nucleus.
- Penicillins undergo a complex series of reactions leading to a variety of inactive degradation products.

- They are extremely susceptible to nucleophilic attack by water or hydroxide ion to form the penicilloic acid. β-Lactamses also cleave the β-lactam ring to give penicilloic acid with a consequent loss of antibacterial activity.
- In strongly acidic solutions (pH < 3), penicillin is protonated at the β-lactam nitrogen, and this is followed by nucleophillic attack of the acyl oxygen atom on the β-lactam carbonyl carbon. The subsequent opening of the β-lactam ring destabilizes the thiazoline ring, which opens to form penicillenic acid that degrades into two major products penicillamine and penilloic acid. A third product, penicilloaldehyde is also formed.
- Acid-catalyzed degradation in the stomach contributes in a major way to the poor oral absorption of penicillin. Thus, efforts to obtain penicillins with improved pharmacokinetic and microbiologic properties have sought to find acyl functionalities that would minimize sensitivity of the β-lactam ring to acid hydrolysis and at the same time, maintain antibacterial activity.
- Substitution of an electron-withdrawing group for the α-position of the benzyl penicillin has stabilized the penicillin to acid catalyzed hydrolysis. The increased stability imparted by such electron-withdrawing groups has been attributed to a decrease in the reactivity of the side chain amide carbonyl oxygen atom towards participation in β-lactam ring opening to form the penicillenic acid.

Mode of action: The cell wall of bacteria is essential for the normal growth and development. Peptidoglycan is a heteropolymeric component of the cell wall that provides rigid mechanism for stability by virtue of its highly cross-linked lattice-wise structure. The peptidoglycan is composed of glycan chains, which are linear strands of two alternating amino sugars (N-acetyl glucosamine and N-acetylmuramic acid) that are cross-linked by peptide chains of an enzyme, transpeptidase. Penicillins inhibit the transpeptidase activity to the synthesis of cell walls. They also block cleavage of terminal D-alanine during the cell wall synthesis. The biosynthesis of peptidoglycan involves three stages (Fig. 4.2).

B-lactam antibiotics inhibit the last step in peptidoglycan synthesis. The transpeptidase enzyme that contains serine is probably acylated by β-lactam antibiotics with the cleavage of -CO-N-bond of the β-lactam ring. This renders the enzyme inoperative and inhibits peptidoglycan synthesis.

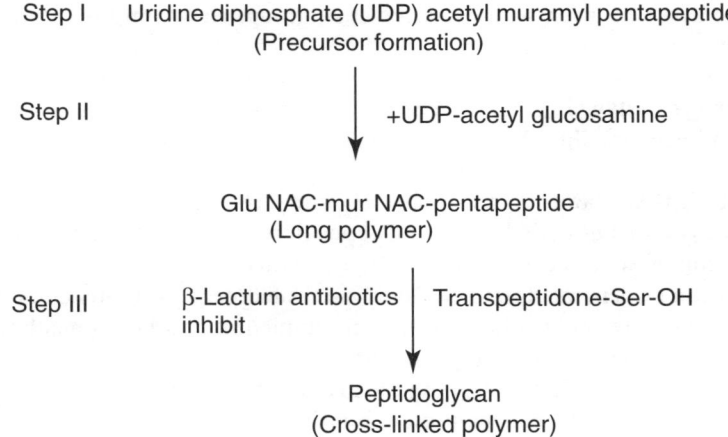

Figure 4.2 Stages involved in the biosynthesis of peptidoglycan.

SAR of Penicillins

6-Acyl side chain: The substitution of R on the primary amine with an electron withdrawing group decreases the electron density on the side chain and protects from acid degradation. Substituents on the α-carbon of the side chain, such as amino (ampicillin), chloro, and guanidine exerts good resistance to inactivation by acids. Benzyl penicillin undergoes acid and alkali degradation and is susceptible to all known β-lactamase. The increased latitude in varying the acyl amino side chain through acylation of 6-APA results with superior biological activity. Substitution of α-aryl of the alkyl group in the side chain gives increased stability and oral absorption.

1. Substitution of bulky groups on α-carbon of the side chain confers β-lactamase resistance. Examples: methicillin, nafcillin, oxacillin, etc. In all these penicillins, an aromatic ring is attached directly to the side chain amide carbonyl, and there is substitution at both positions ortho to the point of attachment. The size of the ring systems play an important role in determining the ability of the ortho substitutent to confer penicillinase resistance.
2. The isomeric forms of penicillins differs in their activity. Example: D-isomer is 2–8 times more active than L-isomer of amoxicillin. The introduction of polar group or ionized molecule into the α-position of the side chain in the benzyl carbon atom of penicillin-G confers against the gram-negative bacilli. Amino, hydroxyl, carboxyl, and sulphonyl increases gram-negative activity. Example: ampicillin and carbenicillin.
3. Replacement of acyl side chain with hydroxymethyl groups shows improved gram-negative activity and introduction of C-6 α-methoxy group produces greater stability against β-lactamase. N-acylated ampicillins (ureidopenicillins) have increased activity against Pseudomonas.
4. Many esters of the carboxyl group attached to C-3 have been prepared as prodrugs to increase lipophilicity and acid stability. Example: Acetoxymethyl ester derivatives are used for preparing prodrugs.
5. The sulphur of the thiazolidine ring with O, CH_2, and CH-β-CH_3 gives broad-spectrum antibacterial activity. The geminal dimethyl group at C-2 position is a characteristic of the penicillin. In general, derivatization of the C-3 carboxylic acid functionality is not tolerated unless the free penicillin carboxylic acid can be generated in vivo. Doubly activated penicillin esters, undergo rapid cleavage in vivo to generate active penicillin. Example: pivampicillin and becampicillin. The antibacterial activity is evidented by N-4 atom at ring junction.
6. In vitro degradation is retarded by keeping the pH of the solution between 6.0 and 8.0. More lipophilic side chain increases the plasma protein binding. Example: Ampicillin: 25% plasma protein bound and phenoxy methyl penicillin: 75% plasma protein bound.

SYNTHESIS AND DRUG PROFILE

I. Penicillinase resistant penicillins

i. Methicillin

2,6-Dimethoxyphenyl penicillin

Synthesis

2,6-Dimethoxybenzoyl chloride + 6-Amino-3,3-dimethyl-7-oxo-4-thia-1-aza-bicyclo[3.2.0]heptane-2-carboxylic acid $\xrightarrow{(C_2H_5)_3N}$ Methicillin

Properties and uses: Methicillin sodium is a white crystalline solid, odourless, soluble in water, slightly soluble in chloroform, but insoluble in ether. It is particularly resistant to inactivation by the penicillinase found in *Staphylococci* and somewhat more resistant than penicillin G to penicillinase from *Bacillus cereus*. Methicillin sodium has been introduced for use in the treatment of *Staphylococci* infections caused by the strains resistant to other penicillins. It is given by IM or by slow IV infusion every 4–6 h.

ii. Oxacillins (Isoxazolyl penicillins)

Properties and uses: Oxacillin sodium monohydrate is a white powder, soluble in water and methanol, insoluble in methylene chloride. The use of oxacillin and other isoxazolyl penicillins should be restricted to the treatment of infections caused by *Staphylococci* that are resistant to penicillin G, although their spectrum of activity is similar to that of penicillin G.

Synthesis

Name	R₁	R₂
Oxacillin	–H	–H
Cloxacillin	–H	–Cl
Dicloxacillin	–Cl	–Cl
Floxacillin	–F	–Cl

Assay: It is assayed by adopting liquid chromatography technique.

II. Penicillinase Susceptible Penicillins
i. Penicillin-V

3, 3-Dimethyl-7-oxo-6[(phenoxy acetylamino]-4-thia-1-azabiclo(3.2.0) heptane-2-carboxylic acid

Synthesis

[Scheme: Synthesis of Penicillin-V]

Phthalimide potassium salt (NK) + BrCH₂COO–t–Bu → N-CH₂COO–t–BU phthalimido derivative

(i) CH₃COOH
(ii) NaNH₂

*t*Butyl-α-phthalimido malonaldehyde + D-Penicillamine (S–CH(CH₃)₂, H₂N–CH–COOH) → Phthalimido ester acid — Thiazolidine

(i) NH₂NH₂
(ii) HCl

An amine hydrochloride: Cl⁻ H₃N⁺–HC—HC(S)(CH₃)(CH₃)—COOBu, HN—COOH

(i) C₆H₅–O–CH₂–C(=O)–Cl
(ii) (C₂H₅)₃N

An ester: C₆H₅–O–CH₂–C(=O)–NH–HC—CH(S)(CH₃)(CH₃), COOBu, HN—COOH

Dry HCl gas at 0°C in pyridine

→ C₆H₅–O–CH₂–C(=O)–NH–HC—HC(S)(CH₃)(CH₃), COOH, HN—COOH

(i) Equivalent KOH
(ii) C₆H₁₁N=C=NC₆H₁₁ (*N,N*-Dicyclohexyl carbodiimide)

→ **Penicillin-V**

Properties and uses: Penicillin V is a white, odourless, crystalline powder with slightly bitter taste and soluble in water. It is more resistant to inactivation by gastric juice than penicillin G and better absorbed from the gastro intestinal (GI) tract. Equivalent oral doses provide two or five times greater plasma concentration than penicillin G. Penicillin V is given to treat 'trench mouth'. It is useful in the treatment of streptococcal pharyngitis, pneumonia, arthritis, meningitis, and endocarditis caused by *S. pyrogenes*.

Dose: Dose of penicillin V by oral route is 125–500 mg six times daily for 10 days. For prophylaxis of rheumatic fever, the dose is 125–250 mg twice daily.

Assay: It is assayed by adopting liquid chromatography technique.

III. Amino penicillins

i. Ampicillin (Amcil, Omnipen)

6[D-α-Aminophenylacetamido] penicillanic acid

Synthesis

Ampicillin

Properties and uses: Ampicillin is a white hygroscopic powder, freely soluble in water, sparingly soluble in acetone, practically insoluble in fatty oils and liquid paraffin. The corresponding product from acylation with 2-azido-4-hydroxyphenyl acetyl chloride is amoxicillin. The protonated α-amino group of ampicillin has a pKa of 7.3 and is thus extensively protonated in acidic media, which explains ampicillin's stability towards acid hydrolysis and instability towards alkaline hydrolysis. The α-amino group plays an important role in the broader activity. It is used to treat urinary tract infections and respiratory tract infections.

Assay: It is assayed by adopting liquid chromatography technique.

Dose: Available as capsules of 250 or 500 mg, as sodium salt for parenteral use, for oral suspension in strengths of 125–500mg/5ml, and in paediatric drops of 100 mg/ml. The consumption dose for adults is 1–4 g per day in divided dose for every 6 h, for children the dose is 100–200 mg/kg per day in three portions.

Dosage forms: Ampicillin capsules I.P., Ampicillin sodium injection I.P., Ampicillin injection B.P.

ii. Pivampicillin

Synthesis

Properties and uses: Pivampicillin is a white crystalline powder, practically insoluble in water, soluble in methanol, ethanol, and dilute acids. It is a produg for ampicillin and in the in vivo esters hydrolyzes back to the parent ampicillin. It is used to treat urinary tract infections and respiratory tract infections.

Assay: It is assayed by adopting liquid chromatography technique.

IV. Antipseudomonal penicillins

i. Carbenicillin

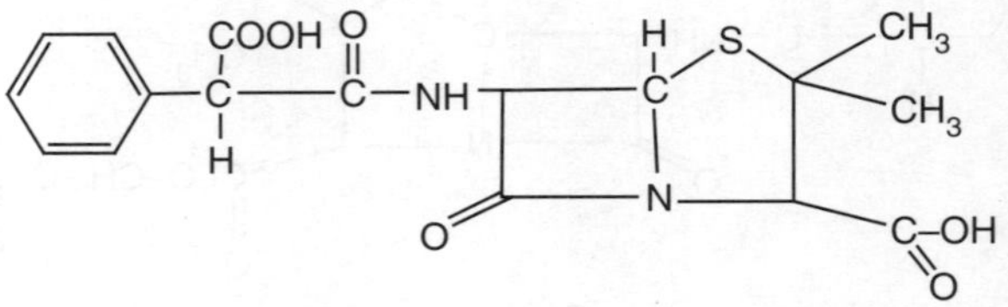

Synthesis

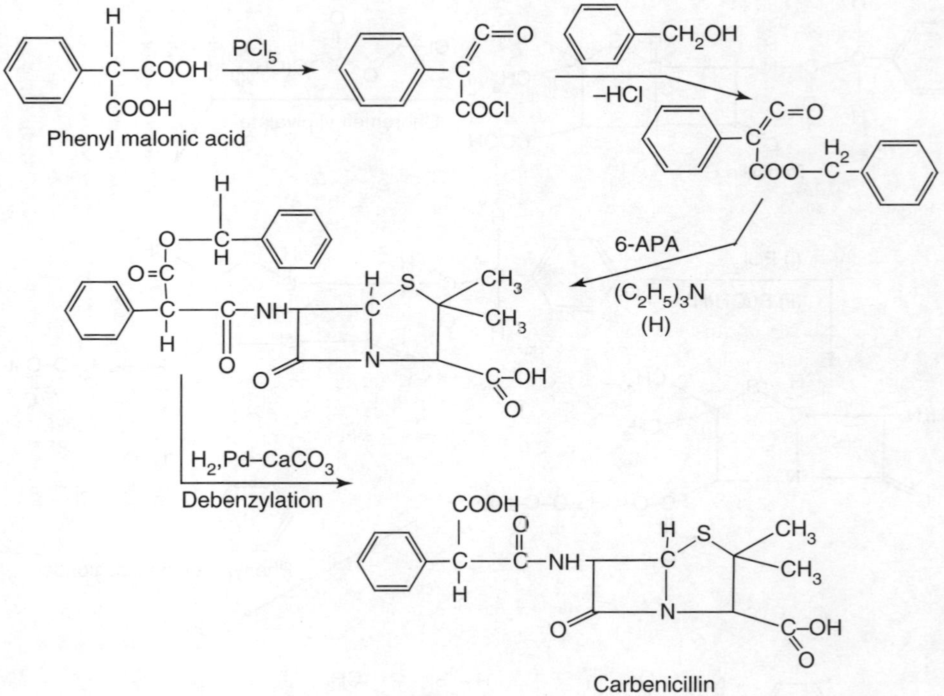

Carbenicillin

Properties and uses: It is a white to off white crystalline powder with bitter taste, hygroscopic in nature, soluble in water or alcohol, insoluble in chloroform or ether. It differs from ampicillin by having an ionizable carboxyl group substituted on the alpha carbon atom of the benzyl side chain rather than an amino group. The carboxyl group is thought to provide improved penetration of the molecule through the cell wall barriers of gram-negative bacilli as compared with other penicillins. A similar sequence starting with

3-thiophenylmalonic acid leads to the ticarcillin. It is acid labile being a malonic acid derivative, it decarboxylates readily to penicillin G. It is effective in the treatment of systemic and urinary tract infections. It has low toxicity, except allergic sensitivity, and the drug interferes with platelet function resulting in bleeding.

V. Ureido penicillins
i. Aziocillin (Azlin)

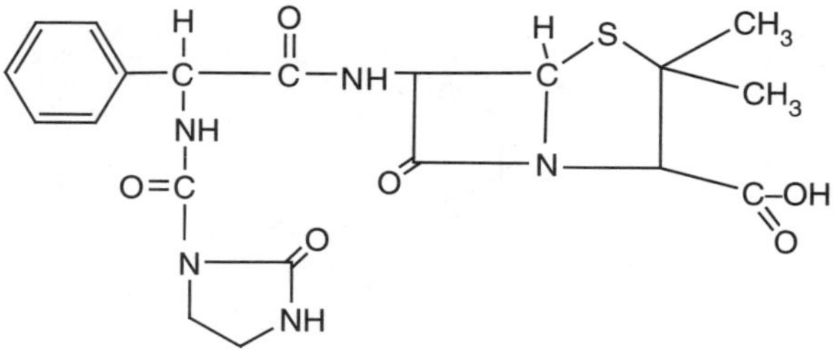

Synthesis

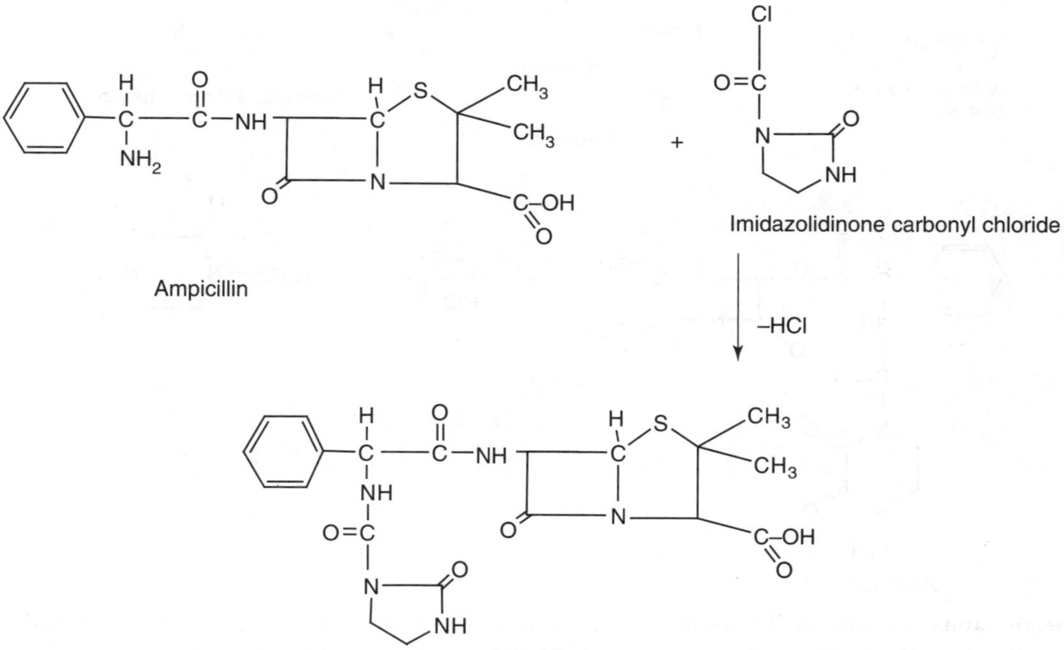

Ampicillin

Imidazolidinone carbonyl chloride

−HCl

Aziocillin

Properties and uses: It is the newest of ureidopenicillins, and is about 10 times more active than carbenicillin against *Pseudomonas* and *Streptococci*.

Dose: The dose is 8–18 g per day in 4–6 divided doses.

ii. Piperacillin (Pipracil, Pracil)
Synthesis

Properties and uses: Piperacillin sodium is a white hygroscopic powder, soluble in water and methanol, practically insoluble in ethyl acetate. It is available as a powder for solubilization and injection. It is best given in combination with an aminoglycoside antibiotic.

Assay: It is assayed by adopting liquid chromatography technique.

Dose: For serious and complicated infections: The adult dose as sodium is 200–300 mg/kg daily in divided doses or 3–4 g per day in divided doses of every 4 or 6 h. For life threatening conditions: especially those caused by *Pseudomonas* or *Klebsiella* spp, the dose is at least 16 g per day; usual maximum dose is 24 g per day. For children: 1 month–12 years, as sodium 100–300 mg/kg daily in 3–4 divided doses. For neonates: The dose for less than 7 days or lesser than 2 kg, that is, 150 mg/kg daily in 3 divided doses; for more than 7 days and more than 2 kg, that is, 300 mg/kg in 3–4 divided doses, IV route is preferred for infants and children. Single dose more than 500 mg should not be given via IM injection.

Parenteral: For mild or uncomplicated infections: The adult dose as sodium is 100–125 mg/kg daily, the usual dose, if given via IV injection/infusion is 2 g every 6 or 8 h or 4 g every 12 h, if given via IM injection the dose is 2 g every 8 or 12 h. Prophylaxis of infection during surgery, for adults: as sodium the dose is 2 g just before the procedure or when the umbilical cord is clamped in caesarean section, followed by at least two doses of 2 g at intervals of 4 or 6 h within 24 h of procedure.

VI. Miscellaneous penicillins
i. Mecillinam (Amdinocillin)

6-β-(Hexahydro-1H-azepin-1-yl)-methylene aminopenicillonic acid

Synthesis

Properties and uses: Mecillinam is particularly active against enterobacteria including some ampicillin resistant strains and to treat urinary tract infections. It is structurally different from other penicillins, in that, it is not an acyl derivative, but rather alkylidene amino-(amidino) derivative of 6-APA, due to this difference, it has significant gram-negative antibacterial activity as compared to gram-positive antibacterial activity.

Cephalosporins

The cephalosporins were isolated from the fungus *Cephalosporium acremonium* in 1948 by Pro Tzu, Newton, and Abraham (1953). The main product being cephalosporin-C, the molecular modification of cephalosporin-C gave origin to semisynthetic substances. They are β-lactam antibiotics with same fundamental structural requirements as penicillins, the main difference between the two is that cephalosporins contain dihydrometathiazine ring, while penicillin contains a tetrahydrothiazole (thiazolidine) ring. The cephalosporins are much more acid stable than the corresponding penicillins and also have a mechanism of action similar to that of penicillins; they mainly inhibit the cross-linking of the peptidoglycan units in bacterial cell walls by inhibiting transpeptidase enzyme. However, they bind in the target proteins other than penicillins binding proteins.

Cephalosporins can be divided into three classes:

1. *Cephalosporin N*: It has a penicillin-like structure being a derivative of 6-aminopenicillanic acid.
2. *Cephalosporin P*: An acidic antibiotic, which is steroidal in nature.
3. *Cephalosporin-C*: It is a true cephalosporin and it is a derivative of 7 amino-cephalosporanic acid.

Generalized formula for cephalosporins
In cephalosporin C

Cepahlosporin C contains a side-chain derived from D-α-aminoadipic acid, which is attached to 7-amino-cephalosporanic acid

In cephalosporin N

Pencillanic acid

A compound structurally similar to cephalosporin P is called fusidic acid

Nomenclatures

Cephalosporins are named in the following ways:

1. *Chemical abstracts*: 5-Thia-1-azobicyclo (4.2.0) octanes. Accordingly, cephalothin is 3-(Acetoxy methyl)-8-oxo-7-(2-thienyl) acetamido-5thia-1-aza-bicyclo[4.2.0]-oct-2ene-2-carboxylic acid.
2. *Cepham derivatives*: Cepham is the name given to the unsubstituted bicyclic lactam.

Cephem Cepham

Classification

Cephalosporins are classified on the basis of their chemical structure, clinical pharmacology, antibacterial spectrum, or penicillinase resistance.

a. Orally administered: cephalexin, cephradine, and cefaclor
b. Parentrally administered: cephalothin, cephapirin, cephacetrile, and cefazedone. These agents are sensitivity to β-lactamase
c. Resistant to β-lactamase and parentrally administered: cefuroxime, cefamandole, cefoxitin
d. Metabolically unstable: cephalothin and cephapirin

Clinically used cephalosporins

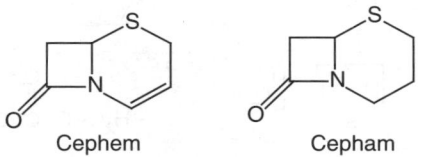

I. First-generation cephalosporins

These drugs have the highest activity against gram-positive bacteria and the lowest activity against gram-negative bacteria (Table 4.1).

II. Second-generation cephalosporins

These drugs are more active against gram-negative bacteria and less active against gram-positive bacteria than first-generation members (Table 4.2).

III. Third-generation cephalosporins

These drugs are less active than first-generation drugs against gram-positive organisms, but have a much-expanded spectrum of activity against gram-negative organisms (Table 4.3).

Table 4.1 First-generation cephalosporins.

Name	R₁	R₂	R₃
Cephaloridine	2-thienyl-CH$_2$–	pyridinium-CH$_2$–	–H
Cephalothin	2-thienyl-CH$_2$–	–H$_2$C–O–CO–CH$_3$	–H
Cephapirin	4-pyridyl-S–CH$_2$–	–H$_2$C–O–CO–CH$_3$	–H
Cephalexin	C$_6$H$_5$–CH(NH$_2$)–	–CH$_3$	–H
Cephaloglycine	C$_6$H$_5$–CH(NH$_2$)–	–H$_2$C–O–CO–CH$_3$	–H
Cefadroxil	4-HO-C$_6$H$_4$–CH(NH$_2$)–	–CH$_3$	–H
Cephradine	1,4-cyclohexadienyl–CH(NH$_2$)–	–CH$_3$	–H
Cefazolin	tetrazolyl-N–CH$_2$–	–H$_2$C–S–(2-methyl-1,3,4-thiadiazol-5-yl)	–H
Cephradine	C$_6$H$_5$–CH(NH$_2$)–	–CH$_3$	–H

Table 4.2 Second-generation cephalosporins.

Name	R₁	R₂	R₃
Cefamandole	C₆H₅–CH(OH)–	–H₂C–S–(1-methyl-1,2,4-triazol-3-yl)	–H
Cefoxitin	(thiophen-2-yl)–CH₂–	–H₂C–O–C(=O)–NH₂	–OCH₃
Cefuroxime	(furan-2-yl)–C(=N–OCH₃)–	–H₂C–O–C(=O)–NH₂	–H
Cefaclor	C₆H₅–CH(NH₂)–	–Cl	–H
Cefonicid	C₆H₅–CH(OH)–	–SCH₂–(1-(CH₂SO₃⁻)-tetrazol-5-yl)	–H

Moxalactam

[Structure: HO–C₆H₄–CH(COONa)–C(=O)–NH– attached to a bicyclic oxacephem nucleus with OCH₃ substituent, COONa group, and –CH₂–S–(1-methyltetrazol-5-yl) side chain]

Chemotherapy

Table 4.3 Third-generation cephalosporins.

Name	R₁	R₂	R₃
Ceftizoxime	2-aminothiazolyl-C(=N-OCH₃)-	–H	–H
Cefotoxime	2-aminothiazolyl-C(=N-OCH₃)-	–H₂C-O-C(=O)-CH₃	–H
Ceftazidime	2-aminothiazolyl-C(=N-O-C(CH₃)₂-COO⁻)-	–CH₂-N⁺(pyridinium)	–H
Ceftriaxone	2-aminothiazolyl-C(=N-OCH₃)-	–H₂C-S-(3-methyl-2,6-dioxo-1,2,5,6-tetrahydro-1,2,4-triazin-5-yl)	–H
Cefmenoxime	2-aminothiazolyl-C(=N-OCH₃)-	H₂C-S-(1-methyl-1H-tetrazol-5-yl)	–H

IV. Fourth-generation cephalosporins

Cefepime and cefpirome are new fourth-generation parenteral cephalosporins with a spectrum of activity which makes them suitable for the treatment of infections caused by a wide variety of bacteria (Table 4.4).

Table 4.4 Fourth-generation cephalosporins.

Name	R₁	R₂	R₃
Cefepime	2-aminothiazolyl-C(=NOCH₃)-	1-methylpyrrolidinium-CH₂–	–H

(Continued)

Name	R₁	R₂	R₃
Cefpirome	(2-aminothiazol-4-yl)-C(=NOCH₃)-	cyclopenta-fused pyridinium-N-CH₂-	-H

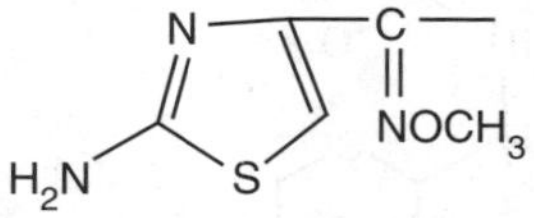

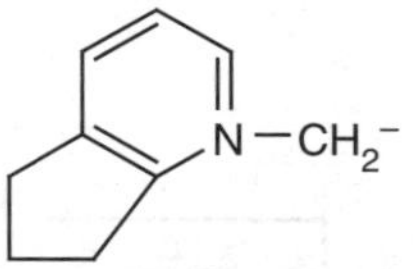

(Continued)

V. Micellaneous

i. Cefaparole

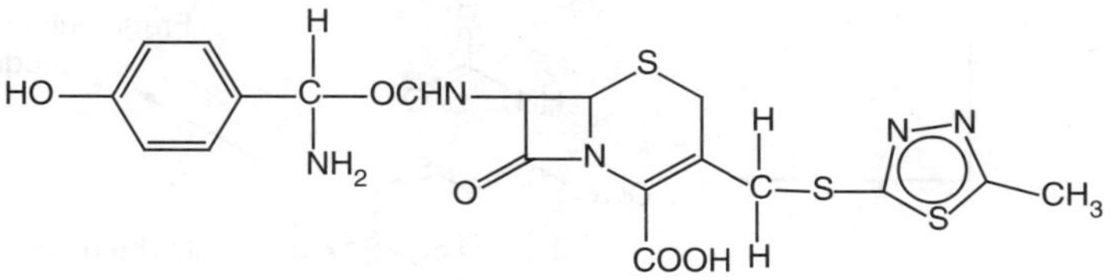

ii. Cefoperazone

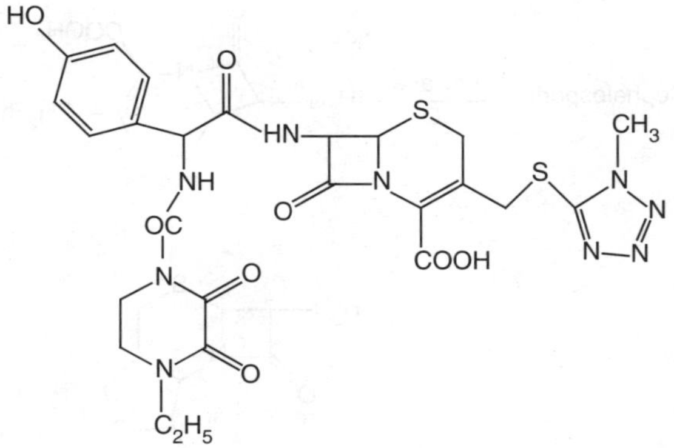

Degradation of Cephalosporins

Cephalosporins experience a variety of hydrolytic degradation reactions.
In strong acid solutions

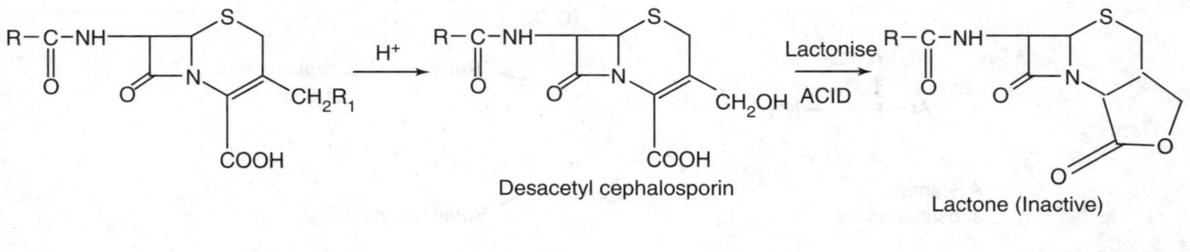

Desacetyl cephalosporin

Lactonise
ACID

Lactone (Inactive)

Chemotherapy

In the presence of β-lactamase

Cephalosporin —β-Lactamase→ Cephalosporic acid → Fragmentation and rearrangement product (Inactive)

→ Anhydro desacetyl cephalosporic acid → Fragmentation and rearrangement product (Inactive)

In the presence of acylase

Cephalosporin —Acylase/H_2O→ 7-ACA —H^+/H_2O→ Desacetyl-7-ACA lactone (Inactive lactone)

SAR of Cephalosporins

- Replacement (O, C)
- Substitution or replacement (O, S, N)
- Acylamino substituents
- Substitution on C-3

1. **7-Acylamino substitution**
   a. The addition of amino group and a hydrogen to α and α_1 position produces basic compound, which is protonated under acidic conditions of stomach. The ammonium ion improves the stability of β-lactum of cephalosporins and make active orally. Activity against positive bacteria is increased and gram negative is decreased by acylation of amino group.
   b. When the new acyl groups are derived from carboxylic acids, it shows good spectrum of antibacterial action for gram-positive bacteria.
   c. Substitutions on the aromatic ring phenyl that increase lipophilicity provide higher gram-positive activity and generally lower gram-negative activity.
   d. The phenyl ring in the side chain can be replaced with other heterocycles with improved spectrum of activity and pharmacokinetic properties; these include thiophene, tetrazole, furan, pyridine, and aminothiazoles.
   e. The L-isomer of an α-amino α_1-hydrogen derivative of cephalosphorins was 30–40 fold stable than D-isomer. Addition of methoxy oxime to α and α_1 increases the stability to nearly 100-fold. The presence of catechol grouping can also enhance activity, particularly, against *Pseudomonas aeruginosa*, and also retain some gram-positive activity, which is unused for a catechol cephalosporin.

These compounds penetrate into the cell by utilizing the bacterial ion β-dependent ion transport system. There is a reduction of Gram negative activity when the lipophilicity of this side chain is increased and effects of polar α-substituents are enhanced (OH, NH_2, SO_3H, COOH).

2. **Modification in the C-3 substitution:** The pharmacokinetic and pharmacodynamics depends on C-3 substituents. Modification at C-3 position has been made to reduce the degradation (lactone of desacetyl cephalosporin) of cephalosporins.

   a. The benzoyl ester displayers improved gram-positive activity, but lowered gram-negative activity.
   b. Pyridine, imidaozle replaced acetoxy group by azide ion yields derivative with relatively low gram-negative activity.
   c. Displacement with aromatic thiols of 3-acetoxy group results in an enhancement of activity against gram-negative bacteria with improved pharmacokinetic properties.
   d. Orally active compounds are produced by replacement of acetoxy group at C-3 position with CH_3 and Cl.

3. Other modifications

a. Methoxy group at C-7, shows higher resistance to hydrolysis by β-lactamase.
b. Oxidation of ring spectrum to sulphoxide or sulphone greatly diminishes or destroys the antibacterial activity.
c. Replacement of sulphur with oxygen leads to oxacepam (latamoxet) with increased antibacterial activity, because of its enhanced acylating power. Similarly, replacement of sulphur with methylene group (loracavet) has greater chemical stability and a longer half-life.
d. The carboxyl group position-4 has been converted into ester prodrugs to increase bioavailability of cephalosporins, and these can be given orally as well.
e. The antibacterial activity depends on the olefinic linkage at C-3 and C-4 position and their activity is lost due to the ionization of double bond to 2nd and 3rd positions.

SYNTHESIS AND DRUG PROFILE

7-Aminocephalosporinic acid (7ACA)

Synthesis

I. First-generation cephalosporins

i. Cephalexin (Keflex, Keforal)

Synthesis

Properties and uses: Cephalexin monohydrate is a white crystalline powder, sparingly soluble in water, and practically insoluble in alcohol. The α-amino group of cephalexin renders it acid stable. The 3-methyl group is responsible for the metabolic stability. It is particularly recommended for urinary tract infection.

Dose: The oral dose for adults is 250–500 mg every 6 h, for children, the dose is 18–25mg/kg every 6 h.

Assay: It is assayed by adopting liquid chromatography technique.
Dosage forms: Cefalexin capsules I.P., B.P., Cefalexin oral suspension I.P., B.P., Cefalexin tablets I.P., B.P.

ii. Cefadroxil (Cefadrox, Droxyl, Codroxil)

7-(2-Amino-2-(4-hydroxyphenyl)acetamido)-3-methyl-8-oxo-5-thia-1-aza-bicyclo[4.2.0]oct-2-ene-2-carboxylic acid

Synthesis

Properties and uses: Cefadroxil monohydrate is a white or almost white powder, slightly soluble in water, and sparingly soluble in ethanol. The antibacterial spectrum of action and therapeutic indications of cefadroxil are very similar to those of cephalexin and cephradine. The D-p-hydroxyphenylglycyl isomer is much more active than the L-isomer.

Assay: It is assayed by adopting liquid chromatography technique.

Dosage forms: Cefadroxil capsules I.P., B.P., Cefadroxil oral suspension I.P., B.P. Cefadroxil tablets I.P.

Dose: In the case of uncomplicated lower urinary tract infections: For adults, the dose is 1–2 g daily as a single or 2 divided doses. For children more than 6 years, the dose is 500 mg twice a day, that is, 1–6 years, 250 mg twice a day; for children less than 1 year, the dose is 25 mg/kg daily in divided doses. In the case of skin and skin structure infections: For adults, the dose is 1g per day in single or divided doses. For children, the dose is 30 mg/kg per day in equally divided doses every 12 h. In the case of pharyngitis and tonsilitis: For adults in the treatment of group A beta-haemolytic streptococcal pharyngitis and tonsilitis, the dose is 1 g per day in single or divided doses for 10 days. In the case of children, 30 mg/kg per day in equally divided doses every 12 h for at least 10 days.

iii. Cephalothin (Keflin)

Synthesis

7-ACA + 2-(Thienyl)acetylchloride $\xrightarrow{\text{Triethylamine}}$ Cephalothin

Properties: Cephalothin is a white, odourless, crystalline powder, insoluble in most organic solvents, soluble in organic solvents and it is acid stable. It is hygroscopic and decomposes on heating, and it has been described as broad-spectrum antibacterial compound, it is not in the same class as the tetracyclines. Its spectrum of activity is broader than that of penicillin G and more similar to that of ampicillin.

Dose: The dose for adults given IM or IV is equivalent to 500 mg–1 g every 4 to 6 h; children the dose is 13–26 mg/kg of body weight every 4 h.

iv. Cefsulodin

Synthesis

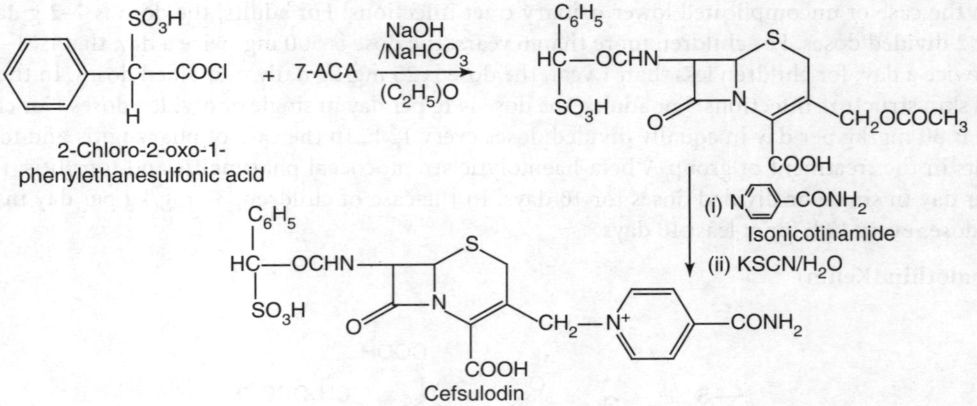

[Reaction scheme: 2-Chloro-2-oxo-1-phenylethanesulfonic acid + 7-ACA → (NaOH/NaHCO$_3$, (C$_2$H$_5$)$_2$O) → intermediate → (i) Isonicotinamide (ii) KSCN/H$_2$O → Cefsulodin]

Properties and uses: It is indicated for use in staphylococcal and pseudomonal infections.

v. Cephradine

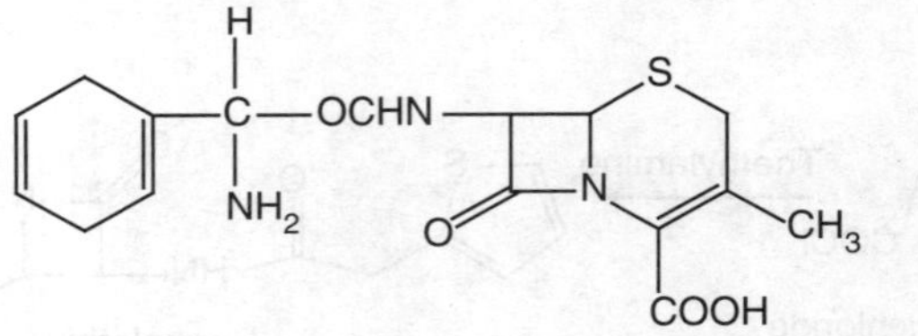

[Structure of Cephradine]

Synthesis

Route-I.

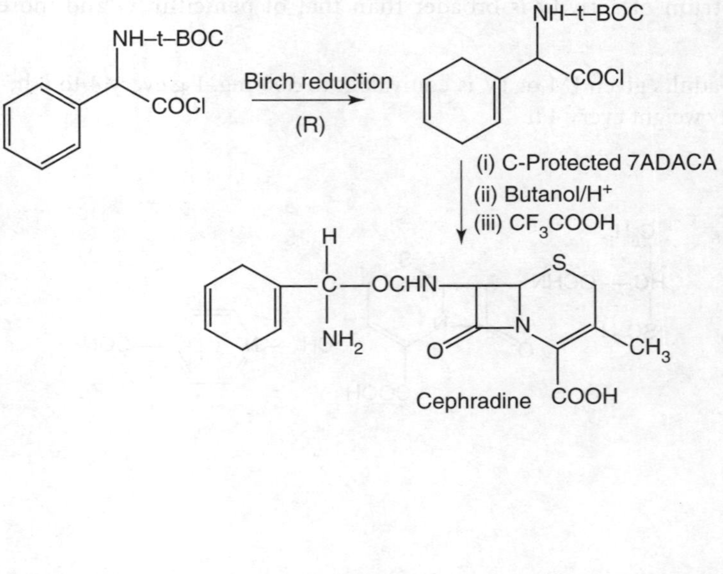

[Reaction scheme: NH–t–BOC phenyl acid chloride → Birch reduction (R) → cyclohexadienyl NH–t–BOC COCl → (i) C-Protected 7ADACA (ii) Butanol/H$^+$ (iii) CF$_3$COOH → Cephradine]

Route-II. From: 2-Amino-2-phenylacetic acid

[Reaction scheme: 2-Amino-2-phenylacetic acid → (Liq. NH₃, C₂H₅OH, Birch reduction) → dihydro intermediate → (i) N-Protection (CH₃)₃CCOCN₃; (ii) COOH Protection CH₃CH₂CHOCOCl / CH₃ → protected intermediate → 7-ADACA → Deblocking → Cephradine]

Properties and uses: Cephradine exists as colourless crystals, soluble in propylene glycol, but slightly soluble in acetone or alcohol. Used as an antibacterial agent.

II. Second-generation cephalosporin

i. Cefaclor

[Structure of Cefaclor]

Properties and uses: Cefaclor is a white or slightly yellow powder, slightly soluble in water, practically insoluble in methanol and methylene chloride. It has chloro group at C-3 position, and hence, stable in acid and achieves sufficient oral absorption. Used in the treatment of upper respiratory tract infections caused by *Streptococcus pneumoniae* and *Haemophilus influenzae*.

Dose: The dose orally for adults is 250–500 mg every 8 h.

Assay: It is assayed by adopting liquid chromatography technique.

Dosage forms: Cefaclor capsules B.P., Cefaclor oral suspension B.P., Prolonged-release Cefaclor tablets B.P.

Synthesis

[Scheme showing synthesis of Cefaclor from a thienylacetamido cephalosporin intermediate: reaction with potassium ethyl thioxanthate (KS-C(=S)-OC₂H₅), then Zn/HCOOH, then (i) O₃ (ii) SO₂, then SOCl₂/DMF, then (i) PCl₅, Pyridine (ii) Isobutanol to give the 7-amino-3-chlorocephem, followed by acylation with N(C₂H₅)₃, C₂H₅COCl and HN—CO—OC(CH₃)₃ / HC—COOH / C₆H₅ side chain, then (i) PTOSOH/CH₃CN (ii) DMF/HCl/Zn to give Cefaclor, where R = —CH₂—C₆H₄—NO₂ (p-nitrobenzyl) or R = O₂N—C₆H₄—CH₂—]

ii. Cefuroxime (Zinacef, Kefurox)

[Structure of Cefuroxime: furan-2-yl-C(=NOCH₃)-CONH- attached to cephem nucleus with -CH₂OCONH₂ at C-3 and COOH at C-4]

Synthesis

[Synthesis scheme for Cefuroxime: 2-Acetylfuran → Furan-2-glyoxalic acid (NaNO₂/HCl) → oxime with O-methyl hydroxylamine (NH₂-OCH₃, HCl) → (i) COCl/COCl (ii) 7-ACA(C₂H₅)₃N → cephem intermediate with CH₂OCOCH₃ and COOCH(C₆H₅)₂ ← (C₆H₅)₂CN₂ (Diphenyl diazo methane) ← cephem with COOH; then Citrus acetyl esterase → CH₂OH intermediate → (i) ClSO₂,NCO, CH₃CN (Chlorosulphonyl isocyanate) (ii) H₂O → CH₂OCONH₂ intermediate → Anisole/CF₃COOH → Cefuroxime]

Properties and uses: Cefiroxime sodium is a white hygroscopic powder, freely soluble in water, and very slightly soluble in ethanol. It has excellent activity against all *gonococci*, hence, is used to treat gonorrhoea. It may be used to treat lower respiratory tract infections caused by *H. influenza* and *Para influenzae*, *Klebsiella* spp. *E.coli*, *Staphylococcus pneumoniae*, and pyrogens.

Assay: It is assayed by adopting liquid chromatography technique.

Dose: The dose is 1.5 g (IM) as a single dose and also available as powder for injection in strengths of 0.75 and 1.5 g.

Dosage forms: Cefuroxime sodium injection I.P., Cefuroxime injection B.P.

iii. Cefoxitin

Synthesis

Properties and uses: Cefoxitin sodium is a white hygroscopic powder, soluble in water and sparingly soluble in alcohol. It is not the drug of choice for any infection, but it is an alternative drug for intra-abdominal infections, colorectal surgery, appendectomy, and ruptured viscus because it is active against most enteric anaerobes, including *Bacteroides fragilis*. It is approved for use in the treatment of bone and joint infections caused by *Staphylococcus aureus*, gynecological and intra-abdominal infections by *Bacteroides* spp.

Assay: It is assayed by adopting liquid chromatography technique.

Dosage forms: Cefoxitin injection B.P.

iv. Cefamandole (Mandol, Kefadol)

Synthesis

Properties and uses: Cefamandole nafate is a white powder, soluble in water, and sparingly soluble in methanol. It is the first compound of second-generation cephalosporin marketed in the United States. Cefamandole nafate is very unstable in solution and hydrolyzes rapidly to release cefamandole and formate. There is no loss of potency; however, these solutions are stored for 24 h at room temperature or up to 96 h by refrigeration.

Assay: It is assayed by adopting liquid chromatography technique.

Dose: IV dose is 0.5–2 g every 4 to 6 h, also available as injection in strength of 0.5 and 1 mg/10ml.

v. Cefonicid

Synthesis

Properties and uses: Cefonicid is a second-generation cephalosporin that is structurally similar to cefamandole, except that it contains a methane sulphonic acid group attached to the N-1 position of the tetrazole ring. Used in the treatment of bacterial infections.

III. Third-generation cephalosporins

i. Cefotaxime Sodium

7-(2-(2-aminothiazol-4-yl)-2-(methoxyimino)acetamido)-3-((1-methyl-1*H*-tetrazol-5-ylthio methyl)-8-oxo-5-thia-1-aza-bicyclo[4.2.0]oct-2-ene-2-carboxylic acid

Synthesis

[Synthesis scheme for Cefotaxime sodium starting from ethyl acetoacetate, via NaNO₂/H₂SO₄, (CH₃O)₂SO₂, Br₂/CH₂Cl₂ (p-TsOH), thiourea condensation, trityl protection, coupling with 7-ACA using DCCD, HCOOH deprotection to give Cefotaxime, then reaction with 1-methyl-1H-tetrazole-5-thiol in H₂O, NaHCO₃ + (C₂H₅)₃N⁺CH₂C₆H₅Br⁻ to give Cefotaxime sodium.]

Properties and uses: Cefotaxime sodium exists as white solid and soluble in water, exhibits broad-spectrum activity against both gram-positive and gram-negative bacteria. Used in genitourinary infection and lower respiratory infection.

ii. Ceftizoxime sodium

[Structure of Ceftizoxime sodium showing 2-aminothiazole with methoxyimino group, connected via amide to cephem nucleus with carboxylic acid.]

Synthesis

7-Phenylacetomido-3-cephem-4-carbonic acid -4-nitrobenzyl ester

Ceftizoxime

Properties and uses: It is a beta lactamase resistant cephalosphorin, used in lower respiratory infection and meningitis.

iii. Ceftriazone disodium

Synthesis

Properties and uses: It exists as white crystals, soluble in water, exhibits broad-spectrum activity against both gram-positive and gram-negative bacteria.

IV. Fourth-generation cephalosporin

i. Cefpirome (Ceform, Ominorm, Taform)

Synthesis

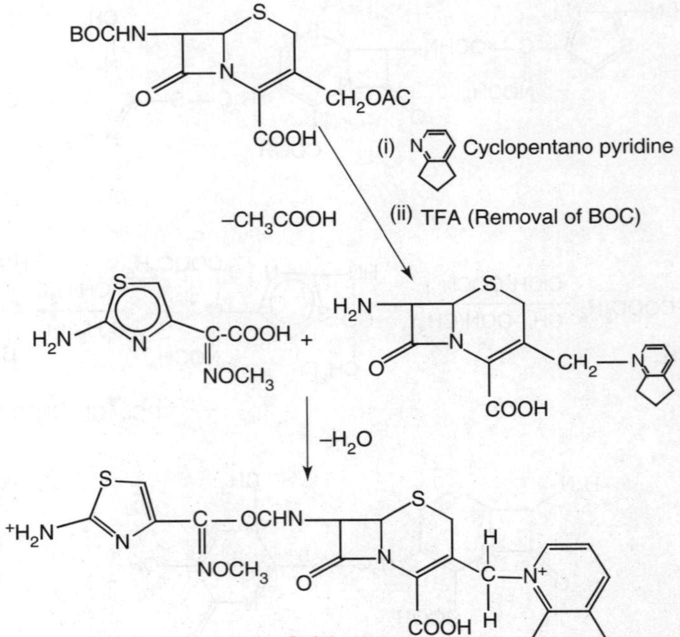

[Structure: BOCHN-cephem-CH₂OAC with COOH]

(i) Cyclopentano pyridine
(ii) TFA (Removal of BOC)
−CH₃COOH

[Aminothiazole-C(=NOCH₃)-COOH] + [H₂N-cephem-CH₂-N(cyclopentano pyridinium)]

−H₂O

[Cefpirome structure: aminothiazole-C(=NOCH₃)-C(O)NH-cephem-CH₂-N⁺(cyclopentanopyridinium)-COOH]

Cefpirome

Properties and uses: Cefpirome is used to treat susceptible infections, including urinary and respiratory tract infections, skin infections, septicaemia, and infections in immuno-compromised patients.

Dose: Intravenous dose for adults as sulphate is 1–2 g every 12 h over 3–5 min or infuse over 20–30 min.

V. Miscellaneous

i. Cefoperazone

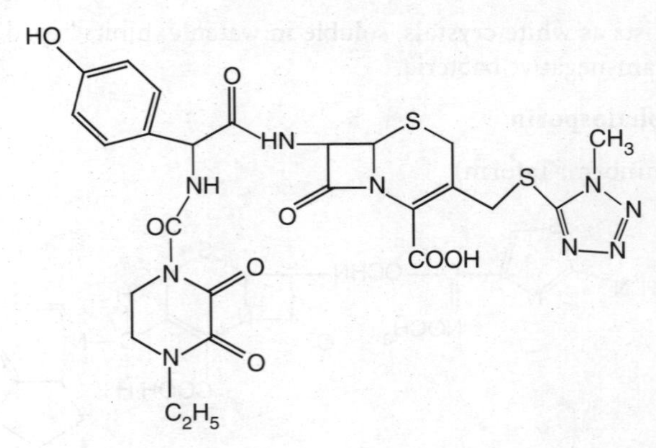

[Structure of Cefoperazone: 4-hydroxyphenyl-CH(NHCO-N-piperazinedione-N-C₂H₅)-CONH-cephem-CH₂-S-(1-methyl-tetrazole), COOH]

Synthesis

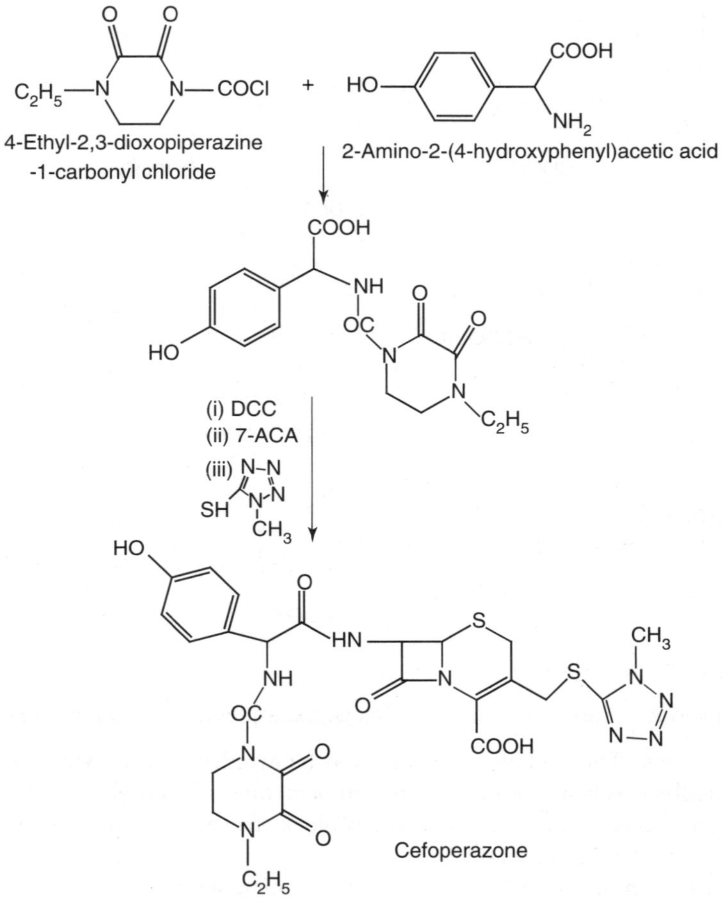

[Structures: 4-Ethyl-2,3-dioxopiperazine-1-carbonyl chloride + 2-Amino-2-(4-hydroxyphenyl)acetic acid → intermediate amide]

Reagents:
(i) DCC
(ii) 7-ACA
(iii) 5-mercapto-1-methyl-1H-tetrazole (SH—tetrazole-CH₃)

[Final structure: Cefoperazone]

Properties and uses: Cefoperazone exists as white powder. It is a third-generation, antipseudomonal cephalosporin that resembles piperacillin, chemically and microbiologically. It is less active than cephalothin against gram-positive bacteria and less active than cefamandole against most of the enterobacteria.

ii. Cefaparole

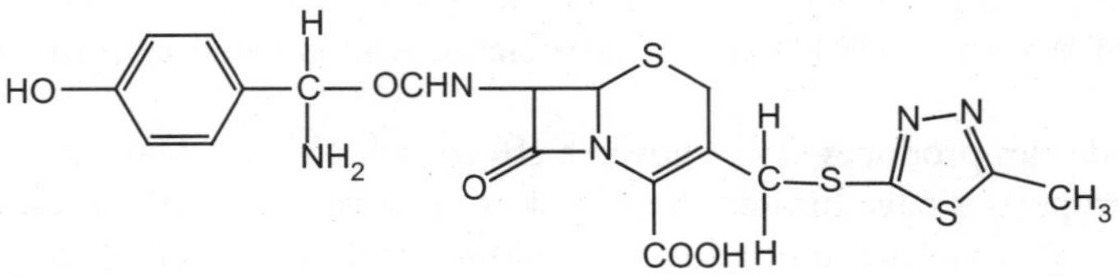

[Structure of Cefaparole]

Synthesis

[Reaction scheme: 7-amino cephalosporin with thiadiazole methylthio side chain + 4-hydroxyphenyl glycine N-Boc protected, coupled with DCC; then deprotection with CF₃COOH in Anisole to give the final hydroxyphenyl glycyl cephalosporin (cefadroxil-type structure).]

Adverse reactions of the cephalosporins

The cephalosporins produce a number of adverse effects. Examples are the following:

i. *Allergic manifestation*: The cephalosporins should be avoided or used with caution in individuals allergic to penicillins. When cefamandole or cefoperazone is ingested with alcohol, a disulphiram-like effect is seen, because these cephalosporins block the second step in alcohol oxidation, which results in the accumulation of acetaldehyde.
ii. *Bleeding*: Bleeding can occur with cefamandole or ceforperazone because of antivitamin K effects. But the administration of the vitamin overcomes this problem.

2. Aminoglycoside antibiotics

The aminoglycoside antibiotics contain one or more amino sugars linked to an aminocytitol ring by glycosidic bonds. These are broad-spectrum antibiotics; in general, they have greater activity against gram-negative than gram-positive bacteria. The development of streptomycin, the first antibiotic of this group, was a well-planned work of Waksman (1944) and his associates, who isolated it from a strain of *Streptomyces griseus*.

The aminoglycoside can produces severe adverse effects, which include nephrotoxity, ototoxicity, and neuro effects. These properties have limited the use of aminoglycoside chemotherapy to serious systemic indications. Some aminoglycosides can be administered for ophthalmic and topical purposes.

Mode of action: The aminoglycosides exhibit bactericidal effects as a result of several phenomena. Ribosomal binding on 30s and 50s subunits as well as the interface produces misreading; this disturbs the normal protein synthesis. Cell membrane damage also plays an integral part in ensuring bacterial cell death. Some examples of aminoglycoside antibiotics are listed in Table 4.1.

Table 4.1 Examples of aminoglycoside antibiotics.

Name	Source
Streptomycin	*Streptomyces griseus*
Neomycin	*S. fradiae*
Kanamycin	*S. kanamyeleticus*
Gentamysin	*Micromonospora purpura*
Netilmicin	*Micromonospora species*
Tobramycin (Nebramycin)	*S. tenebrarius*
Framycetin (Soframycin)	*S. decaris*
Paromomycin	*S. rimosus and S. paramomycinus*
Amikacin	It is 1-L-(-) 4-amino-2-hydroxy butyryl kanamycin

a. Streptomycin and dihydrostreptomycin

Properties and uses: Streptomycin sulphate is a white hygroscopic powder, very soluble in water, and practically insoluble in ethanol. The organism, *S. griseus*, releases the other substances, such as hydroxystreptomycin, mannisidostreptomycin, and cycloheximide, but do not reach up to the required activity/potency level. The development of resistant strains of bacteria and chronic toxicity constitutes major drawbacks of this category. It is an aminoglycoside antibacterial also used as an antitubercular drug.

Assay: It is assayed by microbiological method.

Dosage forms: Streptomycin injection B.P.

b. Gentamycins

Properties and uses: Gentamycin is a mixture of C_1, C_2, and C_1A compounds, obtained commercially from *Micromonospora purpurea*. Gentamycin sulphate exists as white hygroscopic powder, soluble in water, and practically insoluble in alcohol, although it is a broad-spectrum antibiotic. It is used in the treatment of infections caused by gram-negative bacteria of particular interest and has a high degree of activity against *P. aeruginosa*, where the important causative factor is burned skin. It is used topically in the treatment of infected bed-sores, pyodermata, burns, and in the eye infection.

Assay: It is assayed by microbiological method.

Dosage forms: Gentamicin cream B.P., Gentamicin ear drops B.P., Gentamicin and Hydrocortisone acetate ear drops B.P., Gentamicin eye drops B.P., Gentamicin injection B.P., Gentamicin ointment B.P.

c. Neomycin

Properties and uses: Neomycin sulphate is a white or yellowish-white hygroscopic powder, very soluble in water, very slightly soluble in alcohol, and practically insoluble in acetone. Neomycin is a mixture of closely related epimers, neomycin B, and C. Neomycin B differ from neomycin C by the nature of the sugar attached terminally to D-ribose, this sugar called neosamine. B_1 differs from neosamine C in its stereochemistry. In neomycin B_1, the neobiosamine moiety contains. β-L-iodopyranosyl, whereas in neomycin C the configuration is inverted and it is 2-D-glucopyranosyl. It is photosensitive and its main use is in the treatment of the ear, eye, and skin infections; these include burns, wounds, ulcer, and infected dermatoses.

Assay: It is assayed by microbiological method.

Dosage forms: Dexamethasone and Neomycin ear spray B.P., Hydrocortisone and neomycin cream B.P., Hydrocortisone acetate and Neomycin ear drops B.P., Hydrocortisone acetate and Neomycin eye drops B.P., Neomycin eye drops B.P., Hydrocortisone acetate and Neomycin eye ointment B.P., Neomycin eye ointment B.P., Neomycin oral solution B.P., Neomycin tablets B.P.

d. Kanamycin

Kanamycin A = R_1 = NH_2; R_2 = OH
Kanamycin B = R_1 = R_2 = NH_2
Kanamycin C = R_1 = OH; R_2 = NH_2

Properties and uses: Kanamycin sulphate is a white crystalline powder, soluble in water, practically insoluble in acetone and in alcohol. The mixture consists of three related structures, that is, Kanamycin A, B, and C. The kanamycins do not possess D-ribose molecule that is present in neomycins and paramomycins. The use of kanamycins is restricted to infections of the intestinal tract and to systemic infections.

Assay: It is assayed by microbiological method.

e. Amikacin

Properties and uses: Amikacin is a semisynthetic drug derived form kanamycin A. It retains 50% of the original activity of kanamycin A. L-Isomer is more active than D-isomer. It resists attack by most bacterial-inactivating enzyme. Therefore, it is very effective and less ototoxic than other aminoglycosides.

Dosage forms: Amikacin sulphate injection I.P.

f. Tobramycin

Properties and uses: Its activity is similar to gentamycin. The superior activity of tobramycin against *P. aeruginosa* may make it useful in the treatment of bacterial oesteromyelitis, and pneumonia caused by *P. species*.

Dosage forms: Tobramycin injection I.P.

g. Netilmicin (1-*N*-ethylsisomicin)

Properties and uses: Netilimycin sulphate is a white or yellowish-white hygroscopic powder, very soluble in water, practically insoluble in acetone and alcohol. It is similar to gentamycin and tobramycin. The majority of the aminoglycoside inactivating enzymes do not metabolize it. It is useful for the treatment of serious infections due to susceptible enterobacteria and other aerobic gram-negative bacilli.
Assay: It is assayed by microbiological method.

SAR of Aminoglycoside Antibiotics

The aminoglycosides consist of two or more amino sugars joined in glycoside linkage to a highly substituted 1,3-diaminocyclo hexane (aminocyclitol), which is a centrally placed ring. The ring is a 2-deoxy streptamine in all aminoglycosides except streptomycin and dihydrostreptomycin, where it is streptidine.

Thus,

- In kanamycin and gentamycin families, two amino sugars are attached to 2-deoxy streptamine.
- In streptomycin, two amino sugars are attached to strepidine.
- In neomycin family, there are amino sugars attached to 2-deoxy streptamine.

The aminoglycoside antibiotics contain two important structural features. They are amino sugar portion and centrally placed hexose ring, which is either 2-deoxystreptamine or streptidine.

1. Amino sugar portion

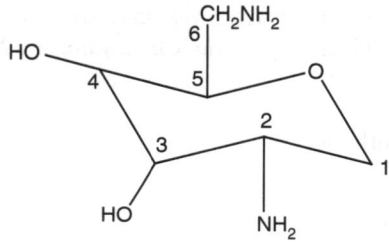

i. The bacterial inactivating enzymes targets C-6 and C-2 position, and the substitution with methyl group at C-6 increases the enzyme resistance.
ii. Cleavage of 3-hydroxyl or the 4-hydroxyl or both groups does not affect the activity.

2. Centrally placed hexose ring (aminocyclitol ring)

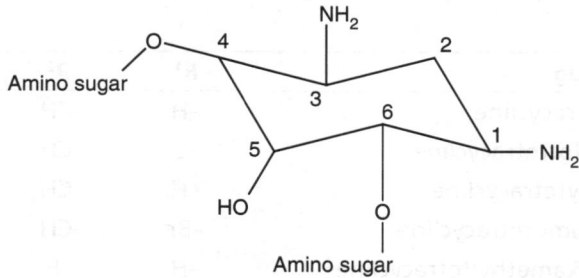

i. Various modifications at C-1 amino group have been tested. The acylation (e.g. amikacyn) and ethylation (e.g. 1-N-ethylsisomycin) though does not increase the activity helps to retain the antibacterial potency.
ii. In sisomicin series, 2-hydroxylation and 5-deoxygenation result in the increased inhibition of bacterial inactivating enzyme systems. Thus, very few modifications of the central ring are possible, which do not violate the activity spectrum of aminoglycosides.

3. Tetracycline antibiotics

Tetracyclines have a ring system of four linear annelated six-membered rings and are characterized by a common octahydronaphthacenes skeleton. They are potent, broad-spectrum antibacterial agents effective against gram-positive and gram-negative aerobic and anaerobic bacteria. As a result, the tetracyclines are drugs of choice or well-accepted alternatives for a variety of infectious diseases. Among these, they also play a role in the treatment of sexually transmitted and gonococcal diseases, urinary tract infections, bronchitis, and sinusitis remain prominent.

The majority of the marketed tetracyclines (tetracycline, chlorotetracycline, oxytetracycline, and demeclocycline) are naturally occurring compounds obtained by the fermentation of *Streptomyces spp.* broths. The semisynthetic tetracyclines (methacycline, doxycycline, minocycline) have the advantage of longer duration of antibacterial action. However, all these tetracyclines exhibit a similar profile in terms of antibacterial potency. In general, their activity encompasses many strains of gram-negative *E. coli, Proteus, Klebsiella, Enterobacter, Niesseria,* and *Serratia* spp., as well as gram-negative *Streptococci* and *Staphylococci* of particular interest is the potency of tetracylines against *Haemophilus, Legionella, Chlamydia,* and *Mycoplasma*.

Classes of tetracyclines

I. Natrual tetracyclines (biosynthetic)
II. Semisynthetic tetracyclines
III. Protetracyclines

I. Natural tetracyclines

S. No.	Drug	R^1	R^2	R^3
1.	Tetracycline	–H	–CH_3	–H
2.	Chlortetracycline	–Cl	–CH_3	–H
3.	Oxytetracycline	–H	–CH_3	–OH
4.	Bromotetracycline	–Br	–CH_3	–H
5.	Dexamethyltetracycline	–H	–H	–H
6.	Dexamethylchlortetracycline	–Cl	–H	–H

II. Semisynthetic tetracyclines

S. No.	Drug	R¹	R²	R³	R⁴
1.	Doxycycline	–OH	–H	–CH$_3$	–H
2.	Minocycline	–H	–H	–H	–N–(CH$_3$)$_2$
3.	Methacycline	–OH	=CH$_2$	–	–H
4.	Meclocycline	–OH	=CH$_2$	–	–Cl
5.	Sancycline	–H	–H	–H	–H

III. Pro-tetracyclines

S. No.	Drug	R
1.	Rolitetracycline	–CH(H)–N(pyrrolidine)
2.	Lymecycline	–CH$_2$–NH(CH$_2$)$_4$–CH(NH$_2$)–COOH
3.	Clomocycline	–CH$_2$–OH
4.	Apicycline	–CH(COOH)–N(piperazine)N–(CH$_2$)$_2$OH
5.	Pipacycline	–CH(H)–N(piperazine)N–(CH$_2$)$_2$OH
6.	Guamecycline	–CH(H)–N(piperazine)N–C(=NH)–NH–C(=NH)–NH$_2$
7.	Meglucycline	–CH(H)–NH–(glucosamine: CH$_2$OH, HO, OH, OH)

General mode of action of tetracyclines: In bacterial protein synthesis, the messenger RNA attaches itself to 30S ribosomes. The initiation complex of mRNA starts the protein synthesis and polysome formation of the nascent peptide that is attached to 50S ribosomes. Its specific tRNA transports the next amino acid to the acceptor site of the ribosome, which is complementary to the base sequence of the next mRNA codon. The nascent peptide is transferred to the newly attached amino acid by peptide bond formation. Tetracyclines bind to 30S ribosomes and the attachment of aminoacyl tRNA to mRNA ribosome complex is interfered.

Physicochemical properties: These are amphoteric due to the acidic and the basic substituents, and have low solubility in water (0.5 mg/ml) with strong acids and bases. They form water-soluble salts in each tetracycline, there are three ionizable groups present: tricarbonyl methane moiety (pKa 3.3), phenol diketone moiety (pKa 7.7), and ammonium cation moiety (pKa 9.7).

Effect of pH on tetracyclines: An interesting property of tetracyclines is their ability to undergo epimerization at C-4 position in solutions of intermediate pH range. These isomers are called epitetracyclines. Under the influence of the acidic conditions, equilibrium is established in about a day consisting of approximately equal amount of isomers. Epitetracyclines exhibit much less activity than natural isomers.

Strong acids and bases attack the tetracyclines having a hydroxyl group on C-6, causing a loss in activity through the modification of C-ring. Strong acids produce dehydration through a reaction involving the C-6 hydroxyl group and C-5a hydrogen. The double bond formed between the positions C-5a and C-6 induces a shift in the position of double bond between C-11a and C-12 to a position between C-11 and C-11a forming the more energetically favoured resonance of the naphthalene group found in the inactive anhydro tetracyclines.

5,6-Anhydrotetracycline

Isotetracycline

Bases promote a reaction between the C-6 hydroxyl group and the ketone group at the C-11 position, causing the bond between the C-11 and C-11a atoms to cleave and to form the lactone ring found in the isotetracycline.

Effect of metals on tetracyclines: Tetracyclines form stable chelate complexes with many metals, including calcium, magnesium, and iron. The chelates thus formed are insoluble in water accounting for the impairment in absorption of most of the tetracyclines in the presence of milk, calcium, magnesium, and aluminium containing antacids and iron salts.

The affinity of tetracyclines for calcium causes them to be laid down in newly formed bones and teeth as tetracycline calcium orthophosphate complexes. Deposits of these antibiotics in tooth cause yellow discolouration that darkens because of photochemical reaction. Tetracyclines are distributed into the milk of lactating mothers and also cross the placenta into the foetus. The possible effect of these agents on bones and teeth of the child should be taken into consideration before they are used during pregnancy or in children under eight years of age.

II. Semisynthetic tetracyclines

i. Methacycline

4-(Dimethylamino)-3,5,10,12,12a-pentahydroxy-6-methylene-1,11-dioxo-1,4,4a,5,5a,6,11,12a-octahydrotetracene-2-carboxamide

Synthesis

[Reaction scheme: Oxy tetracycline → (N-Chlorosuccinimide, Cis 1,2-dimethoxy ethane) → 11a-chlorotetracycline 6,12-hemiketal → (HF anhydrous) → 11a-Chloro-6-methylene tetracycline → (NaHSO$_3$) → Methacycline]

Properties and uses: Methacycline is a yellow crystalline powder, sparingly soluble in water. It is obtained by the chemical modification of oxytetracycline. It has an antibiotic spectrum similar to tetracyclines, but greater potency; about 600 mg of methacycline is equivalent to 1 g of tetracycline.

ii. Doxycycline (Vibramycin)

4-(Dimethylamino)-3,5,10,12,12a-pentahydroxy-6-methyl-1,11-dioxo-1,4,4a,5,5a,6,11,12a-octahydrotetracene-2-carboxamide

Synthesis

Methacycline → (Cata [H] Rhodium, Reduction at the 6th methylene group) → Doxycycline

Properties and uses: It was first obtained in small yields by a chemical transformation of oxytetracycline. The 6α-methyl epimer is more than three times as active as its β epimer.

Dose: In adults, the oral dosage is 100 mg every 12 h.

Dosage forms: Doxcycline HCl capsules I.P., Doxcycline HCl tablets I.P.

iii. Minocycline (Cynomycin, Minolox)

Synthesis

Properties and uses: It is a yellow crystalline powder with slightly bitter taste, soluble in water. It is very active against gram-positive bacteria. It is especially effective against *Mycobacterium marinum*. As a prophylactic against streptococcal infections, it is the drug of choice. It lacks the 6-hydroxyl group, therefore, it is stable to acids and does not dehydrate or rearrange to anhydro or lactone forms.

Dose: The dose orally for adults is 200 mg.

iv. Rolitetracycline

Synthesis

SAR of Tetracyclines

The key structural feature is a linearly fused tetracyclic nucleus and each ring needs to be six membered and purely carbocyclic. A tetracyclic backbone skeleton is essential for activity.

- The D-ring needs to be aromatic and the A-ring must be appropriately substituted at each of its carbon atoms for notable activity.
- The B-ring and the C-ring tolerate certain substitutent changes as long as the keto-enol systems (at C-11, 12, 12a) remain intact and conjugated to the phenolic D-ring.
- The D, C, B-ring phenol, keto-enol system is imperative and the A-ring must also contain a conjugated keto enol system.

- Specifically, the A-ring contains a tricarbonyl derived keto-enol array at positions C-1, 2, and -3. Other structural requirements for good antibacterial activity include a basic amine function at C-4 position of the A-ring.

Modification of C-1 and C-3 position: The keto-enol tautomerism of ring A in carbon atom 1 and 3 is a common feature to all biologically active tetracyclines, blocking this system by forming derivatives at C-1 and C-3 results in loss of antibacterial activity A–C = O, a function of C-1 and C-3 is essential for activity. In addition, equilibrium between non-ionized and Zwitterionic structure of tetracycline is essential for activity.

Modification of C-2 position: The antibacterial activity resides on the carboxamide moiety. The amide is best left unsubstituted or monosubstitution is acceptable in the form of activated alkylaminomethyl amide (Mannich bases). An example includes rolitetracycline large alkyl group on the carboxamide that may alter the normal keto-enol equilibrium of the C-1, 2, and 3 conjugated systems and diminishes inherent antibacterial activity. The replacement of carboxamide group or dehydration of carboxamide to the corresponding nitrile results in a loss of activity.

Modification of C-4 position: The keto-enolic character of the A-ring is due to the α-C-4 dimethyl amino substituent. Loss of activity is exerted when dimethyl amino group is replaced with hydrazone oxime or hydroxyl group.

Modification of C-4a position: The α-hydrogen at C-4a position of tetracyclines is necessary for useful antibacterial activity.

Modification of the C-5 and C-5a positions: Alkylation of the C-5 hydroxyl group results in loss of activity. Naturally occurring antibacterial tetracyclines have an unsubstituted methylene moiety at the C-5 position. However, oxytetracycline contains C-5 α-hydroxyl group, was found to be a potent compound, and has been modified chemically to some semisynthetic tetracyclines. Esterification is only acceptable if the free oxytetracycline can be liberated in vivo; only small alkyl esters are useful. Epimerization is detrimental to antibacterial activity.

Modification at the C-6 position: The C-6 methyl group contributes little to the activity of tetracycline. The C-6 position is tolerant to a variety of substituents. The majority of tetracyclines have α-methyl group and α β-hydroxyl group at this position. Demeclocyclin is a naturally occurring C-6 demethylated chlortetracycline with an excellent activity. Removal of C-6 hydroxyl group affords doxycycline, which exerts good antibacterial activity.

C-7 and C-9 substituents: The nature of the aromatic D-ring predisposes the C-7 position to electrophilic substitution. Substitution with electron withdrawing group such as nitro and halogen groups are introduced in some C-7 tetracyclines, which produces the most potent of all the tetracyclines in vitro, but their are compounds are potentially toxic and carcinogenic. The C-7 acetoxy, azido, and hydroxyl tetracyclines are inferior in terms of antibacterial activity.

C-10 substituents: The C-10 phenolic moiety is necessary for antibacterial activity. C-10 substitution with para or ortho hydrogen group activates the C-9 and C-7.

C-11 substituents: The C-11 carbonyl moiety is a part of one of the conjugated keto-enol system required for antibacterial activity.

C-11a substituents: No stable tetracyclines are formed by modifications at the C-11a position.

C-12/12a substituents: Esterification of the hydroxyl group leads to the incorporation of drug with the tissues due to the enhanced lipophilicity and it should undergo hydrolysis to leave the active tetracycline with hydroxyl group at 12a position, which is necessary to produce good antibacterial action. The transport and binding of these drugs depends on keto-enol system.

4. Polypeptide antibiotics

The compounds have complex polypeptide structure. These are resistant to animal and plant proteases. These contain lipid moieties besides amino acids that are not found in peptides of animal and plant origins. Examples: bacitracin, polymycin, amphomycin, tyrothricin, and vancomycin.

i. Bacitracin

Properties and uses: Bacitracin is a white hygroscopic powder, soluble in water and alcohol. Bacitracin antibiotic is isolated from the fermentation broth of a culture of tracyl-1 strain of *Bacillus subtilis*. It is found to be a complex mixture of at least 10 polypeptides (A, A_1, B, C, D, E, F_1, F_2, F_3, and G), of which bacitracin A fraction is believed to be the most abundant and the most potent. A divalent ion Zn^{++} enhances its activity. Although bacitracin is occasionally employed for topical application (often in combination with neomycin, polymycin, and tyrothicin) for the treatment of burns, ulcer, and wounds, it can cause serious necrosis of the kidney tubules; if it is given systematically (i.e. I.V route) an oral administration is not feasible due to its lack of absorption from the GI tract. A variety of gram-positive *cocci* and *bacilli* are sensitive to bacitracin. It should be stored in airtight containers due to its hygroscopic nature.

Assay: It is assayed by microbiological method.

ii. Polymyxin

```
                                            → L-DAB-D-Phe-L-Leu
                                           /          |
                                          /           ↓
R-L-DAB ──→ L-THR ──→ L-DAB-L-DAB
                                          \
                                           \
                                            → L-THR-L-DAB-L-DAB
```

PolymyxinB$_1$:R = (+)-6-methyloctanoyl

PolymyxinB$_2$:R = 6-methylpeptanoyl

DAB = α–γ–Diaminobutyric acid

Properties and uses: Polymycin sulphate is a white hygroscopic powder, soluble in water, and slightly soluble in ethanol. The polymyxins are cyclic peptides holding a fatty acid side chain. This is a group of relatively simple basic, cationic, detergent peptides that are produced by *Bacillus polymyxia*. At least, five polymyxins (A, B, C, D, and E) are known, but only polymyxin B and polymyxin E are of clinical utility. Both polymyxin B and polymyxin E (colistin) are mixtures of two components and is used in the treatment of bacterial meningitis, urinary tract infection, burns, wounds, and gastroenteritis. Polymyxin may affect renal tubules and central nervous system (CNS), and because of their nephrotoxicity associated with their systemic use, they are primarily employed to treat topical infections.

Assay: It is assayed by adopting liquid chromatography technique.

5. Macrolide antibiotics

The macrolide antibacterial agents are extremely useful chemotherapeutic agents for the treatment of a variety of infectious disorders and diseases caused by a host of gram-positive bacteria, both *cocci* and *bacilli*; they also exhibit useful effectiveness against gram-negative *cocci*, specially, *neisseria* spp. The macrolides are commonly administered for respiratory, skin, tissue, and genitourinary infections caused by these pathogens.

Chemistry: They are characterized by five common chemical features.

1. A macrocyclic lactone usually has 12–17 atoms, hence the name macrolide.
2. A ketone group.
3. One or two amino sugars glycosidically linked to the nucleus.
4. A neutral sugar linked either to amine sugar or to nucleus.
5. The presence of dimethyl amino moiety on the sugar residue, which explains the basicity of these compounds, and consequently the formation of salts. The antibacterial spectrum of activity of the more potent macrolides resembles that of penicillin. Examples: erythromycin, oleandomycin, clarithromycin, flurithromycin, dirithomycin, azithromycin.

i. Azithromycin

Properties and uses: Azithromycin is a white powder, practically insoluble in water, soluble in anhydrous ethanol and methylene chloride. It is very stable under acidic conditions, is less active against *Streptococci* and *Staphylococci* than erythromycin, and is far more active against respiratory infections due to *H. influenzae* and *Chlamydia trachomatis*.

Name	R	R_1
Erythromycin	=O	–H
Roxithromycin	$CH_3OCH_2CH_2OCH_2O-$	–H
Clarithromycin	=O	$-CH_3$

Acid degradation of erythromycin

Erythromycin is unstable in the acid media. The C-6 hydroxyl group reversibly attacks the C-9 ketone giving rise to a hemiketal intermediate. Dehydration prevents regeneration of the parent erythromycin and the C-12 hydroxyl group can subsequently add to produce a spiroketal species. The cladinose group is cleaved from the macrocycle and more harsh conditions lead to the release of desosamine. Useful antibacterial activity last till the dehydration of the hemiketal and the spiroketal is weakly active.

Mode of action: Macrolide antibiotics are bacteriostatic agents that inhibit protein synthesis by binding irreversibly to a site on the 50S subunits of the bacterial ribosome. Thus, inhibiting the translocation steps of protein synthesis at varying stages of peptide chain elongation (hinder the translocation of elongated peptide chain back from 'A' site to 'P' site). The macrolides inhibit ribosomal peptidyl transferase activity. Some macrolides also inhibit the translocation of the ribosome along with the mRNA template.

6. Lincomycins

Lincomycin R = OH
Clindamycin R = Cl

Properties and uses: The antibiotic lincomycin is obtained from *Actinomycetes, Streptomyces,* and *Lincolnensis*. The ability of lincomycin to penetrate into bones, adds to its qualities and it gets promoted in the chemotherapy of bone and joint infections by penicillin resistant strains of *S. aureus*. Variation of the substituents on pyrrolidine portion and C-5 side chain affects the activity. Some of the examples are as follows:

i. *N*-demethylation imparts activity against gram-negative bacteria.
ii. Increase in the chain length of the propyl substitutent at C-4 position in pyrrolidine moiety up to *n*-hexyl increase *in vivo* activity.
iii. The thiomethyl ether of α-thiolincosamide moiety is essential for activity.
iv. Structural modifications at C-7 position, such as introduction of 7S chloro or 7R-OCH$_3$, change the physiochemical parameters of the drug (i.e. partition coefficient), and thus, alter the activity spectrum and pharmacokinetic properties. The usual side effects include skin rashes, nausea, vomiting, and diarrhoea.

Dosage forms: Lincomycin HCl capsules I.P.

7. Other antibiotics

Examples of other antibiotics are chloramphenicol, rifampicin and mupirocin.

i. Chloramphenicol or chloromycetin

Chloramphenicol has a spectrum of activity resembling that of the tetracyclines except that it exhibits a bit less activity against some gram-positive bacteria. It is isolated from *Salmonella venezuelae* by Ehrlich et al in 1947. It contains chlorine and is obtained from an actinomycete, and thus, named as chloromycetin. It is specifically recommended for the treatment of serious infections caused by *H. influnzae, S. typhi* (typhoid), *S. pneumoniae,* and *N. meningitides*. Its ability to penetrate into the CNS presents an alternative therapy for meningitis and exhibits antirickettsial activity.

Structure

$$O_2N-C_6H_4-\underset{\underset{OH}{|}}{\overset{\overset{H}{|}}{C}}-\underset{\underset{H}{|}}{\overset{\overset{NHCOCHCl_2}{|}}{C}}-CH_2OH$$

N-(1,3-Dihydroxy-1-(4-nitrophenyl)propan-2-yl)dichloroacetamide

Properties and uses: Chlorampenicol is a white or greyish-white or yellowish-white crystalline powder or fine crystals, slightly soluble in water, soluble in alcohol and propylene glycol. It was the first, and still is the only therapeutically important antibiotic to be produced in competition with microbiological processes. It contains a nitrobenzene moiety and is a derivative of dichloroacetic acid. Since it has two chiral centres, four isomers are possible. The D-(-) threo is the biologically active form. It is used in the treatment of typhoid fever caused by *S. typhi*. The most serious adverse effect of chloramphenicol is bone marrow depression and fatal blood dyscrasias.

Assay: Dissolve the sample in water, dilute with the same solvent, and measure the absorbance at the maximum of 278 nm using ultraviolet spectrophotometer.

Dose: Usual adult dose is 500 mg every 6 h.

Dosage forms: Chloramphenicol capsules I.P., B.P., Chloramphenicol ear drops I.P., B.P., Chloramphenicol eye ointment I.P., B.P., Chloramphenicol eye drops B.P.

Synthesis

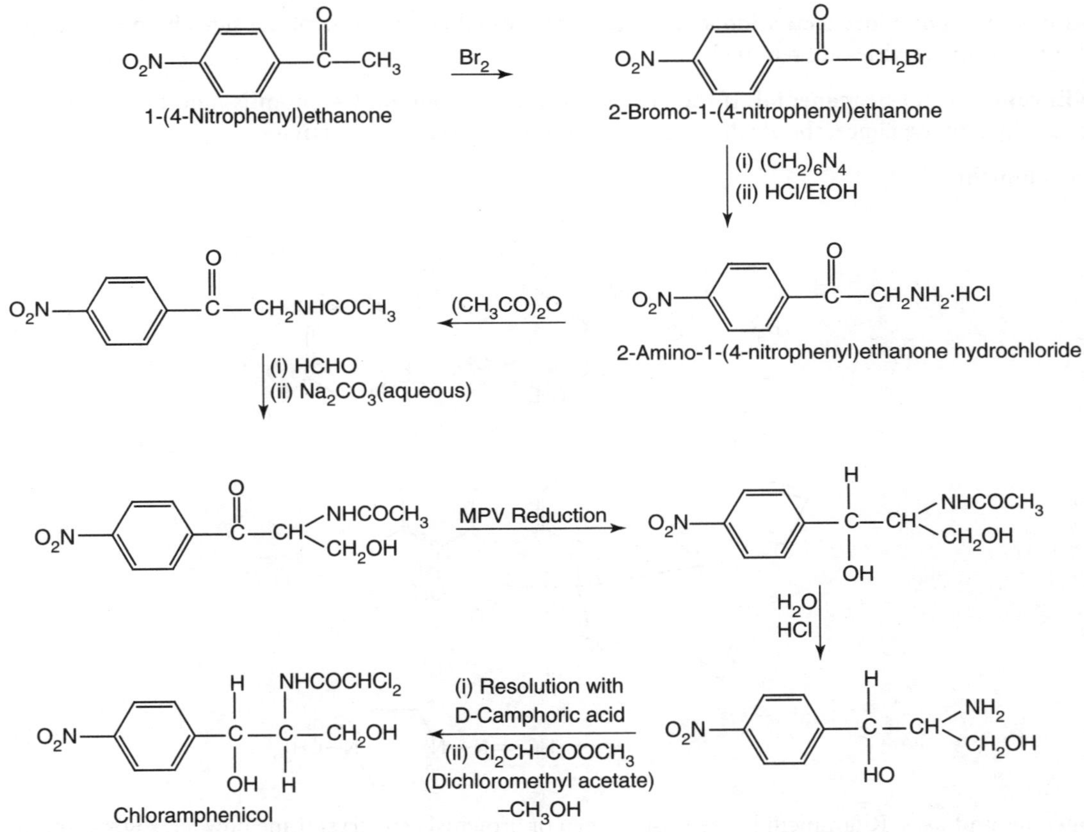

1-(4-Nitrophenyl)ethanone → (Br$_2$) → 2-Bromo-1-(4-nitrophenyl)ethanone

(i) $(CH_2)_6N_4$
(ii) HCl/EtOH

→ 2-Amino-1-(4-nitrophenyl)ethanone hydrochloride

→ $(CH_3CO)_2O$ → O_2N-C$_6$H$_4$-CO-CH$_2$NHCOCH$_3$

(i) HCHO
(ii) Na$_2$CO$_3$ (aqueous)

→ O_2N-C$_6$H$_4$-CO-CH(NHCOCH$_3$)(CH$_2$OH) → MPV Reduction → O_2N-C$_6$H$_4$-CH(OH)-CH(NHCOCH$_3$)(CH$_2$OH)

H$_2$O / HCl

→ O_2N-C$_6$H$_4$-CH(OH)-CH(NH$_2$)(CH$_2$OH)

(i) Resolution with D-Camphoric acid
(ii) Cl$_2$CH–COOCH$_3$ (Dichloromethyl acetate)
–CH$_3$OH

→ **Chloramphenicol**: O_2N-C$_6$H$_4$-CH(OH)-CH(NHCOCHCl$_2$)-CH$_2$OH

SAR of Chloramphenicol

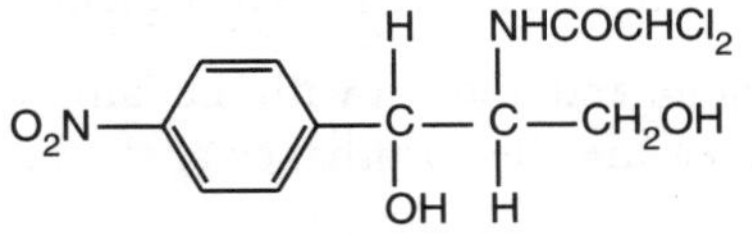

O_2N-C$_6$H$_4$-CH(OH)-CH(NHCOCHCl$_2$)-CH$_2$OH

a. Modification of *p*-nitrophenyl group.
b. Modification of dichloroacetamide side chain.
c. Modification of 1, 3-prepanediol.

Modification of *p*-nitrophenyl group: The *p*-nitrophenyl group may be modified through the following ways:

  a. Replacement of the nitro group by other substituents leads to a reduction in activity.
  b. Shifting of the nitro group from the para position also reduces the antibacterial activity.
  c. Replacement of phenyl group by the alicyclic moieties results in less potent compounds.

Modification of dichloroacetamido side chain: Other dihalo derivatives of the side chain are less potent although major activities are retained.

Modification of 1,3-propanediol: If the primary alcoholic group on C-1 atom is modified, it results in a decrease in activity; hence, the alcoholic group seems to be essential for activity.

ii. Rifampicin

$R= -HC=N-NN-CH_3$

Properties and uses: Rifampicin is a reddish-brown or brownish-red crystalline powder, slightly soluble in water, acetone, and alcohol and soluble in methanol. It is a broad-spectrum bactericidal antibiotic, structurally similar to complex macrocyclic antibiotic obtained from *S. mediterrani*. They belong to a new class of antibiotics called as ansamycins. Five types, that is, rifampicin A, B, C, D, and E are present. It penetrates well into cerebrospinal fluid and is, therefore, used in the treatment of tuberculous meningitis.

Assay: Dissolve the sample in methanol and dilute it with the same solvent. Dilute the solution with phosphate buffer solution pH 7.4 and measure the absorbance at the maximum at 475 nm, using phosphate buffer solution pH 7.4 as blank.

PROBABLE QUESTIONS

1. What are penicillins? Classify with suitable examples and write the SAR of penicillins.
2. What are the cardinal requirements of a substance to be called as an antibiotic? Draw the structure, chemical name, and other names of the naturally occurring penicillins.
3. Explain the synthesis and the uses of phenoxy methyl penicillin and amoxycillin.
4. Draw the structure, chemical name, and uses of the following:
   (a) Penicillins related to ampicillin (b) Esters of ampicillin
5. Write short notes on the degradation of penicillins.
6. Write the structure, chemical name, uses, and synthesis of the given category of penicillins.
   (a) Acid-resistant penicillins (b) Betalactamase-resistant penicillins.
7. What are cephalosporins? Explain how it differs from penicillins chemically. Write the SAR of cephalosporins in detail.
8. Write a comprehensive account of cephalosporins with suitable examples.
9. What are aminoglycoside antibiotics? Write the mode of action, structure, and uses of three potent drugs of this category.
10. Name any five aminoglycoside antibiotics and mention their source.
11. What are the reasons for recognizing chlorapmphenicol as a potent antibiotic? Write in detail about the SAR and stereochemistry of chloramphenicol. Describe the synthesis of chloramphenicol.
12. Explain the salient features of the tetracylines. Write a brief account on the SAR of tetracylines.
13. What are the five common characterized chemical features of macrolide antibiotics? Write its mode of action.
14. Write short notes on the semisynthetic tetracyclines.
15. Elaborate the characteristics of the tetracylines with specific reference to their
    (a) Effect on metals and (b) Effect on strong acids and bases.

SUGGESTED READINGS

1. Abraham DJ (ed). *Burger's Medicinal Chemistry and Drug Discovery* (6th edn). New Jersey: John Wiley, 1995.
2. Barnes WG and Hodges GR (eds). *The Aminoglycoside Antibiotics: A Guide to Therapy.* Boca Raton, FL: CRC, 1984.
3. *British Pharmacopoeia*. Medicines and Healthcare Products Regulatory Agency. London, 2008.
4. Bruntan LL, Lazo JS, and Parker KL. *Goodman and Gilman's: The Pharmacological Basis of Therapeutics* (11th edn). New York: McGraw Hill, 2006.
5. Bryker AJ, Butzler JP, Neu HC, and Tulken PM (eds). *Macrolides, Chemistry, Pharmacology and Clinical Uses.* Paris: Arnate Blackwell, 1993.
6. Coute JE. *Manual of Antibiotics and Infectious Diseases* (8th edn). Baltimore: Williams & Wilkins, 1995.
7. Ehrlich J, Bartz QR, Smith RM, Joslyn DA, Burkholder PR. 'Chloromycetin: A new antibiotic from a soil actinomycete'. *Science* 106: 417, 1947.

8. Gennaro AR. *Remington: The Science And Practice of Pharmacy* (21st edn). New York: Lippincot Williams and Wilkins, 2006.
9. Havaka JJ and Boothe JH (eds). *The Tetracyclines*. New York: Springer-Verlag, 1985.
10. *Indian Pharmacopoeia*. Ministry of Health and Family Welfare. New Delhi, 1996.
11. Kirsk HA. 'Dirithromycin'. *Drugs of Today* 31: 1–10, 1995.
12. Lednicer D and Mitscher LA. *The Organic Chemistry of Drug Synthesis*. New York: John Wiley, 1995.
13. Lemke TL and William DA. *Foye's Principle of Medicinal Chemistry* (6th edn). New York: Lippincott Williams and Wilkins, 2008.
14. Mandell GL, Douglas RG (Jr), and Bennett JE (eds). *Principles and Practice of Infectious Diseases* Vol. 1 (4th edn). New York: Churchill-Livingstone, 1995.
15. Mitscher LA. *The Chemistry of Tetracycline Antibiotics*. New York: Marcell Dekker, 1978.
16. Neu HC, Young LS, and Zinner SH. *The New Macrolides*. New York: Marcel Dekker, 1995.
17. Omura S (ed). *Macrolide Antibiotics*. Orland, FL: Academic Press, 1984.
18. Progdeu RN and Peters DH. 'Diithromycin: A review'. *Drugs* 48: 599–616, 1994.
19. Schatz A, Bugie E, and Waksman S. 'Streptomycin, a substance exhibiting antibiotic activity against gram-positive and gram-negative bacteria'. *Proc Soc Exptl Biol Med* 55: 66–69, 1944.

Chapter 5

Antitubercular Agents

INTRODUCTION

Tuberculosis is the most prevalent infectious disease worldwide and a leading killer caused by a single infectious agent, that is, *Mycobacterium tuberculosis*. According to World Health Organization (WHO) report, *M. tuberculosis*, currently infects over 2 billion people worldwide, with 30 million new cases reported every year. This intracellular infection accounts for at least 3 million deaths annually. Common infection sites of the tuberculosis are lungs (primary site), brain, bone, liver, and kidney. The main symptoms are cough, tachycardia, cyanosis, and respiratory failure. Depending upon the site of infection, the disease can be categorized as follows:

- Pulmonary tuberculosis (respiratory tract).
- Genitourinary tuberculosis (genitourinary tract).
- Tuberculous meningitis (nervous system).
- Miliary tuberculosis (a widespread infection).

Drugs used in the treatment of tuberculosis can be divided into two major categories (Fig. 4.1):

1. First-line drugs: Isoniazid, streptomycin, rifampicin, ethambutol, and pyrazinamide.
2. Second-line drugs: Ethionamide, *p*-amino salicylic acid, ofloxacin, ciprofloxacin, cycloserine, amikacin, kanamycin, viomycin, and capreomycin.

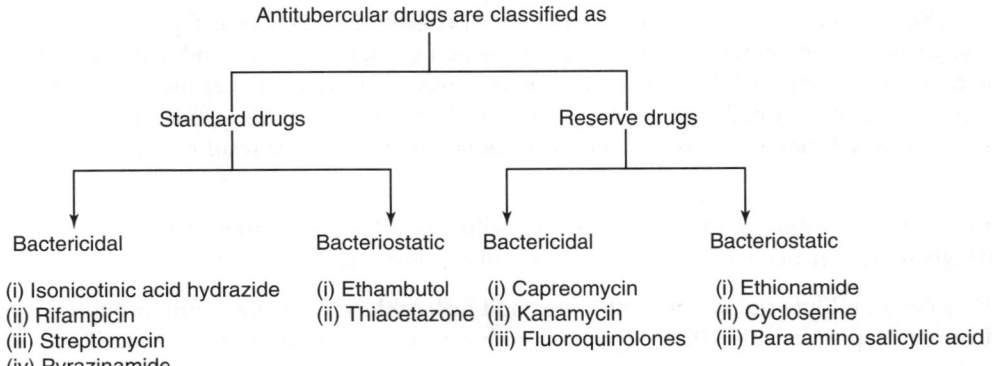

Figure 4.1 Classification of antitubular drugs.

The majority of the patients with tuberculosis are treated with first-line drugs and shows excellent results with a 6-month course of treatment. For the first 2 months, isoniazid, rifampicin, and pyrazinamide are given, followed by isoniazid and rifampicin for the remaining 4 months. Second-line drugs are used mainly to treat multidrug resistant *M. tuberculosis* infections.

SYNTHESIS AND DRUG PROFILE

I. Standard drugs
i. Isoniazid (Continazin, Laniazid, Isonex, Ipcazide, INH, Isokin))

Isonicotinic acid hydrazide (INH)

Synthesis

4-Picoline $\xrightarrow{(O), KMnO_4}$ isonicotinic acid $\xrightarrow{C_2H_5OH, H_2SO_4}$ ethyl isonicotinate $\xrightarrow{NH_2NH_2}$ Isoniazid

Mode of action: Isoniazid is a prodrug that is activated on the surface of *M. tuberculosis* by katG enzyme to isonicotinic acid. Isonicotinic acid inhibits the bacterial cell wall mycolic acid, thereby making *M. tuberculosis* susceptible to reactive oxygen radicals. Isoniazid may be bacteriostatic or bactericidal in action, depending on the concentration of the drug attained at the site of infection and the susceptibility of the infecting organism. The drug is active against susceptible bacteria only during bacterial cell division.

Metabolism: Isoniazid is extensively metabolized to inactive metabolites. The major metabolite is *N*-acetyl isoniazid. The enzyme responsible for acetylation is cytosolic *N*-acetyl transferase. Other metabolites include isonicotinic acid, which is found in the urine as a glycine conjugate and hydrazine. Isonicotinic acid also may result from hydrolysis of acetyl isoniazid, but in this case, the second product of hydrolysis is acetyl hydrazine. Acetyl hydrazine is acetylated by *N*-acetyl transferase to inactive diacetyl product. It has been suggested that a hydroxylamine intermediate is formed that results in an active acetylating agent.

Properties and uses: Isoniazid exists as white crystalline powder or colourless crystals, soluble in water, and sparingly soluble in alcohol. It is used as an antituberculosis drug.

Assay: Dissolve and dilute the sample with water, add hydrochloric acid, potassium bromide, and methyl red and titrate drop wise with 0.0167 M potassium bromate, shaking continuously, until the red colour disappears.

Antitubercular Agents

[Metabolism scheme of isoniazid showing formation of N-acetyl isoniazid, isonicotinic acid + hydrazine, and related metabolites including acetyl hydrazine and diacetyl hydrazine]

Dose: For the prophylaxis in case of adults is 5 mg/kg, with a maximum of 300 mg. For children: 10–20 mg/kg daily. Combination therapy Isoniazid, Rifampin and Pyrazinamide for 2 months followed by Isoniazid (15 mg/kg orally) with. Rifampin (10 mg/kg upto 600 mg per dose) twice/week for 4 months.

Dose: For the prophylaxis in case of adults 5 mg/kg, with a maximum of 300 mg.

Dosage forms: Isoniazid tablets I.P., B.P. Isoniazid injection B.P.

ii. Pyrazinamide

Pyrazine-2-carboxamide

Synthesis

Route I. From: Pyrazine-2, 3-dicarboxylic acid

Pyrazine-2,3-dicarboxylic acid + Urea $\xrightarrow{-2CO_2, -NH_3}$ Pyrazinamide

Route II. From: Pyrazine-2, 3-diamine

Pyrazine-2,3-diamine + Glyoxal → Quinoxaline

KMnO₄ | (O)

Quinoxaline-2,3-dicarboxylic acid (pyrazine with two COOH groups)

(i) –CO₂
(ii) C_2H_5OH/H^+

→ Pyrazine-2-carboxylic acid ethyl ester ($COOC_2H_5$)

↓ NH_3

Pyrazinamide ($CONH_2$)

Metabolism: The metabolic route constitutes of hydrolysis by hepatic microsomal pyrazinamidase into pyrazinoic acid, which may be then, oxidized by xanthine oxidase to 5-hydroxy pyrazinoic acid. The later compound may appear free either in the urine or as a conjugate with glycine.

Pyrazinamide → Pyrazinoic acid → 5-Hydroxy pyrazinoic acid

Properties and uses: Pyrazinamide is a white crystalline powder, sparingly soluble in water, slightly soluble in alcohol and in methylene chloride. It is a prodrug and is activated by *M. tuberculosis* amidase enzyme into pyrazine carboxylic acid, which has bactericidal activity. Pyrazinamide has recently been elevated to first-line status in the short-term treatment of tuberculosis regimens because of its tuberculocidal activity and comparatively less short-term toxicity. Pyrazinamide is maximally effective in the low pH environment that exists in macrophages (monocytes). It is used to treat tuberculosis and meningitis. The drug should be used with great caution in patients with hyperuricaemia or gout.

Assay: Dissolve the sample in acetic anhydride and titrate with 0.1 M perchloric acid. Determine the end point potentiometrically.

Dose: Daily administered dose is 20–35 mg/kg in 3–4 equally spaced doses and maximum is 3 g daily.

Dosage forms: Pyrazinamide tablets B.P.

iii. Ethambutol HCl (Myambutol)

$$\begin{array}{c} H_2C-NH-\overset{C_2H_5}{\underset{|}{CH}}CH_2OH \\ | \\ H_2C-NH-\overset{C_2H_5}{\underset{|}{CH}} \\ | \\ CH_2OH \end{array} \cdot HCl$$

2,2′-Ethylene (diamine) di-(2-butyl-1-ol)

Synthesis

Route I. From: 1,2-Dichloroethane

$$\underset{\text{1,2-Dichloroethane}}{\begin{array}{c} CH_2Cl \\ | \\ CH_2Cl \end{array}} + 2\;\underset{\text{2-Aminobutan-1-ol}}{\begin{array}{c} C_2H_5 \\ | \\ HC-NH_2 \\ | \\ CH_2OH \end{array}} \xrightarrow[-2\,HCl]{\Delta} \underset{\text{Ethambutol}\cdot HCl}{\begin{array}{c} H_2C-NH-CHCH_2OH \\ | \quad\quad\quad C_2H_5 \\ H_2C-NH-CH \\ | \\ CH_2OH \end{array}} \cdot HCl$$

Route II. From: Nitropropane

$$2\;CH_3-CH_2-CH_2-NO_2 \xrightarrow[NH_4OH]{HCHO} \underset{\text{2-Nitro butanol}}{2\;CH_3-CH_2-\underset{|}{CH}-NO_2} \xrightarrow{Sn/HCl} \underset{\substack{(\pm)\;\text{Racemic mixture of}\\ \text{2-Amino butanol}}}{2\;CH_3-CH_2-\underset{|}{CH}-NH_2}$$
$$\quad\quad\quad\quad\quad\quad\quad\quad\quad\quad\quad\quad\quad\quad\quad\quad CH_2OH \quad\quad\quad\quad\quad\quad\quad\quad\quad CH_2OH$$

$$\underset{\text{Ethambutol}}{\begin{array}{c} H_2C-NH-\overset{C_2H_5}{\underset{|}{CH}}CH_2OH \\ | \\ H_2C-NH-\overset{C_2H_5}{\underset{|}{CH}} \\ | \\ CH_2OH \end{array}} \xleftarrow[-2\,HCl]{\begin{array}{c} Cl-CH_2CH_2-Cl \\ \text{Dichloro ethane} \end{array}} \underset{\text{Dextro rotatory compound}}{\begin{array}{c} 2\;CH_3-CH_2-CH-NH_2 \\ | \\ CH_2OH \end{array}} \;\Bigg\uparrow\text{Resolve}$$

Metabolism: The majority of the administered ethambutol is excreted unchanged (73%), with not more than 15% appearing in the urine as a metabolite, which are devoid of biological activity.

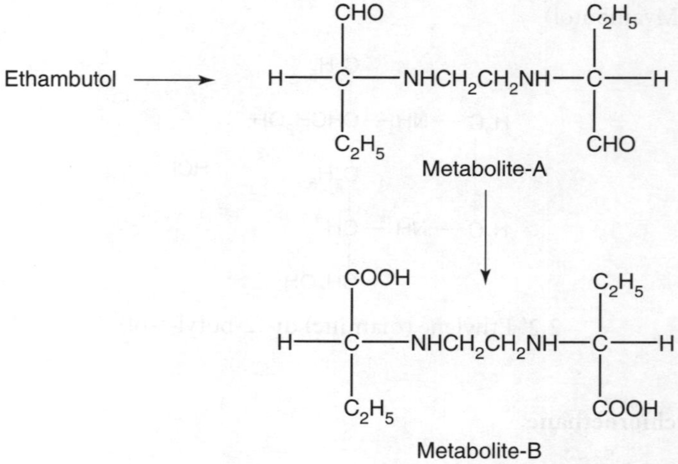

Ethambutol ⟶

Metabolite-A: H—C(CHO)(C₂H₅)—NHCH₂CH₂NH—C(C₂H₅)(CHO)—H

↓

Metabolite-B: H—C(COOH)(C₂H₅)—NHCH₂CH₂NH—C(C₂H₅)(COOH)—H

Mode of action: It is a bacteriostatic drug that inhibits the incorporation of mycolic acid into the mycobacterium cell wall.

Properties and uses: Ethambutol hydrochloride is a white crystalline powder, soluble in water and in alcohol. It is not recommended for use as a single drug, but used in combinations with other antitubercular drugs in the chemotherapy of pulmonary tuberculosis.

Assay: Dissolve and dilute the sample with solution of dilute ammonia, copper sulphate solution, and dilute sodium hydroxide, and measure the angle of optical rotation of the solution at 436 nm.

Dose: The administered dose is 15–25 mg/kg once a day; low doses for new cases, and high doses for use in patients who have had previous antitubercular therapy.

Dosage forms: Ethambutol HCl tablets I.P., Ethambutol tablets B.P.

iv. Rifampicin

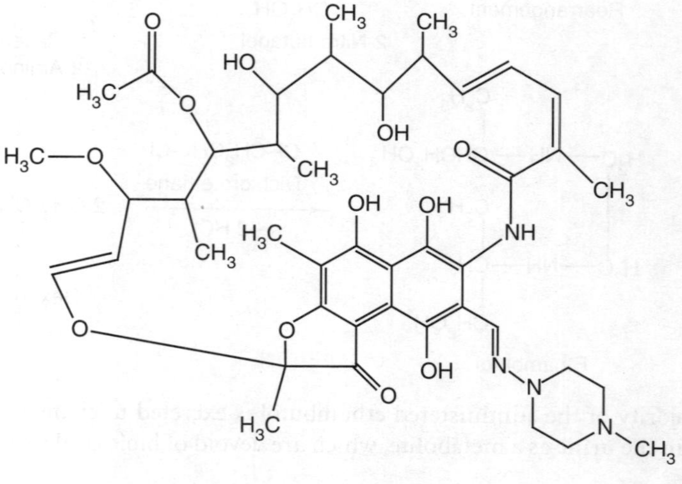

Mode of action: It is an antibiotic obtained from *Streptomyces mediterranei*. Rifampicin inhibits DNA-dependent RNA polymerase of mycobacteria by forming a stable drug enzyme complex, leading to suppression of initiation of chain formation in RNA synthesis and acts as a bactericidal drug.

Metabolism: The major metabolism of rifampicin and rifapentine is deacetylation, which occurs at the C-25 acetate. The resulting products, desacetyl rifampin, and desacetyl rifampentine are still active antibacterial agents. 3-Formylrifamycin has been reported as a second metabolite following both rifampicin and rifampentine administration.

Properties and uses: Rifampicin is a reddish-brown or brownish-red crystalline powder, slightly soluble in water, acetone, alcohol, and soluble in methanol. Rifampicin is the most active agent in clinical use for the treatment of tuberculosis. It is used only in combination with other antitubercular drugs, and it is ordinarily not recommended for the treatment of other bacterial infections when alternative antibacterial agents are available.

Assay: Dissolve and dilute the sample in methanol. Dilute the solution with phosphate buffer solution pH 7.4 and measure the absorbance at the maxima of 475 nm, using phosphate buffer solution pH 7.4 as blank.

Dosage forms: Rifampicin tablets I.P, Rifampicin capsules I.P, B.P., Rifampicin oral suspension B.P.

v. Rifabutin

It is a semisynthetic rifamycin, structurally similar to rifampicin. It is used against *M. avium*, one of the most common causes of disseminated infections, with patients suffering with Human Immunodeficiency Virus (HIV). In vitro activity is attributed to rifabutin's lipophilic nature and its ability to penetrate the cell wall of the organism more effectively than other agents.

Properties and uses: Rifabutin is a reddish-violet amorphous powder, slightly soluble in water and alcohol, soluble in methanol. It is used as an antitubercular drug.

Assay: It is assayed by adopting liquid chromatography technique.

vi. Streptomycin sulphate

Metabolism: The enzymes responsible for inactivation are adenyltransferase, which catalyzes adenylation of the C-3 hydroxyl group in the *N*-methyl glucosamine moiety to give the *O*-3-adenylated metabolite and phosphotransferase, which phosphorylates the same C-3 hydroxyl to give *O*-3 phosphorylated metabolite.

Properties and uses: Streptomycin is a white hygroscopic powder, very soluble in water, and practically insoluble in ethanol. It was the first effective drug for the treatment of tuberculosis. It is most often used in combination with other drugs, such as ethambutol and isoniazid, to treat pulmonary infections in patients with organisms that are known to be resistant. There has been an increasing tendency to reserve streptomycin products for the treatment of tuberculosis.

Assay: It is assayed by adopting microbiological assay method.

Dosage forms: Streptomycin sulphate injection I.P., Streptomycin sulphate tablets I.P., Streptomycin injection B.P.

II. Reserve drugs

i. Ethionamide (Tridocin)

2-Ethylpyridine-4-carbothioamide

Synthesis

Route I. From: 2-Ethyl-4-cyanopyridine

2-Ethyl-4-cyano pyridine →(Partial hydrolysis)→ [amide intermediate] →(H₂S)→ Ethionamide

Route II. From: Ethyl propionyl pyruvate

Ethyl Propionyl pyruvate + 2-Cyanoacetamide → 2-Ethyl-4-carbethoxy-5-cyano-6-pyridone →(i) Partial hydrolysis (ii) –CO₂→ [intermediate] →(H₂O/H⁺)→ [COOH pyridone] →(POCl₃/PCl₅)→ [COCl chloropyridine] →(C₂H₅OH)→ [carbethoxy chloropyridine] →(H₂/Ni)→ [carbethoxy ethyl pyridine] →(NH₃)→ [CONH₂ intermediate] →(POCl₃, –H₂O)→ [CN intermediate] →(C₂H₅OH, H₂S)→ Ethionamide

Mode of action: The antimycobacterial action of ethionamide seems to be due to an inhibitory effect on the mycolic acid synthesis.

Metabolism: Less than 1% of the drug is excreted in the free form, and remainder of the drug appear as six metabolites. Among the metabolites, ethionamide sulphoxide, 2-ethyl-isonicotinamide, and the N-methylated-6-oxo-dihydropyridines are the few.

Properties and uses: Ethionamide is a yellow crystalline powder or crystals, practically insoluble in water, soluble in methanol, and sparingly soluble in alcohol. It is used as antitubercular drug.

Assay: Dissolve the sample in anhydrous acetic acid and titrate with 0.1 M perchloric. Determine the end point potentiometrically.

Dose: The dose to be administered is 500 mg–1 g per day in three or four divided doses with meals.

ii. Para-amino-salicylic acid (PAS, Tubacin)

Mode of action: Aminosalicylic acid is an inhibitor of bacterial folate metabolism in a manner similar to the sulphonamide antibacterials.

Properties and uses: Aminosalicylic acid is bacteriostatic and highly specific for *M. tuberculosis*. Side effects are anorexia, nausea, epigastric pain, diarrhoea, and making poor compliance.

Dose: Dose administered orally 14–16 g daily after meals in three to four divided doses.

Synthesis

Route I. From: Anthranilic acid

Anthranilic acid →[HNO₃ / H₂SO₄]→ 2-amino-4-nitrobenzoic acid →[(i) NaNO₂/HCl (ii) H₂O, Boil]→ 2-hydroxy-4-nitrobenzoic acid →[Sn / HCl]→ *p*-Amino salicylic acid

Route II. From: m-Nitrophenol

3-Nitrophenol →[CO₂ at Controlled pressure Ammonium carbonate]→ 4-nitrosalicylic acid →[Reduction Ni/(H)]→ *p*-Amino salicylic acid

iii. Amikacin

Properties and uses: Amikacin is a white powder, soluble in water, practically insoluble in acetone and in ethanol. It is a semisynthetic aminoglycoside that was first prepared in Japan. It is extremely active against several mycobacterial species, and may become the drug of choice for treatment of diseases caused by nontuberculous mycobacteria.

Assay: It is assayed by adopting liquid chromatography technique.

Dosage forms: Amikacin sulphate injection I.P., Amikacin injection B.P.

iv. Thiacetazone

1-(4-Acetamidobenzylidene)thiosemicarbazide

Synthesis

Uses: It is used as an antitubercular agent.

PROBABLE QUESTIONS

1. What is tuberculosis? How will you categorize it according to the site of infection? Define antitubercular drugs and classify them with suitable examples.
2. Name the pyridine containing antitubercular agents. Outline the synthesis, mode of action, metabolism, dose, and dosage forms available for any one of them.
3. Write the structure, chemical name, and uses of at least two most potent drugs from standard drugs and reserve drugs category.
4. Write a detailed account on pyrazinamide along with its synthesis, mode of action, dosage forms available, and uses.

5. Write the following synthesis:
   (a) Ethambutol (b) Thiacetazone (c) PAS
6. Write a note on antibiotics used in tuberculosis.

SUGGESTED READINGS

1. Abraham DJ (ed). *Burger's Medicinal Chemistry and Drug Discovery* (6th edn). New Jersey: John Wiley, 2007.
2. Banerjee A, Dubnau E, Quemard A, Balasubramanian V, Um KS, Wilson T, Collins D, de Lisle G, Jacobs WR Jr. 'inhA: A gene encoding a target for isoniazid and ethionamide in *Mycobacterium tuberculosis*'. *Science* 263: 227–30, 1994.
3. *British Pharmacopoeia*. Medicines and Healthcare Products Regulatory Agency. London. 2008.
4. Bruntan LL, Lazo JS, and Parker KL. *Goodman and Gilman's: The Pharmacological Basis of Therapeutics*, (11th edn). New York: McGraw Hill, 2006.
5. Gennaro AR. *Remington: The Science and Practice of Pharmacy* (21st edn). New York: Lippincot Williams and Wilkins, 2006.
6. Goldberger MJ. 'Antituberculous agents'. *Med Clin North Am* 72: 661, 1988.
7. Holdiners MR. 'Management of tuberculosis meningitis'. *Drugs* 39: 224, 1990.
8. *Indian Pharmacopoeia*. Ministry of Health and Family Welfare. New Delhi, 1996.
9. Lane HC, Laughon BE, Falloon J, Kovacs JA, Davey RT Jr, Polis MA, and Masur H. 'Recent advances in the management of AIDS-related opportunistic infections'. *Ann Intern Med* 120: 945–955, 1994.
10. Lednicer D and Mitscher LA. *The Organic Chemistry of Drug Synthesis*. New York: John Wiley, 1995.
11. Lemke TL and William DA. *Foye's Principle of Medicinal Chemistry* (6th edn). New York: Lippincott Williams and Wilkins, 2008.
12. Mendell GL, Douglas RG Jr, and Bennett JE (eds). *Principles and Practice of Infections Diseases* (3rd edn), pp. 295–303. New York: Churchill Livingstone, 1990.
13. Wallace RJ Jr, Bedsole G, and Sumter G. 'Activities of ciprofloxacin and ofloxacin against rapidly growing mycobacteria with demonstration of acquired resistance following single-drug therapy'. *Antimicrob Agents Chemother* 34(1): 65–70, 1990.

Chapter 6

Antifungal Agents

INTRODUCTION

Human-fungi-parasitic relationship result in mycotic illnesses. Most fungal infections (mycoses) involve superficial invasion of the skin or mucous membrane of the body orifices. These diseases can usually be controlled by local application of the antifungal agents. Fungi have different shapes and sizes. Some are large while others are minute, parasitic, and saprophytic cells. They differ from the following organisms in some important aspects:

- Algae by lack of photosynthetic ability.
- Protozoa by the lack of motility, possession of chitinuous cell wall, and ease of culture on simple media.
- Bacteria by greater size and having certain intracellular structure such as mitochondria and nuclear membrane.

CLASSIFICATION

On the basis of some differences, fungi may be classified as follows:

a. Phyco myelitis (algae-like)
b. Asco myelitis (sac-like)
c. Basidio myelitis (mushrooms)
d. Duetero myelitis

The potentially effective antifungal compounds are listed in Table 5.1.

Classification Based on the Chemical Structure, Action, and Source

The antifungal agents can be divided into the following classes, based on their chemical structure, mechanism of action, and source:

I. Antibiotics: Amphotericin B, Nystatin, Griseofulvin
II. Azoles (imidazole, triazole derivates)

Table 5.1 Potentially effective antifungal compounds.

Disease	Compounds
Dermatophytoses	Azoles (Butoconazole, Clotrimazole, Econazole, Itraconazole, Miconazole, Oxiconazole, Sulconazole), Griseofulvin, Naftifine, Terbinafine, Tolnaftate
Aspergillosis	Amphotericin B, 5-Fluorocytosin, Itraconazole
Blastomycosis	Amphotericin B, Itraconazole, Ketoconazole
Candidiasis	Amphotercin B, 5-Fluorocytosine, Nystatin Azoles (Butaconazole, Clotrimazole, Econazole, Fluconazole, Itraconazole, Ketoconazole, Miconazole, Terconazole, Tioconazole)
Chromomycosis	5-Fluorocytosine, Itraconazole, Ketocanozole
Coccidiodomycosis	Amphotericin B, Fluconazole, Itraconazolel, Ketoconazole
Cryptococcosis	Amphotericin B, Fluconazole
Histoplasmosis	Amphrotericin B, Itraconazole, Ketoconazole
Mucormycosis	Amyphotericin B
Paracoccidioidomicosis	Itraconazole, Ketoconazole
Pneumocytosis	Trimethoprim, Sulphamethoazole, Pentamidine, ecothionate
Pseudallescheriasis	Amphotericin B, Miconazole
Sporotrichosis	Amphotericin B, Itraconazole, Potassium iodide

      Triazoles—Fluconazole, Itraconzole, Terconazole
      Imidazoles—Clotrimazole, Ketoconazole, Miconazole, Bifonazole, Butoconazole, and Zinoconazole
III. Fluorinated pyrimidines: Flucytosine
IV. Chitin synthetase inhibitors: Nikomycin Z
V. Peptides/proteins: Cispentacin
VI. Miscellaneous: Ciclopirox, Tolnaftate, Naftifine, and Terbinafine

Classification Based on the Route of Administration

I. Drugs for subcutaneous and systemic mycoses: Amphotericin B, Fluconazole, Flucytosine, Itraconazole, Ketoconazole.
II. Drugs for superficial mycoses: Clotrimazole, Econazole, Griseofluvin, Miconazole, Nystatin.

SYNTHESIS AND DRUG PROFILE

I. Antibiotics
1. Amphotericin B

Mode of action: The antifungal activity of this drug depends, at least, in part, on its binding to a sterol moiety. Primarily, ergosterol that is present in the membrane of sensitive fungi, by virtue of their interaction with the sterols of cell membranes and polyenes, appear to form pores or channels. The result is an increase in the permeability of the membrane, allowing leakage of a variety of small molecules, such as intracellular potassium, magnesium, sugars, and metabolites leading to cellular death.

Properties and uses: It is polyene antibiotic obtained from *Streptomyces nodosus*. It is an amphoteric compound that consists of seven-conjugated double bond, an internal ester, a free carbonyl group, and a glycoside side chain with a primary amino group. The carbohydrate moiety is D-mycosamine. The conjugated systems are usually of all *trans* configurations, so that the ring contains a planner lipophilic segment and a less rigid hydrophilic portion. Amphotericin B is an amphoteric, forming soluble salts in both basic and acidic environments, and due to extensive unsaturation, it is unstable, primarily used as antifungal agents.

2. Griseofulvin (Fulvicin)

Mode of action: Griseofulvin is a fungi-static drug that causes disruption of the mitotic spindle by interacting with polymerized microtubules.

Properties and uses: Griseofulvin is a white or yellowish-white microfine powder, practically insoluble in water, freely soluble in dimethylformamide and tetrachloroethane, slightly soluble in ethanol and methanol. Used as an antifungal agent.

Synthesis

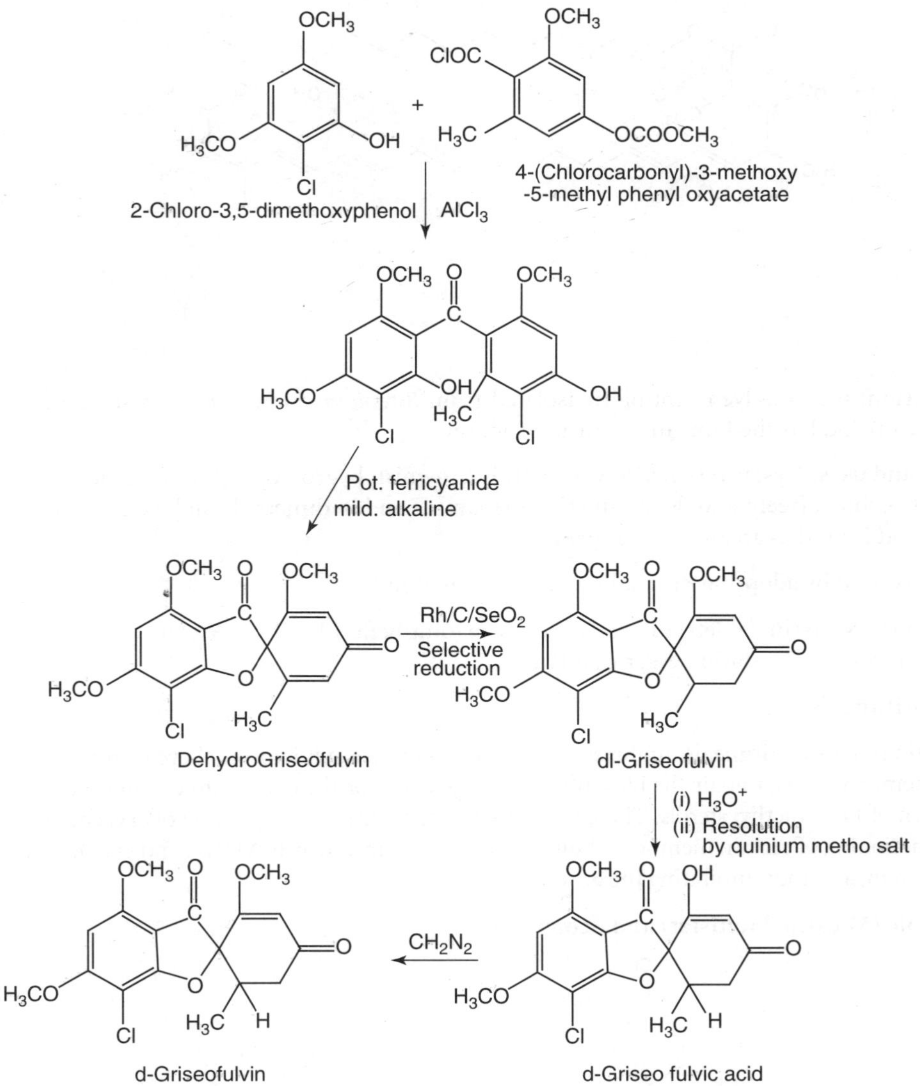

[Scheme: 2-Chloro-3,5-dimethoxyphenol + 4-(Chlorocarbonyl)-3-methoxy-5-methyl phenyl oxyacetate → (AlCl₃) → benzophenone intermediate → (Pot. ferricyanide, mild alkaline) → DehydroGriseofulvin → (Rh/C/SeO₂, Selective reduction) → dl-Griseofulvin → (i) H₃O⁺ (ii) Resolution by quinium metho salt → d-Griseo fulvic acid → (CH₂N₂) → d-Griseofulvin]

Assay: Dissolve the sample in ethanol and measure the absorbance after dilution with ethanol at the maxima of 291 nm using ultraviolet spectrophotometer.

Dose: As an oral suspension, the administered dose is 125 mg/5 ml; as capsules, 250 or 500 mg as tablets. For adults, in divided doses, the dose is 500 mg/day.

Dosage forms: Griseofulvin tablets I.P., B.P.

3. Nystatin

Mode of action: It is a polyene antibiotic isolated from *Streptomyces noursei*. It is structurally similar to amphotericin B and has the same mechanism of action.

Properties and uses: Nystatin is a yellow or slightly brownish hygroscopic powder, practically insoluble in water and in alcohol, freely soluble in dimethylformamide and in dimethyl sulphoxide, and slightly soluble in methanol. It is used as an antifungal agent.

Assay: It is assayed by adopting microbiological assay method.

Dosage forms: Nystatin tablets I.P., B.P., Nystatin ointment I.P., B.P., Nystatin oral suspension B.P., Nystatin pastilles B.P., Nystatin pessaries B.P.

II. Azole antifungals

Mode of action: Azole antifungals inhibit sterol 14-α-demethylase, a microsomal cytochrome P450-dependent enzyme system, and thus, impair the biosynthesis of ergosterol for the cytoplasmic membrane and lead to the accumulation of 14-α-methyl sterols. These methylsterols may disrupt the packing of aryl chains of phospholipids, the functioning of certain membrane bound enzyme systems, such as ATPase and enzymes of the electron transport system, and thus, inhibiting the growth of fungi.

1. Miconazole (Micatin, Monistat) and Econazole

Miconazole

Econazole

Synthesis

Synthesis of Miconazole and Econazole

Properties and uses of Miconazole: Miconazole is a white or almost white powder, very slightly soluble in water, sparingly soluble in methanol, and slightly soluble in alcohol. It is used as an antifungal agent.

Assay: Dissolve the sample in anhydrous acetic acid, with slight heating, if necessary, and titrate with 0.1 M perchloric acid. Determine the end point potentiometrically.

Dose: It is to be applied in the vagina at bedtime for seven days, and 200 mg vaginal suppositories for three days therapy.

Dosage forms: Miconazole cream I.P., B.P., Miconazole pessaries I.P., Miconazole tablets I.P., Miconazole and Hydrocortisone cream B.P., Miconazole and Hydrocortisone acetate cream B.P., Miconazole and Hydrocortisone ointment B.P.

Properties and uses of Econazole: Econazole is white or almost white crystalline powder, very slightly soluble in water, soluble in methanol, sparingly soluble in methylene chloride, and slightly soluble in alcohol. It is used as antifungal agent.

Assay: Dissolve the sample in anhydrous acetic acid and titrate with 0.1 M perchloric acid. Determine the end point potentiometrically.

Dose: It is available as a water insoluble cream (1%) to be applied twice a day.

Dosage forms: Econazole cream B.P., Econazole pessaries B.P.

2. Ketoconazole (Nizoral) and Terconazole

Ketoconazole

Terconazole

Metabolism of Ketoconazole: It is extensively metabolized by deacetylase of the microsomal enzymes and all the metabolites are inactive.

Properties and uses of Ketoconazole: Ketoconazole is a white powder, practically insoluble in water, soluble in methylene chloride and in methanol, sparingly soluble in alcohol. It is a racemic compound, consisting of the *cis*-2S, 4R, and *cis*-2R, 4S isomers. An investigation of the relative potencies of the four possible diastereomers of ketoconazole against rat lanosterol 1,4α-demethylase indicated that the 2S, 4R isomer was 2.5 times more active than its 2R, 4S enantiomer and the *trans* isomers, 2S, 4S, and 2R, 4R are much less active. Ketoconazole is an imidazole antifungal agent, which is a highly lipophilic compound. This property leads to high concentrations of ketoconazole in fatty tissues and purulent exudates. Ketoconazole is active against *Candida* spp and *Cryptococcus neoformans*.

Assay of Ketoconazole: Dissolve the sample in a mixture of anhydrous acetic acid and methyl ethyl ketone (1:7) and titrate with 0.1 M perchloric acid. Determine the end point potentiometrically.

Dose: It is administered as 200 mg scored tablets and 2% topical cream.

Synthesis

2,4-Dichloro acetophenone → (Glycerol, Tosic acid) → dioxolane intermediate → (Br₂/30°C) → bromomethyl dioxolane → (i) C₆H₅COCl/Pyridine; (ii) C₂H₅OH → benzoate ester with CH₂Br → (imidazole/triazole) → azole-substituted benzoate → (i) NaOH; (ii) CH₃SO₂Cl → mesylate → (NaO–C₆H₄–piperazine–N–R) →

Ketaconazole R=COCH₃, X=CH
Terconazole R=CH(CH₃)₂, X=N

Metabolism of Terconzole: It is metabolized by CYP3A4 on oral administration.

Properties and uses of Terconzole: Terconazole is a white powder, practically insoluble in water, soluble in methylene chloride and in acetone, sparingly soluble in alcohol. It is a triazole derivative that is used exclusively for the control of *Vulvovaginal moniliasis* caused by *Candida albicans* and other *Candida spp*.

Assay of Terconzole: Dissolve the sample in a mixture of anhydrous acetic acid and volumes of methyl ethyl ketone (1:7) and titrate with 0.1 M perchloric acid. Determine the end point potentiometrically at the second point of inflexion.

Dose: The administered dose is 80 gm vaginal suppository at bedtime for three days; and 0.4% as vaginal cream for seven days.

3. Clotrimazole (Clotrimin, Mycelex)

1-((2-Chlorophenyl)diphenylmethyl)-1*H*-imidazole

Synthesis

1-[(2-Chlorophenyl)diphenyl]methyl chloride + Imidazole $\xrightarrow{-HCl}$ Clotrimazole

Properties and uses: Clotrimazole is a white or pale yellow crystalline powder, practically insoluble in water, soluble in alcohol and in methylene chloride. It is used as an antifungal agent.

Assay: Dissolve the sample in anhydrous acetic acid and titrate with 0.1 M perchloric acid using naphtholbenzein as indicator until the colour changes from brownish-yellow to green.

Dose: The administered dose is usually as 100 mg tablet per day at bedtime for seven days for vaginal infection.

Dosage forms: Clotrimazole cream I.P., B.P., Clotrimazole pessaries I.P., B.P.

4. Fluconazole (Syscan, Zocon, Flucos)

2-(2,4-Difluorophenyl)-1,3-di(1H-1,2,4-triazol-1-yl)propan-2-ol

Synthesis

3-Chloro-1-(2,4-difluorophenyl)propan-1-one + 1H-1,2,4-triazole $\xrightarrow{-HCl}$ [intermediate] $\xrightarrow{NaH \mid Me_3Si^{\oplus\ominus}}$ [epoxide]

1H-1,2,4-Triazole + [epoxide] $\xrightarrow{HCl}$ Fluconazole

Properties and uses: Flucanazole is a white hygroscopic crystalline powder, slightly soluble in water, and soluble in methanol and in acetone. It is a widely used *bis*-triazole antifungal agent. It is generally considered to be a fungi-static agent, and it is principally active against *Candida* spp and *Cryptococcus* spp. Fluconazole has useful activity against *Coccidioides immitis,* and is often used to suppress the meningitis produced by the fungus.

Assay: Dissolve the sample in anhydrous acetic acid and titrate with 0.1 M perchloric acid. Determine the end point potentiometrically.

Dose: The administered dose for superficial mucosal candidiasis for adults is 50 mg daily, which is increased to 100 mg daily. Recommended treatment duration is 7–14 days; in the case of oropharyngeal candidiasis, 14 days for atrophic oral candidiasis associated with dentures, 14–30 days for other mucosal candidal infections, including oesophagitis. In the case of children, more than 4 weeks the loading dose is 6 mg/kg followed by 3 mg/kg daily.

The administered dose for dermatophytosis, pityriasis versicolor, and candida infections for adults is 50 mg daily for up to 6 weeks.

The administered dose for cryptococcal infections, including meningitis, systemic candidasis for adults, initially is 400 mg followed by 200–400 mg daily; the maximum dose is 800 mg daily in the case of severe infections. In the case of cryptococcal meningitis, usual treatment duration is at least 6–8 weeks and may also be given via IV infusion. For children more than 4 weeks the dose is 6–12 mg/kg daily; same doses may be given every 72 h in neonates up to 2 weeks and every 48 h in neonates 2–4weeks old; the maximum dose is 400 mg daily.

5. Butoconazole

1-(4-(4-Chlorophenyl)-2-(2,6-dichlorophenylthio)butyl)-1*H*-imidazole

Synthesis

6. Bifonazole

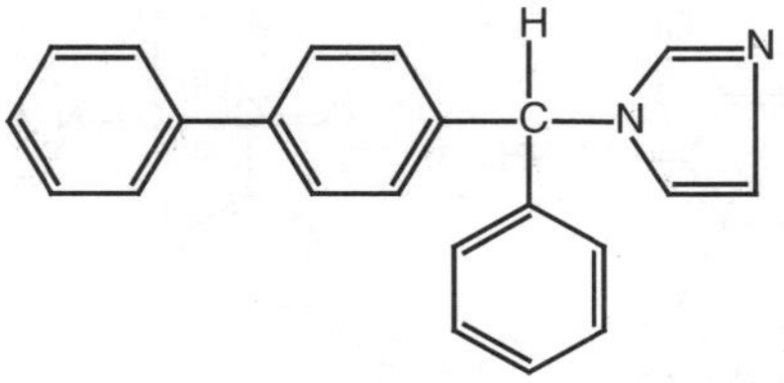

Synthesis

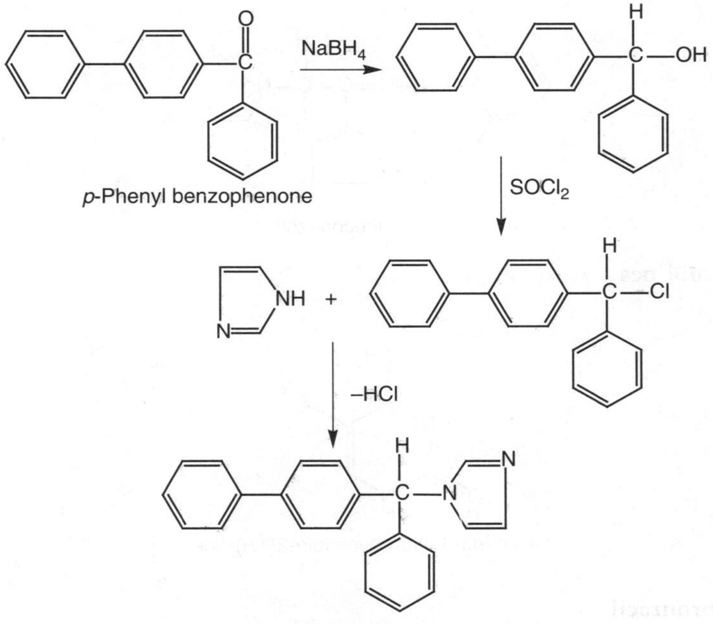
NaBH4
p-Phenyl benzophenone
SOCl2
–HCl
Bifonazole

Properties and uses: Bifonazole is a white crystalline powder, practically insoluble in water, and sparingly soluble in anhydrous ethanol. It is used as an antifungal agent.

Assay: Dissolve the sample in anhydrous acetic acid and titrate with 0.1 M perchloric acid. Determine the end point potentiometrically.

7. Zinoconazole

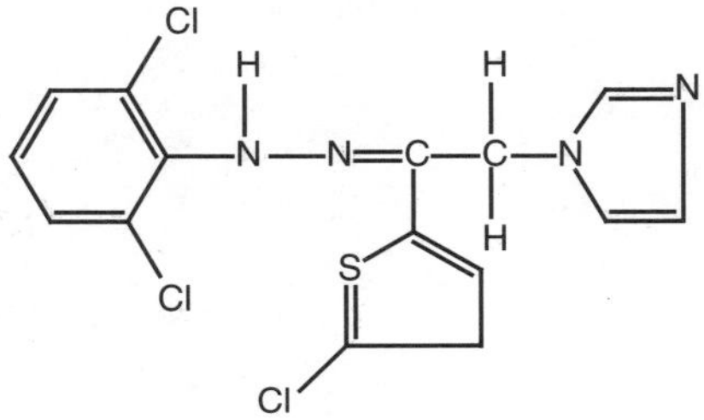

Synthesis:

[2,6-Dichloro phenyl hydrazine] + [imidazole-thiophene ketone] → **Zinoconazole**

III. Fluorinated pyrimidines

1. Flucytosine

4-Amino-5-fluoropyrimidin-2(1H)-one

Synthesis
Route I. From: 5-Fluorouracil

5-Fluoro uracil →(P_2S_5)→ 5-Fluoro pyrimidine-2-one-4-thione →($SOCl_2$)→ [4-chloro-5-fluoro intermediate] →(NH_3)→ **Flucytosine**

Route II. From: 5-Fluorouracil

Mode of action: Flucytosine is converted by cytosine deaminase into 5-flurouracil (5-FU), then, 5-fluoro deoxyuridylic acid is formed. This false nucleotide inhibits thymidylate synthetase, thus, depriving the organism of thymidylic acid, an essential DNA component. It is a potent antimetabolite, which replaces uracil in the pyrimidine pool and thus, disrupts protein synthesis. Mammalian cells do not convert flucytosine to fluorouracil. This fact is crucial for the selective action of this compound. In addition, 5-fluorouracil is metabolized into 5-fluoro uridylic acid by the enzyme uridine monophosphate (UMP) pyrophosphorylase. It is either incorporated into the DNA (via synthesis of 5-fluorouridine triphosphate) or would be metabolized into 5-fluoro deoxyuridylic acid, which is a potent inhibitor of thymidylate synthetase.

Metabolism: It is metabolized to 5-FU by fungal cytidine deaminase.

Then 5-FU is converted into 5-fluorodeoxyuridine, which is a thymidylate synthase inhibitor and interferes with both protein and RNA biosynthesis.

Properties and uses: Flucytosine is a white crystalline powder, sparingly soluble in water, and slightly soluble in ethanol. Flucytosine is the only available antimetabolite drug having antifungal activity.

Assay: Dissolve the sample in anhydrous acetic acid, add acetic anhydride, and titrate with 0.1 M perchloric acid. Determine the end point potentiometrically.

Dosage forms: Flucytosine tablets B.P.

IV. Chitin synthetase inhibitors

1. Nikomycin

Mode of action: Nikomycin competitively inhibits the chitin synthase, mimicking its substrate uridine diphosphate-*N*-acetyl glucosamine of fungi with *C. albicans* as the primary target organism. The enzyme is an integral membrane protein. Nikomycin Z has shown to act synergistically in vitro with fluconazole, ketoconzole, and tioconazole against *C. albicans* at minimum inhibitory concentration (MIC) levels of azoles.

Properties and uses: Nikomycin is a nucleoside peptide antibiotic that is produced by soil strains of *Steptomyces tendae*. It is found to be more potent than most azoles in inhibiting highly chitinous, dimorphic fungal pathogens, such as *Coccidiodes imitis* and *Blastomyces dermatidis*.

V. Peptides\proteins

Examples—L-Norvalyl FMIP, Cispentacin

i. L-Norvalyl—FMIP

(*E*)-2-(2-Aminopentanamido)-3-(4-methoxy-4-oxobut-2-enamido) propanoic acid

Mode of action: The inhibitors of glucosamine-6-phosphate synthase delivered through peptide transport systems have been reported as having anticandidal activity.

ii. *cis* Pentacin

2-Aminocyclopentane carboxylic acid

Properties and uses: It is dipeptide analogue that is shown in vitro and in vivo activity against *C. albicans*.

VI. Miscellaneous agents

1. Naftifine (Nabtin)

N-Methyl-*N*-(naphthalen-1-yl-methyl)-3-phenylprop-2-en-1-amine

Synthesis

N-methyl-(1-naphthyl)-methylamine + Cinnamyl chloride $\xrightarrow{Na_2CO_3}$ Naftifine

Mode of action: The drug has fungicidal activity against *Tinea cruris* and *Corporis* spp. This inhibits squalene 2,3-epoxidase and thus, inhibits fungal biosynthesis of ergosterol.

Dose: It is administered as 1% cream twice daily.

2. Ciclopirox

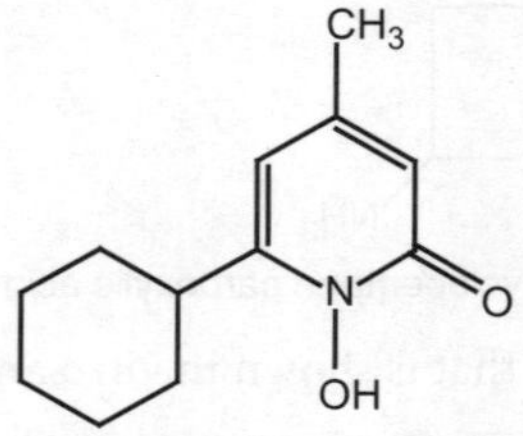

6-Cyclohexyl-1-hydroxy-4-methylpyridin-2(1H)-one

Synthesis

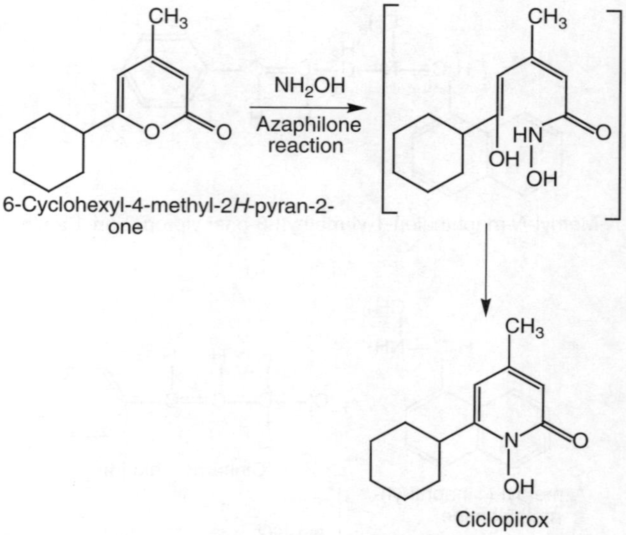

6-Cyclohexyl-4-methyl-2H-pyran-2-one

NH_2OH
Azaphilone reaction

Ciclopirox

Properties and uses: Ciclopirox is a white or yellowish-white crystalline powder, slightly soluble in water, soluble in ethanol and in methylene chloride. It is available as 1% cream on cotton for the treatment of cutaneous candidiasis and for *Tinea corporis, T. cruris, T. pedis,* and *Pityriasis versicolour*.

Assay: Dissolve the sample in methanol, add water, and titrate with 0.1 M sodium hydroxide. Determine the end point potentiometrically.

4. Tolnaftate

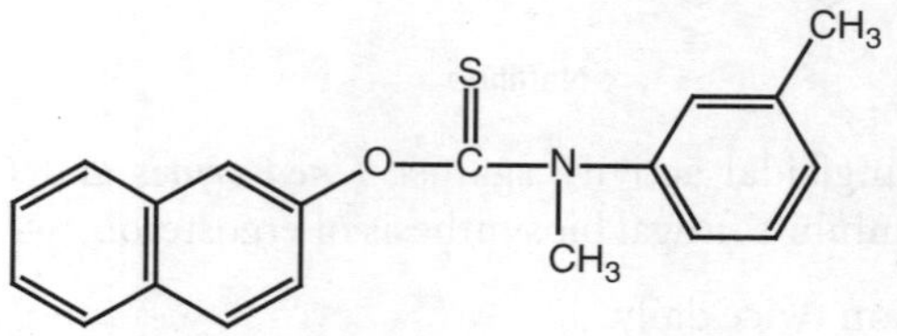

O-(Naphthalen-2-yl)*N*-methyl(*m*-tolyl)carbamothioate

Synthesis

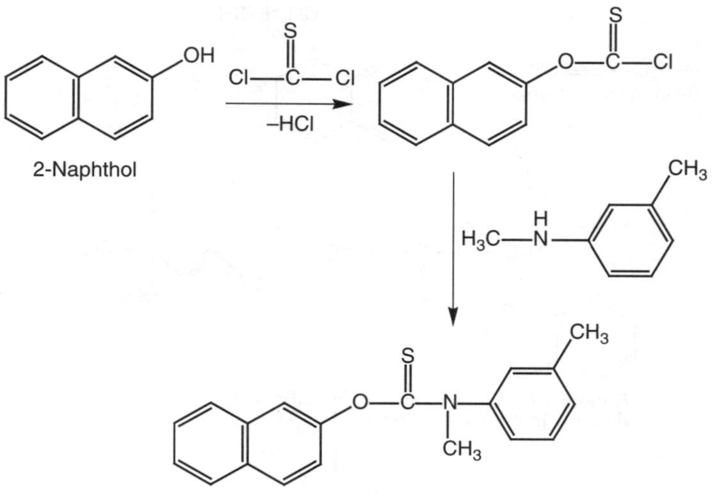

2-Naphthol

Tolnaflate

Properties and uses: Tolnaftate is a white or yellowish-white powder practically insoluble in water, soluble in acetone and in methylene chloride, and very slightly soluble in alcohol. It is effective for the treatment of most cutaneous mycoses, such as *Trichophyton rubrum* and *Microsporum canis*. Replacement of the aromatic methyl group by hydroxy or methoxy or its removal does not affect potency. Replacement of the complete tolyl group by a α-napthyl or a β-napthyl substituent does not decrease its potency. It is nontoxic.

Dose: The administered dose is 1% as a cream, gel, powder, aerosol powder, and topical solution, applied locally twice a day.

Assay: Dissolve the sample in methanol, measure the absorbance, after its dilution with methanol, at the maxima at 257 nm, using ultraviolet spectrophotometer.

5. Terbinafine

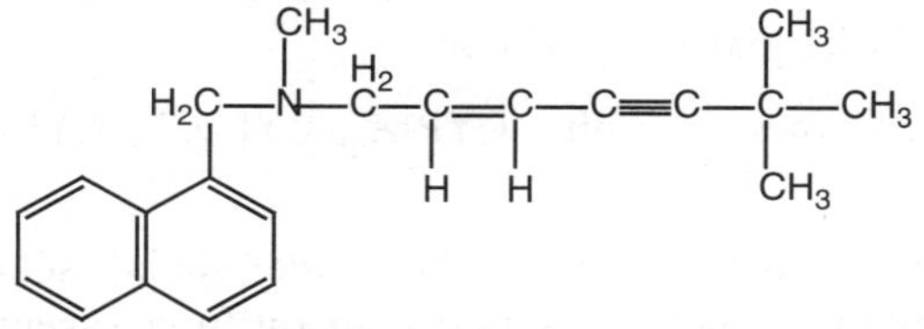

N,6,6-Trimethyl-N-(naphthalen-1-yl methyl)hept-2-en-4-yn-1-amine

Synthesis

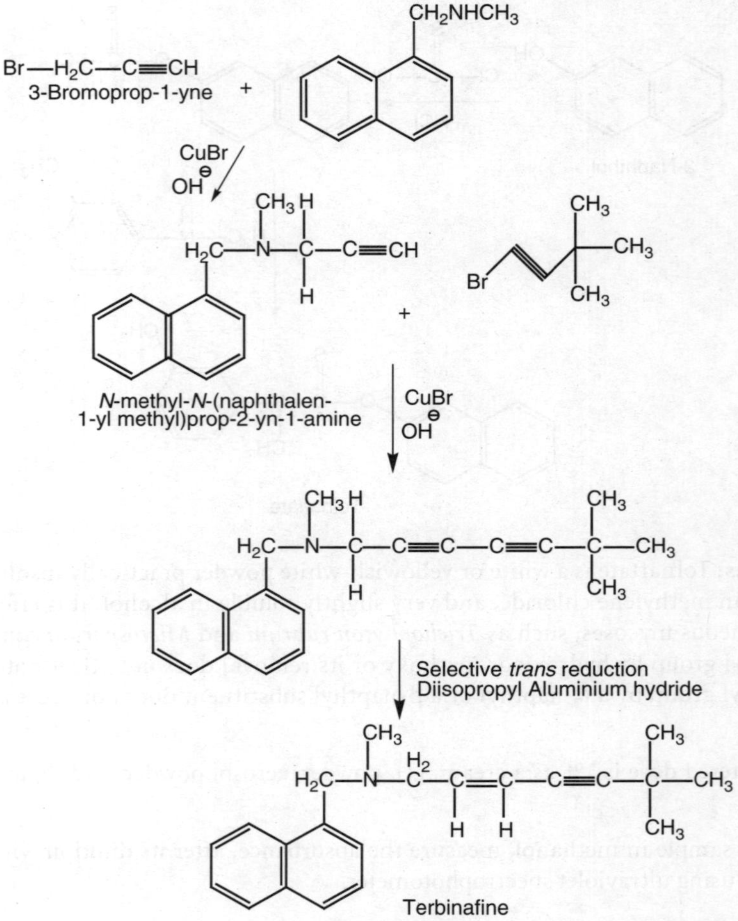

[Scheme: 3-Bromoprop-1-yne (Br—H₂C—C≡CH) + N-methylaminomethyl naphthalene (naphthalene with CH₂NHCH₃) → with CuBr / OH⁻ → N-methyl-N-(naphthalen-1-yl methyl)prop-2-yn-1-amine + 1-bromo-3-methyl-3-methyl-but-1-ene (Br—CH=CH—C(CH₃)₂—CH₃) → with CuBr / OH⁻ → diyne intermediate → Selective *trans* reduction, Diisopropyl Aluminium hydride → Terbinafine]

Mode of action: The uses and mechanism of action of terbinafine are the same as those of naffine. It is active by virtue of its ability to block squalene epoxidase.

Metabolism: Several CYP450 enzymes, including $CYP1A_2$, $CYP2C1_9$, $CYP2C_9$, $CYP2C_8$, $CYP3A_4$, and $CYP2B_6$, extensively metabolize it.

Properties and uses: Terbinafine hydrochloride is a white powder, slightly soluble in water and in acetone, soluble in anhydrous ethanol and in methanol. It is used as an antifungal agent.

Assay: Dissolve the sample in ethanol, add 0.01 M hydrochloric acid, and titrate with 0.1 M sodium hydroxide. Determine the end point potentiometrically.

PROBABLE QUESTIONS

1. Define and classify antifungal agents. Write the synthesis and uses of any two of them.
2. Enumerate the various fungal diseases and mention the drugs used against those diseases.
3. Write a note on azoles used in fungal infection.
4. Write the synthesis and uses of tolnaftate, clotrimazole, and griseofulvin.

SUGGESTED READINGS

1. Abraham DJ (ed). *Burger's Medicinal Chemistry and Drug Discovery* (6th edn). New Jersey: John Wiley, 2007.
2. Barrett JF and Klaubert DH. 'Recent advances in antifungal agents'. *Ann Rept Med Chem* 27: 149–58, 1992.
3. *British Pharmacopoeia*, Medicines and Healthcare Products Regulatory Agency. London 2008.
4. Bruntan LL, Lazo JS, and Parker KL. *Goodman and Gilman's: The Pharmacological Basis of Therapeutics* (11th edn). New York: McGraw Hill, 2006.
5. Cohen J. 'Antifungal chemotherapy'. *Lancet* 2: 532, 1982.
6. Debono M and Goordee RS. 'Antibiotics that inhibit fungal cell wall development'. *Annu Rev Microbiol* 48: 471–497, 1994.
7. Gennaro AR. *Remington: The Science and Practice of Pharmacy* (21st edn). New York: Lippincot Williams and Wilkins, 2006.
8. *Indian Pharmacopoeia*, Ministry of Health and Family Welfare. New Delhi. 1996.
9. Kobayashi GS and Medoff G. 'Antifungal agents—recent developments'. *Ann Rev Microbiol* 31: 291–308, 1977.
10. Lemke TL and William DA. *Foye's Principle of Medicinal Chemistry* (6th edn). New York: Lippincott Williams and Wilkins, 2008.
11. Lednicer D and Mitscher LA. *The Organic Chemistry of Drug Synthesis*, New York: John Wiley, 1995.
12. Lyman CA and Walgh TJ. 'Systemically administered antifungal agents'. *Drugs* 44(1): 9–35, 1992.
13. McKinley DS and Rapp RP. 'Selecting the right antifungal agent'. *US Pharma* 34–36, 1992.
14. Zervos M and Meunier F. 'Flucoazole—a review'. *Int J Antimicrob Agents* 3: 147–70, 1993.

Chapter 7

Antiviral Agents

INTRODUCTION

Antiviral agents are substances used in the treatment and prophylaxis of diseases caused by viruses. Viral diseases include influenza, rabies, yellow fever, poliomyelitis, ornithosis, mumps, measles, ebola, human immuno deficiency virus (HIV), herpes, warts, and small pox. Viruses are not proper living things, but consists of a genome; they are smaller in size with simple chemical composition, sometimes a few enzymes stored in a capsule made up of protein and rarely covered with a lipid layer. The viruses only replicate within the host cell and the viral replication depends primarily on the metabolic processes of the invaded cell. Viruses does not possess cell wall, but they have RNA or DNA enclosed in a shell of protein known as capsid. The capsid is composed of several subunits known as capsomers. In certain cases, capsid may be surrounded by an outer protein or lipoprotein envelope. One group of RNA virus that deserves special mention are reteroviruses. They are responsible for acquired immuno deficiency syndrome (AIDS) and T-leukaemias. Reteroviruses contain reverse transcriptase (RT) enzyme activity that makes a DNA copy of the viral RNA template. Then, the DNA copy is integrated into the host genome, at which it is referred to as provirus and is transcribed into both the genomic RNA and mRNA for translocation into the viral proteins, giving generation to new virus particles. Viral life cycle varies according to the species, but they all share a general pattern that can be sequenced as follows (Fig. 7.1):

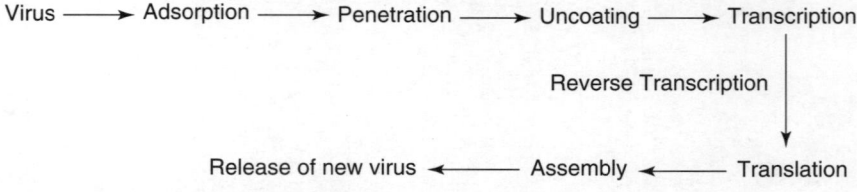

Figure 7.1 Life cycle of virus.

- **Adsorption:** Attachment of the virus to the host cell.
- **Penetration:** Penetration of virus into the cell.
- **Uncoating:** The genetic material or viral genome (DNA or RNA) passes into the host cell leaving the capsid covering outside the host cell.

- **Transcription:** Production of the viral mRNA from the viral genome.
- **Translation:** The viral genome enters the cytoplasm or the nucleoplasma and directs or utilizes the host nucleic acid machinery for the synthesis of the new viral protein and for the production of more viral genome. The viral protein modifies the host cell and allows the viral genome to replicate by using host and viral enzyme. This is often the stage at which the cell is irreversibly modified and eventually killed.
- **Assembly of the viral particle:** New viral coat protein assembles into capsid and viral genomes.
- Release of the mature virus from the cell and the budding process or rupture of the cell and repeat of the process, in a fresh host cell.

Since the host cell machinery is totally utilized for the production of new virions, the normal cell function is affected. Antiviral agents have been developed to act at various stages in the viral replication cycle, such as attachments, replication, and release of the virus.

Some virus types together with diseases that they cause are listed in Table 7.1.

Table 7.1 Examples of viruses with diseases.

Virus	Diseases
DNA virus	
Pox virus	Small pox
Herpes virus	Chicken pox, Shingles herpes, Glandulan fever
Adenovirus	Sore throat, Conjunctivitis
Papilloma virus	Warts
Parvo virus	Canine distemper
RNA viruses	
Orthomyxovirus	Influenza
Paramn virus	Measles, mumps, rabies
Rhabdo virus	Colds, meningitis
Picor virus	Poliomyelitis
Retrovirus	AIDS, T-cell leukaemia
Arena virus	Meningitis, Lassa fever
Hepadna virus	Serum hepatitis
Reo virus	Diarrhoea
Filo virus	Ebola, Marburg
Bunya virus	Encephalitis, haemorrhagic fever

CLASSIFICATION

Classification According to its Mechanism of Action

Antiviral drugs may be classified on the basis of its mechanism of action as follows:

I. Nucleoside RT inhibitors
a. Purine nucleosides and nucleotides

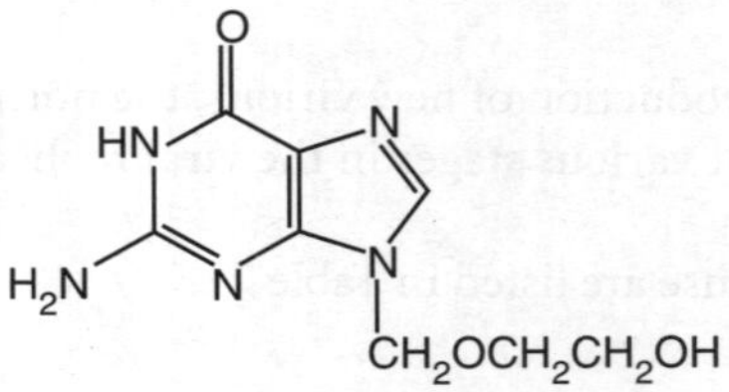

Aciclovir

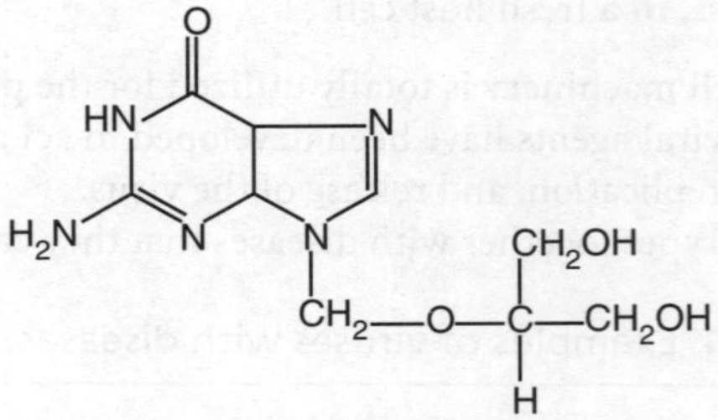

Ganciclovir

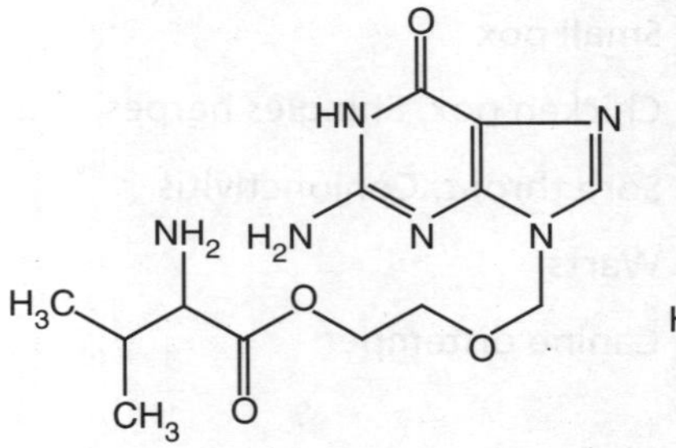

Valaciclovir

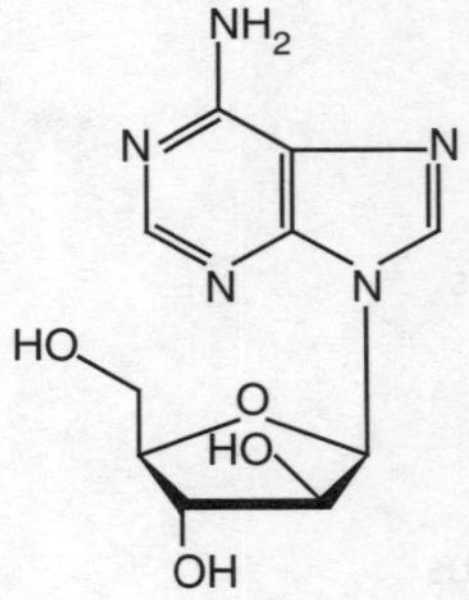

Vidarabine

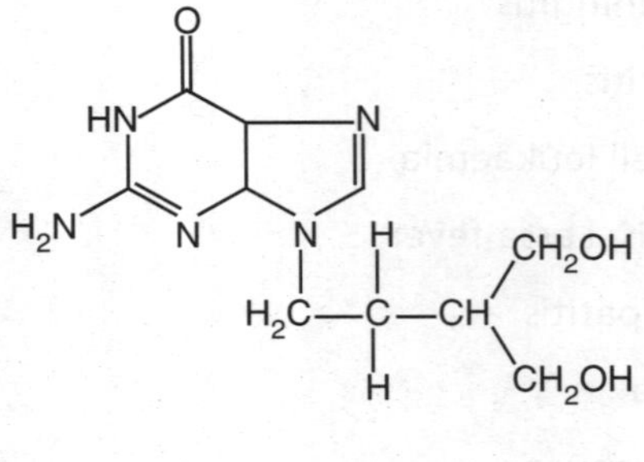

Penciclovir

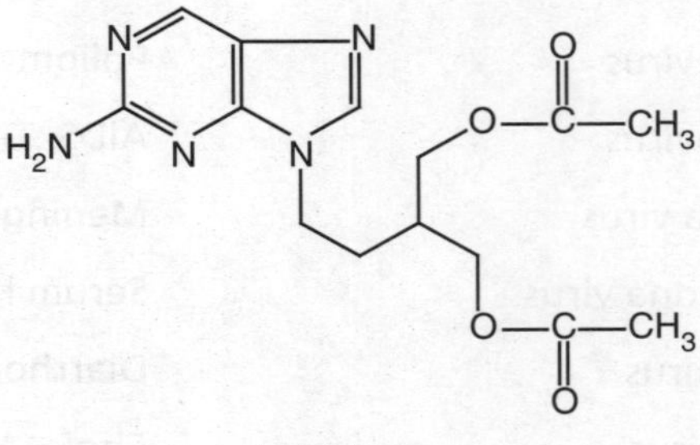

Famciclovir

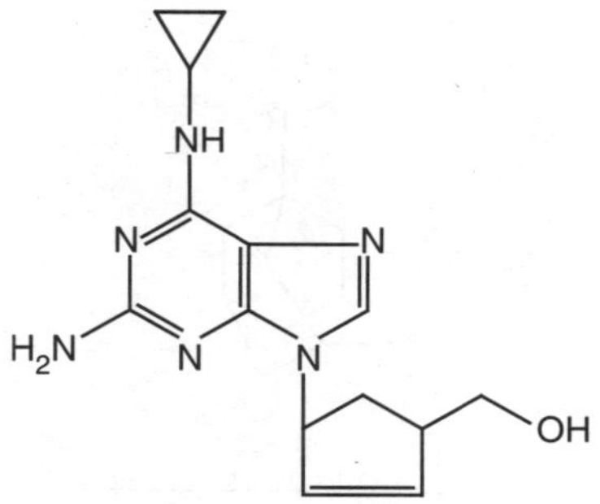

Abacavir

b. Pyrimidine nucleosides and nucleotides

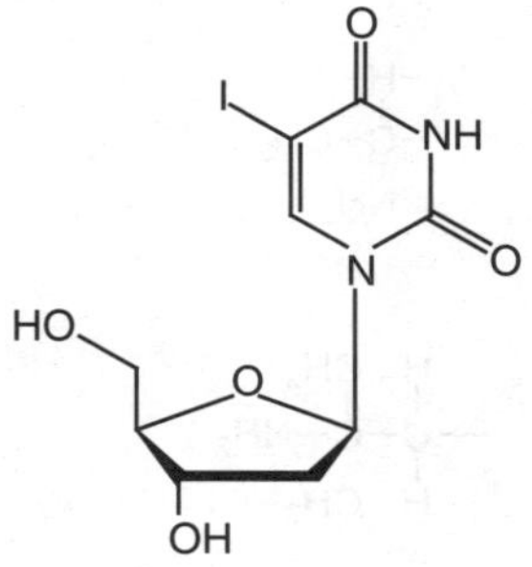

Iodoxuridine

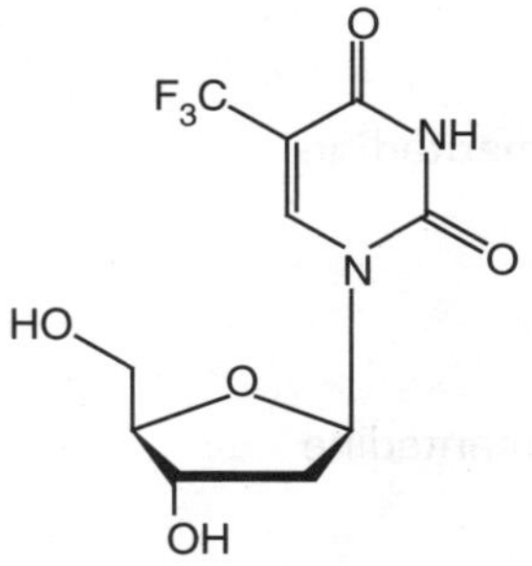

Trifluridine

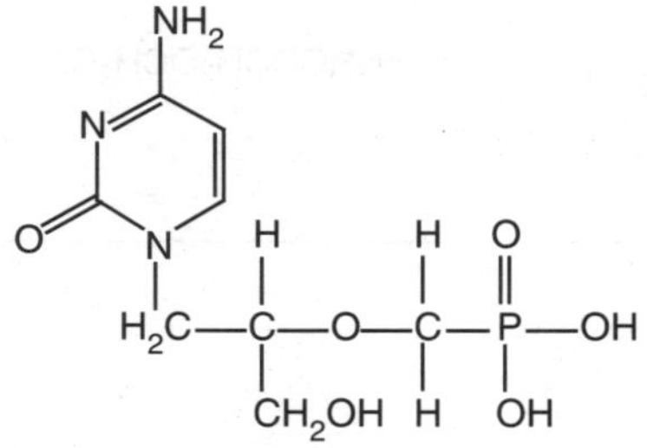

Cidofovir

c. Thiosemicarbazones

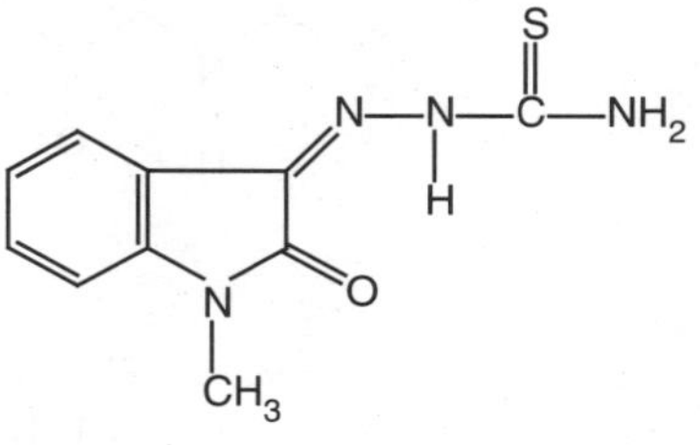

Methisazone

d. Adamantane amines

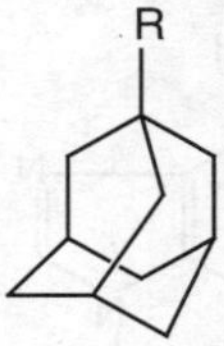

Name	R
Amantadine	$-NH_2$
Rimantadine	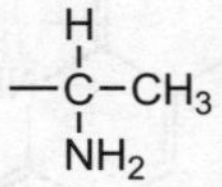 $-\underset{NH_2}{\overset{H}{C}}-CH_3$
Somantadine	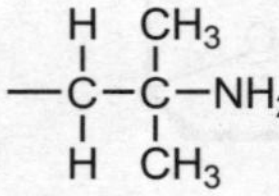 $-\underset{H}{\overset{H}{C}}-\underset{CH_3}{\overset{CH_3}{C}}-NH_2$
Tromantadine	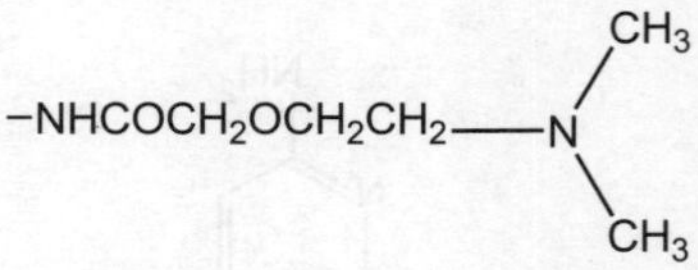 $-NHCOCH_2OCH_2CH_2-N(CH_3)_2$

II. Non-nucleoside RT inhibitors

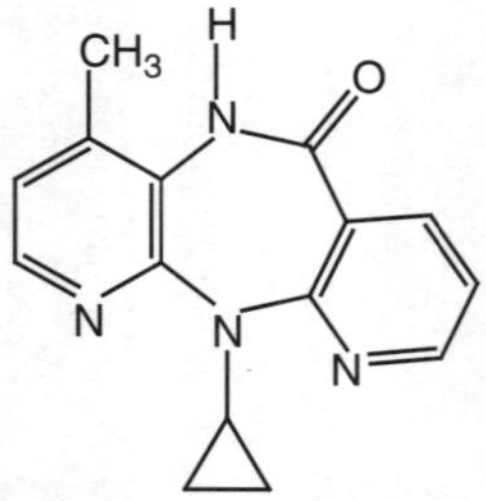

Nevirapine

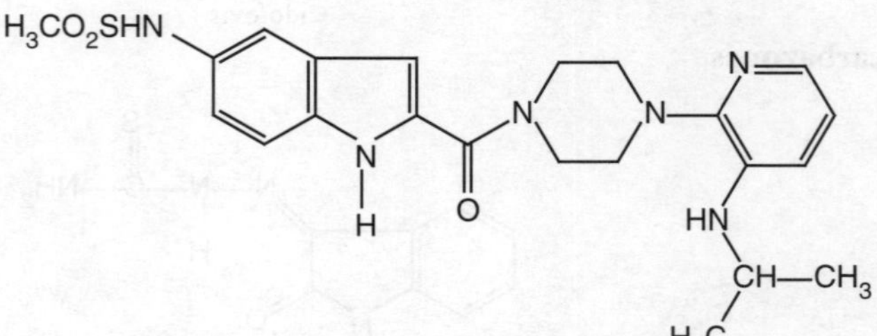

Delavirdine

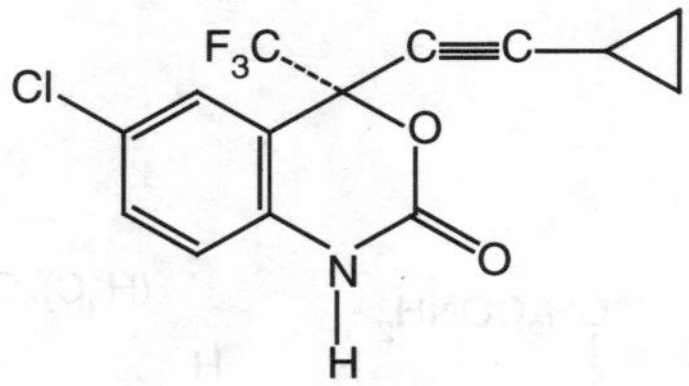

Efavirenz

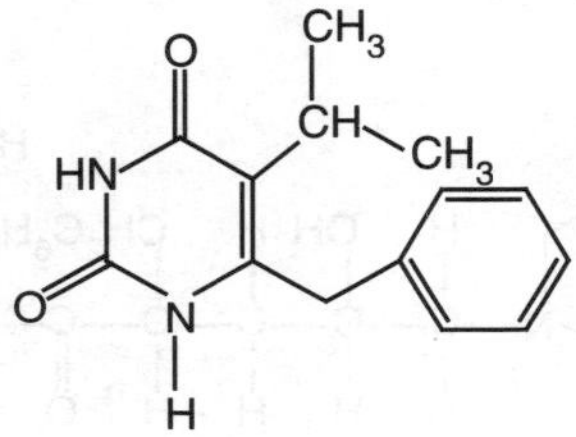

Emivirine

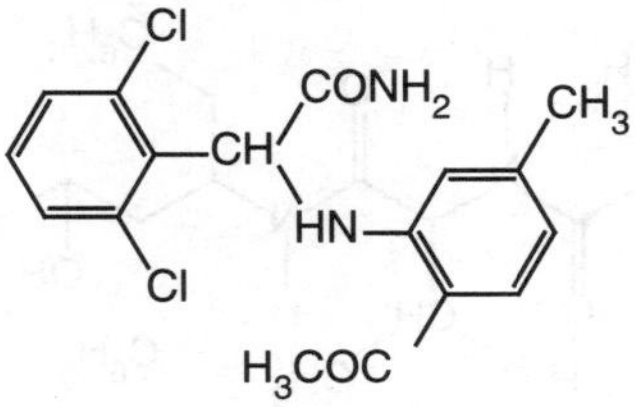

Loviride

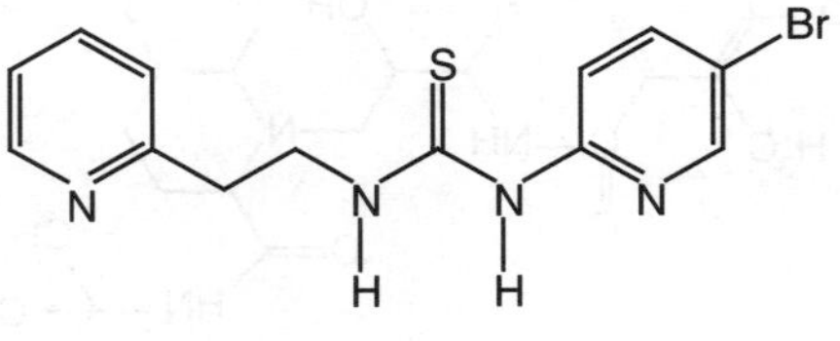

Trovirdine

III. HIV protease inhibitors
a. Saquinavir

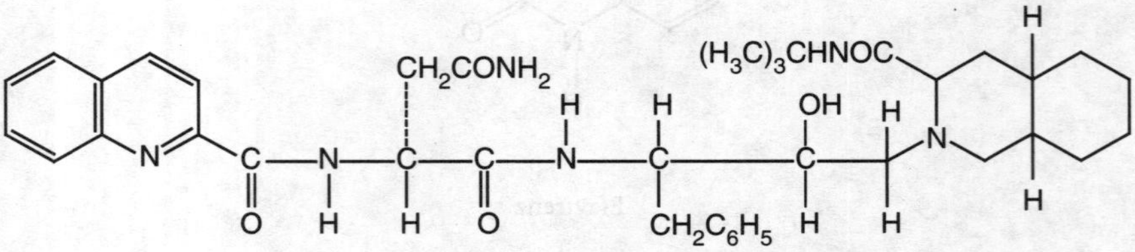

b. Indinavir

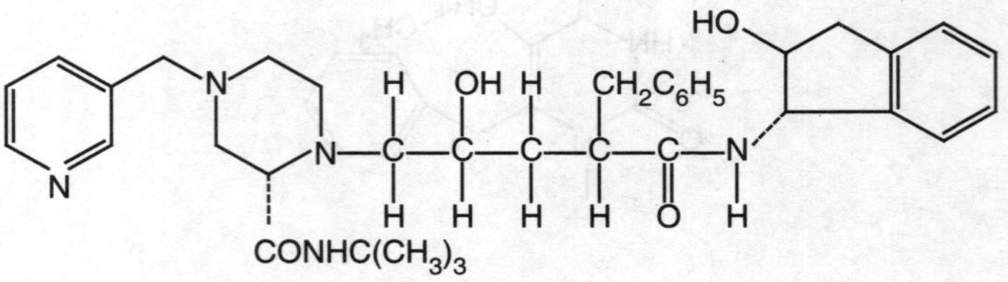

c. Ritonavir

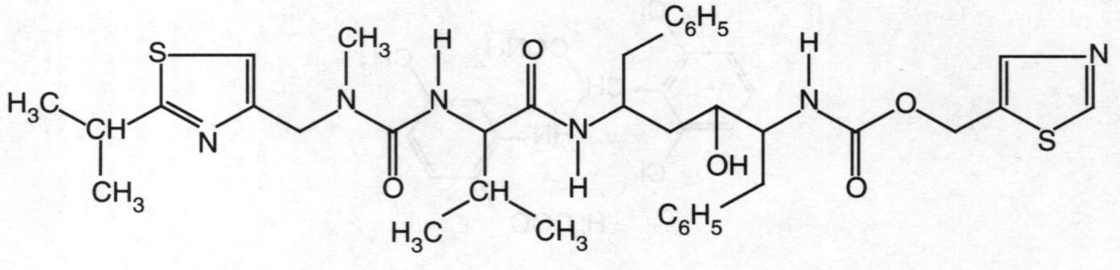

d. Nelfinavir

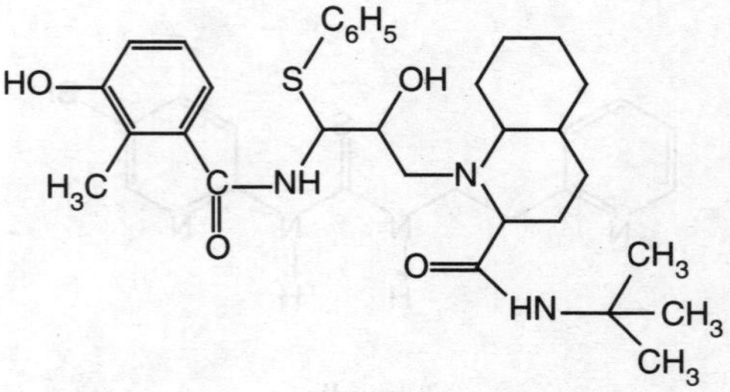

IV. Miscellaneous

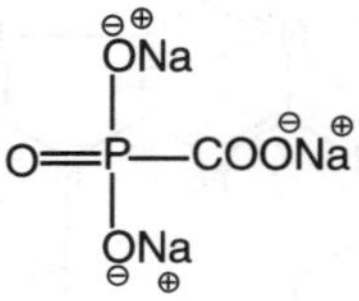

Foscarnet sodium

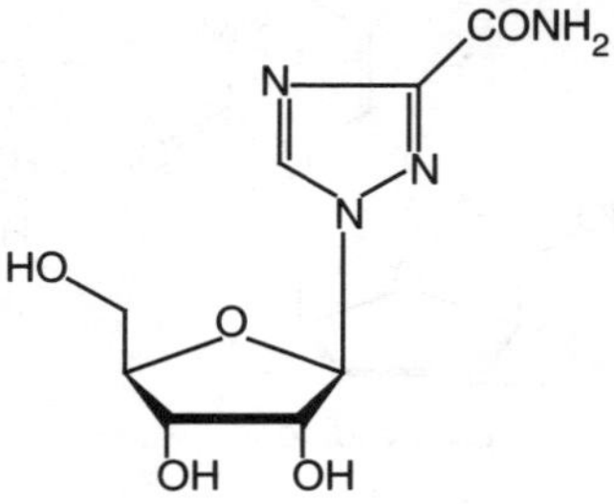

Ribavirin

Classification According to the Enzyme Inhibiton

According to the enzyme inhibition, antiviral agents are classified as follows.

  i. DNA polymerase inhibitors: Idoxuridine, Trifluridine, Vidarabine
 ii. RT inhibitors:

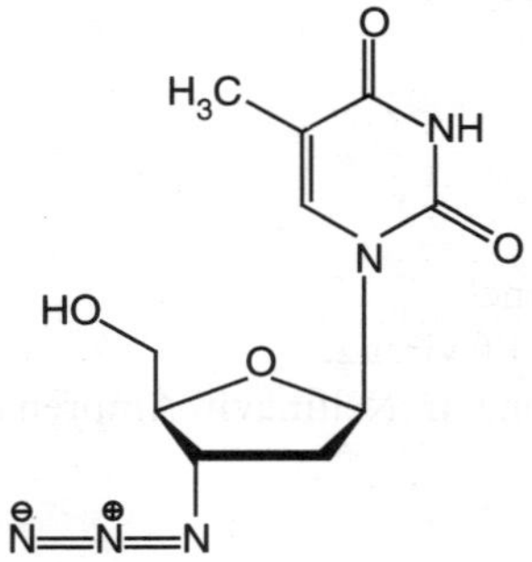

Zidovudine

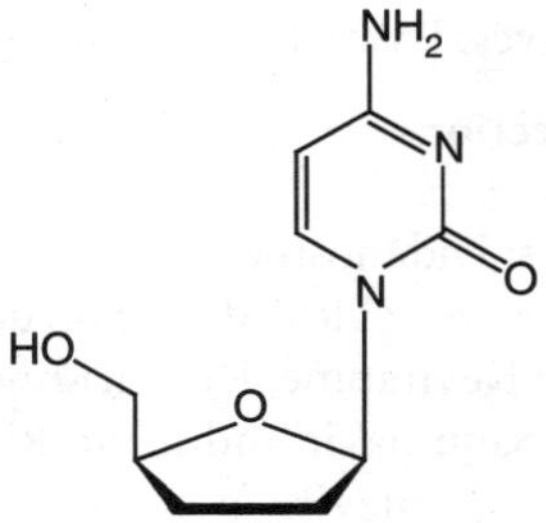

Zalcitabine

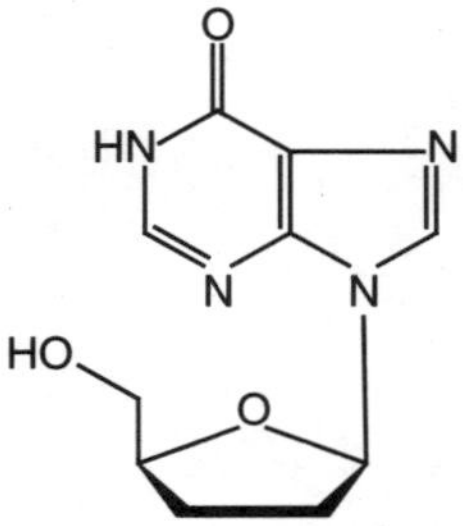

Didanosine

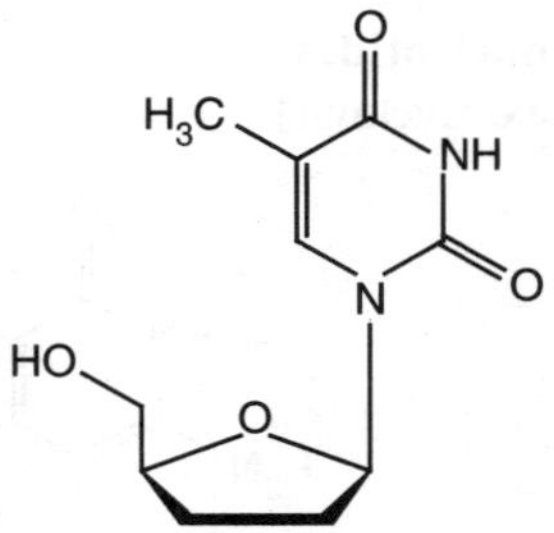

Stavudine

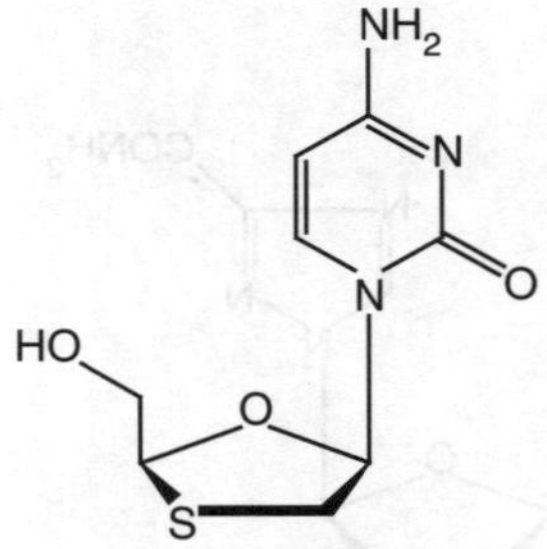

Lamivudine

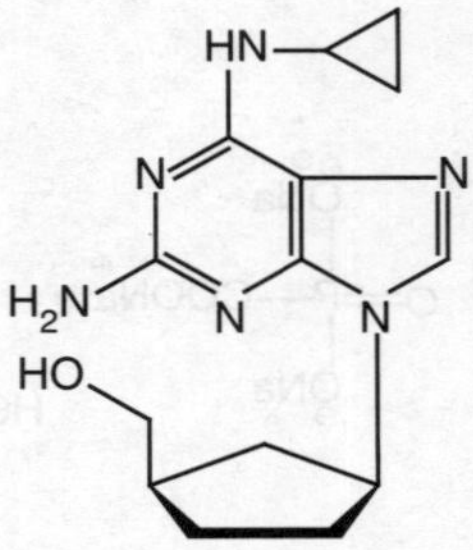

Abacavir

Classification According to the Treatment Protocol

According to the treatment protocol antiviral agents are classified as follows:

I. **Treatment of respiratory virus infection**
Adamantane derivatives: Amantadine, Rimantadine

II. **Treatment of herpes and cytomegalo viruses infection.**
   a. Purine nucleotides: Acyclovir, Ganciclovir, Vidarabine.
   b. Pyrimidine nucleosides: Trifluouridine, Idoxuridine.
   c. Phosphorus derivatives: Foscarnet sodium.

III. **Treatment of HIV infections**
   a. RT inhibition.
      1. Purine derivatives: Didanosine.
      2. Pyrimidine derivative: Zidovudine, Stavudine.
      3. Non-nucleosides: Nevirapine, Delaviridine, Efavirenz.
   b. Protease inhibition: Saquinavir, Indinavir, Ritonavir, Nelfinavir, Amprenavir, Lopinavir.
   c. Integration inhibition: Zintevir.

SYNTHESIS AND DRUG PROFILE

I. Nucleotide analogues
a. Purine nucleosides and nucleotides
i. **Acyclovir** (Ocuvir, Zovirax, Cyclovir)

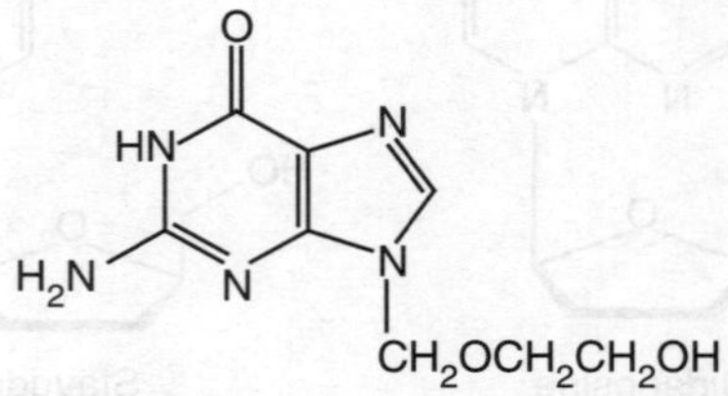

2-Amino-9-((2-hydroxyethoxy)methyl)-1*H*-purin-6(9*H*)-one

Synthesis

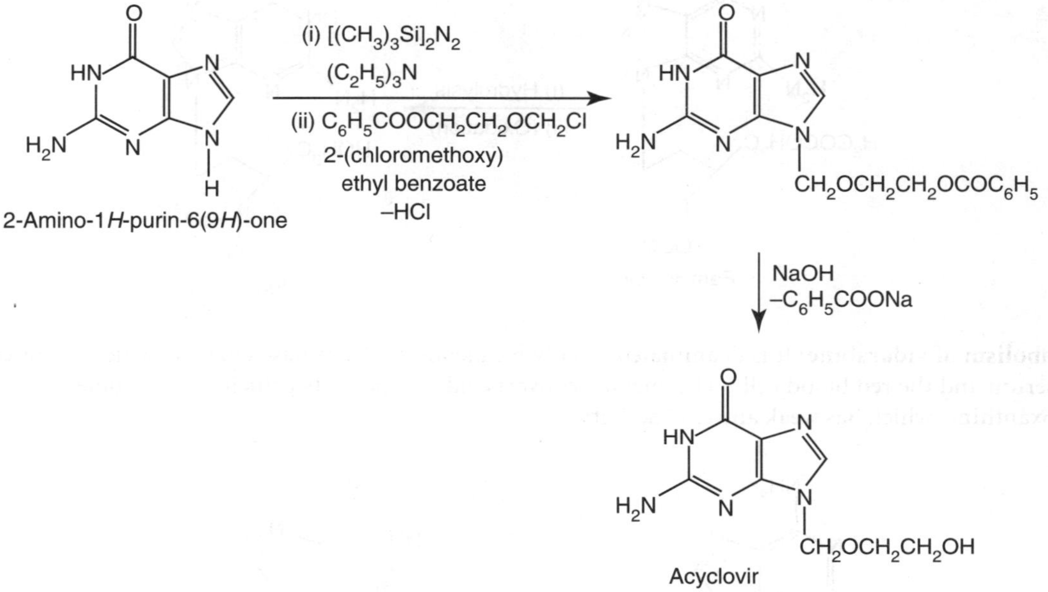

[Scheme: 2-Amino-1H-purin-6(9H)-one reacts with (i) [(CH₃)₃Si]₂N₂, (C₂H₅)₃N; (ii) C₆H₅COOCH₂CH₂OCH₂Cl 2-(chloromethoxy) ethyl benzoate, –HCl to give the N9-alkylated intermediate with CH₂OCH₂CH₂OCOC₆H₅ group. Then NaOH, –C₆H₅COONa gives Acyclovir with CH₂OCH₂CH₂OH group.]

Metabolism: The bioavailability of acyclovir is 15%–30 % and it is metabolized to 9-carboxy-methoxymethyl guanine, which is inactive.

Properties and uses: Acyclovir is a white crystalline powder, slightly soluble in water, soluble in dimethyl sulphoxide and in dilute mineral acids and alkali hydroxides, and very slightly soluble in ethanol. It is a purine nucleoside analogue, used as antiviral agent against herpes viruses.

Assay: Dissolve the sample in anhydrous acetic acid and titrate with 0.1 M perchloric acid. Determine the end point potentiometrically. Perform a blank titration.

Dose: For herpes virus infections the administered dose for immuno-suppressed patients is up to 10 mg/kg body weight every 8 h.

Dosage forms: Acyclovir cream B.P., Acyclovir eye ointment B.P., Acyclovir intravenous infusion B.P., Acyclovir oral suspension B.P., Acyclovir tablets B.P., Dispersible acyclovir tablets B.P.

Metabolism of Valacyclovir: The related analogue 6-deoxy acyclovir is a prodrug form of acyclovir that is activated through metabolism by xanthine oxidase.

Metabolism of Cidofovir: It is metabolized by phosphorylation and it gives cidofovir diphosphate.

Metabolism of Famciclovir: It is a prodrug of penciclovir, which is formed in vivo by hydrolysis of acetyl groups and oxidation at the 6th position by the mixed function oxidase. Penciclovir and its metabolite penciclovir triphosphate posseses antiviral activity.

Famciclovir → (i) Hydrolysis (ii) (Oxidation) → **Penciclovir**

Metabolism of vidarabine: It is deaminated rapidly by adenosine deaminase enzyme, which is present in the serum and the red blood cells. The enzyme converts vidarabine to its principal metabolite, arabinosyl hypoxanthine, which has weak antiviral activity.

Vidarabine → **Arabinofuranosylhypoxanthine**

Uses: It is used for the short-term treatment of herpes simplex and chicken pox caused by varicella-zoster virus (VZV).

ii. Ganciclovir (Ganguard)

2-Amino-9-((1,3-dihydroxypropan-2-yloxy)methyl)-1H-purin-6-one

Synthesis

[Scheme: Epichlorhydrin + C₆H₅CH₂OH (Benzyl alcohol) → (−HCl) → 2-(Benzyloxymethyl)oxirane → (C₆H₅CH₂OH) → 1,3-bis(Benzyloxy)propan-2-ol → (HCHO/HCl, Chloro methylation) → chloromethyl ether intermediate + silylated guanine (OSiMe₃, Me₃SiHN, SiMe₃) → (HCl) → benzyl-protected ganciclovir → (Na / liq. NH₃) → Ganciclovir]

Properties and uses: Ganciclovir is a white powder, soluble in water and it is used as an antiviral agent.

Dose: The recommended dose is 5 mg/kg 1 h for infusion every 12 h for 14 days.

I. b. Pyrimidine nucleoside and nucleotide inhibitors

iii. Idoxuridine (Antizona, Dendrid)

5-Iodo-2-deoxyuridine

Synthesis

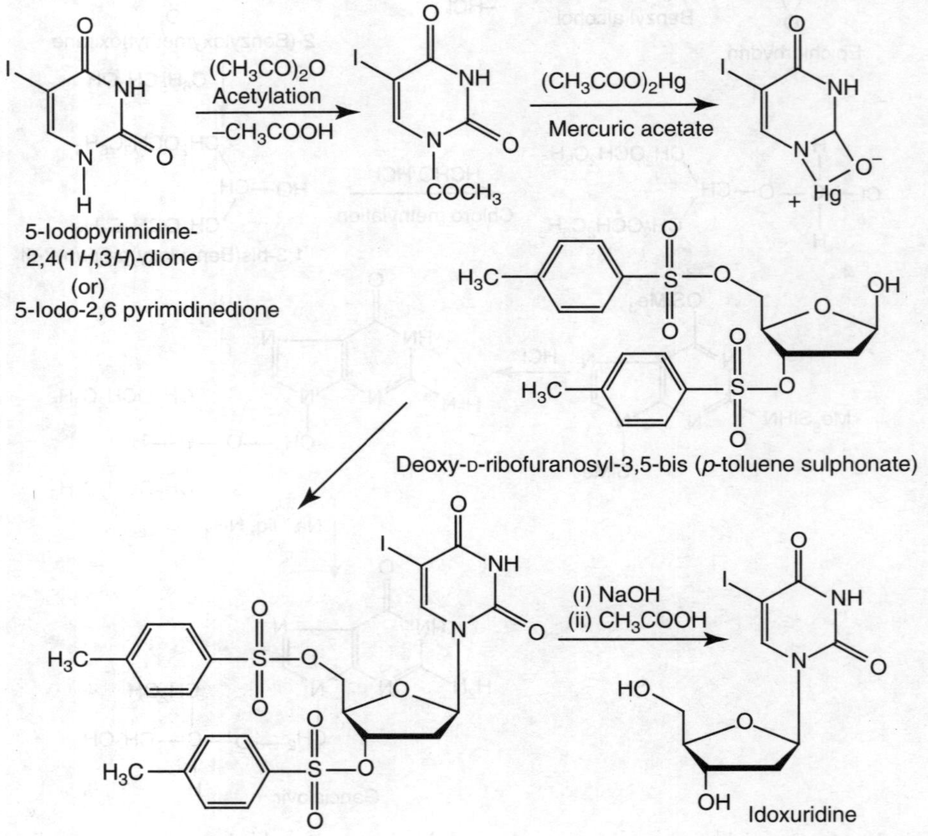

[Scheme: 5-Iodopyrimidine-2,4(1H,3H)-dione (or) 5-Iodo-2,6 pyrimidinedione → (CH₃CO)₂O Acetylation, –CH₃COOH → N-acetyl intermediate → (CH₃COO)₂Hg Mercuric acetate → mercurated intermediate + Deoxy-D-ribofuranosyl-3,5-bis (p-toluene sulphonate) → ditosylated nucleoside → (i) NaOH (ii) CH₃COOH → Idoxuridine]

Metabolism: It has a plasma half-life of 30 min and it is rapidly metabolized in the blood to idoxuracil and uracil.

Properties and uses: Idoxuridine is a white crystalline powder, slightly soluble in water and in alcohol. It dissolves in dilute solutions of alkali hydroxides. It is a pyrimidine nucleoside analogue and used as an antiviral agent against herpes virus.

Assay: Dissolve the sample in dimethylformamide and titrate with 0.1 M tetrabutyl ammonium hydroxide. Determine the end point potentiometrically.

Dose: The administered dose topically as a ointment is 0.5%, 4–16 times a day or 0.1 ml of a 0.1% solution every 1 to 2 h into the conjunctiva.

Dosage forms: Idoxuridine eye drops B.P.

I. c. Thiosemicarbazones
iv. Methisazone (Marboran)

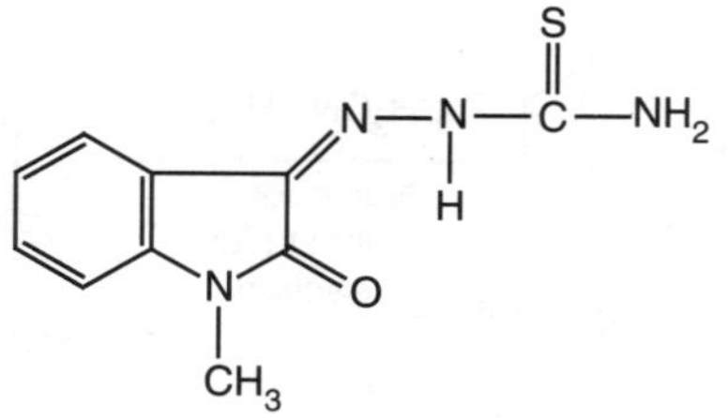

(Z)-1-(1-Methyl-2-oxoindolin-3-ylidene)thiosemicarbazide

Synthesis

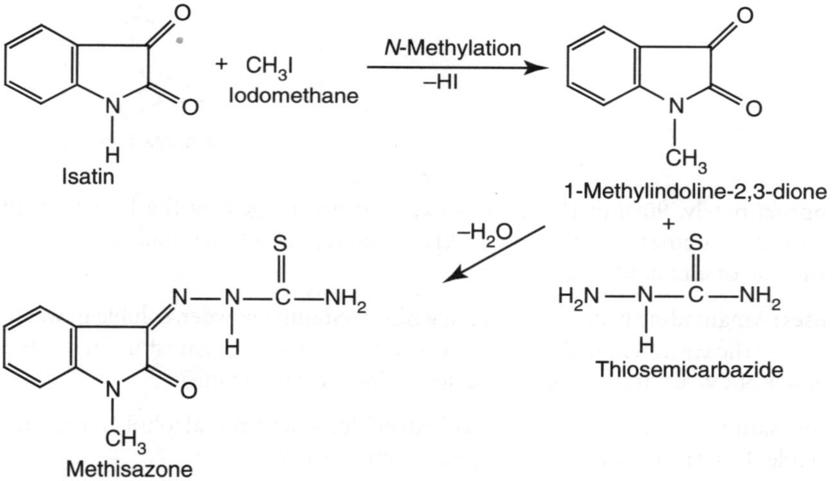

Isatin + CH$_3$I (Iodomethane) → [N-Methylation, –HI] → 1-Methylindoline-2,3-dione

1-Methylindoline-2,3-dione + Thiosemicarbazide (H$_2$N—NH—C(=S)—NH$_2$) → [–H$_2$O] → Methisazone

Dose: The recommended oral dose is 1.5–3.0 g twice daily for four days. As a prophylactic against small pox, it should be administered before the 8th or 9th day of the 12-day incubation period.

Uses: Used in the treatment of viral infection.

I. d. Adamantane amines
1. Amantadine (Symmetrel)

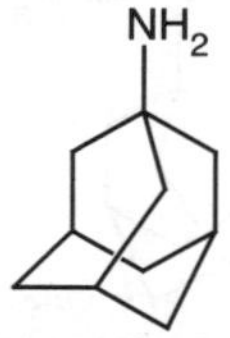

1-Amino adamantane

Synthesis

Adamantane →(Br₂/AlCl₃, −HBr)→ 1-Bromo adamantane →(CH₃CN / H₂SO₄, Nucleophilic substitution reaction)→ 1-Acetyl adamantane (NHCOCH₃) →(NaOH)→ Amantadine (NH₂)

Metabolism: Approximately, 90% of the drug is excreted unchanged by the kidney, primarily through glomerular filtration and tubular secretion, and there are no reports of metabolic products. Acidification of urine increases the rate of amantadine excretion.

Properties and uses: Amantadine hydrochloride is a white crystalline powder, soluble in water and in alcohol. Amantadine is used in the treatment of Parkinson's disease. It is effective against influenza type-A virus, para influenza, and some RNA virus. It is also used as a dopamine receptor agonist.

Assay: Dissolve the sample in a mixture of 0.01 M hydrochloric acid and alcohol (1:10) and titrate with 0.1 M sodium hydroxide. Determine the end point potentiometrically.

Dose: The usual recommended dose is 100 mg twice daily. For children 1–9 years of age the administered dose is 4–9 mg/kg and 9–12 years of age 100 mg twice daily.

Dosage forms: Amantadine capsules I.P., B.P., Amantadine oral solution B.P.

2. Rimantadine

α-Methyl-1-adamatane methylamine

Synthesis

Metabolism: Rimantadine is metabolized in the liver and approximately 20% is excreted unchanged as hydroxylated compound.

Properties and uses: Rimantadine is a white to off-white crystals, soluble in water. It is used for the prevention of infection caused by various strains of influenza virus-A.

Dose: The recommended dose usually is 300 mg.

Miscellaneous

i. Ribavirin (Virazole)

1-(3,4-Dihydroxy-5-(hydroxymethyl)-tetrahydrofuran-2-yl)-1H-1,2,4-triazole-3-carboxamide

Synthesis

Properties and uses: Ribavirin is a white crystalline powder, soluble in water, slightly soluble in ethanol and in methylene chloride. It is used in the treatment of influenza type-A and -B, hepatitis, genital herpes, and Lassa fever.

Assay: It is assayed by adopting liquid chromatography technique.

Dose: For viral hepatitis, influenza, and herpes virus infections, the recommended dose is up to 1g per day in divided doses.

Dosage forms: Ribavirin nebulizer solution B.P.

II. Non-nucleoside RT inhibitors

i. Nevirapine (Neve, Nevipan, Nevimune)

Synthesis

[Synthesis scheme: 2-Chloro-4-methyl pyridin-3-amine + 2-Chloronicotinoyl chloride → (NaH) → intermediate → (Cyclopropylamine) → N-(2-chloro-4-methylpyridin-3-yl)-2-(cyclopropylamino)nicotinamide → (Cyclisation, NaH, –HCl) → Nevirapine]

Metabolism: Nevirapine is metabolized as a glucuronide conjugation to form hydroxylated metabolites and excreted in urine.

Properties and uses: Nevirapine is a white powder, practically insoluble in water, slightly soluble in methylene chloride and in methanol. It is a HIV non-nucleoside RT inhibitor, used as an anti-HIV agent. It causes rash fever, nausea, and headache.

Assay: It is assayed by adopting liquid chromatography technique.

Dose: The recommended dose for HIV infection combined with other antiretrovirals in the case of adults is 200 mg once daily for the first 14 days; then, to increase to 200 mg two times/day if rash does not develop. Interrupting the treatment for more than 7 days necessitates reintroduction of the medicine at a lower dose for the first 14 days. For children 2 months to 8 years the dose is 4 mg /kg once daily for the first 14 days, and increase to 7 mg/kg twice a day, if no rash is present. In the case of patients 8–16 years, the dose is 4 mg/kg once daily for 14 days followed by 4 mg/kg twice/day. Maximum dose that can be administered is 400 mg daily. Interrupting the treatment for more than 7 days necessitates reintroduction at a lower dose for the first 14 days.

ii. Delavirdine

[Structure of Delavirdine]

N-(2-(1-(3-(isopropylamino)pyridin-2-yl)piperazine-4-carbonyl)-1H-indol-5-yl methanesulfonamide

Synthesis

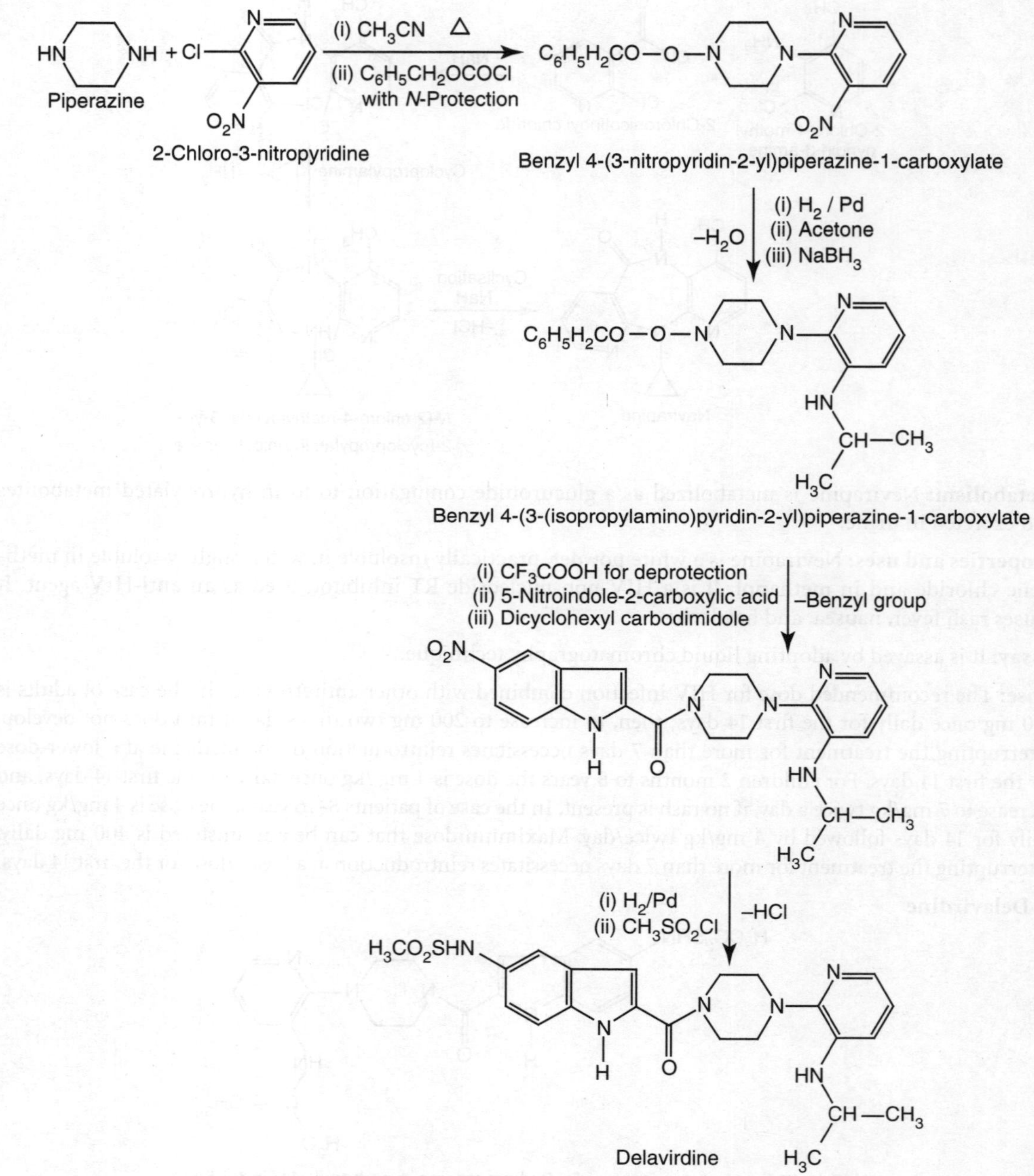

Piperazine + 2-Chloro-3-nitropyridine
(i) CH$_3$CN, Δ
(ii) C$_6$H$_5$CH$_2$OCOCl with N-Protection
→ Benzyl 4-(3-nitropyridin-2-yl)piperazine-1-carboxylate

(i) H$_2$/Pd
(ii) Acetone
(iii) NaBH$_3$
−H$_2$O
→ Benzyl 4-(3-(isopropylamino)pyridin-2-yl)piperazine-1-carboxylate

(i) CF$_3$COOH for deprotection
(ii) 5-Nitroindole-2-carboxylic acid
(iii) Dicyclohexyl carbodimidole
−Benzyl group

(i) H$_2$/Pd
(ii) CH$_3$SO$_2$Cl
−HCl
→ **Delavirdine**

Metabolism: Delavirdine is metabolized to N-desisopropyl metabolite in the liver and the pharmacokinetics is nonlinear.

iii. Emivirine

6-Benzyl-5-isopropyl-hexahydropyrimidine-2,4-dione

Synthesis

II. d. α-Anilinophenylacetamide
i. Loviride

2-(2-Acetyl-5-methylphenylamino)-2-(2,6-dichlorophenyl)acetamide

Synthesis

2,6-Dichlorobenzaldehyde + NaCN + 1-(2-Amino-4-methylphenyl)ethanone

→ (intermediate α-amino nitrile) $\xrightarrow{H_2SO_4}$ Loviride

II. e. Pyridyl ethyl thiourea
i. Trovirdine

1-(5-Bromopyridin-2-yl)-3-(2-(pyridin-2-yl)ethyl)thiourea

Synthesis:

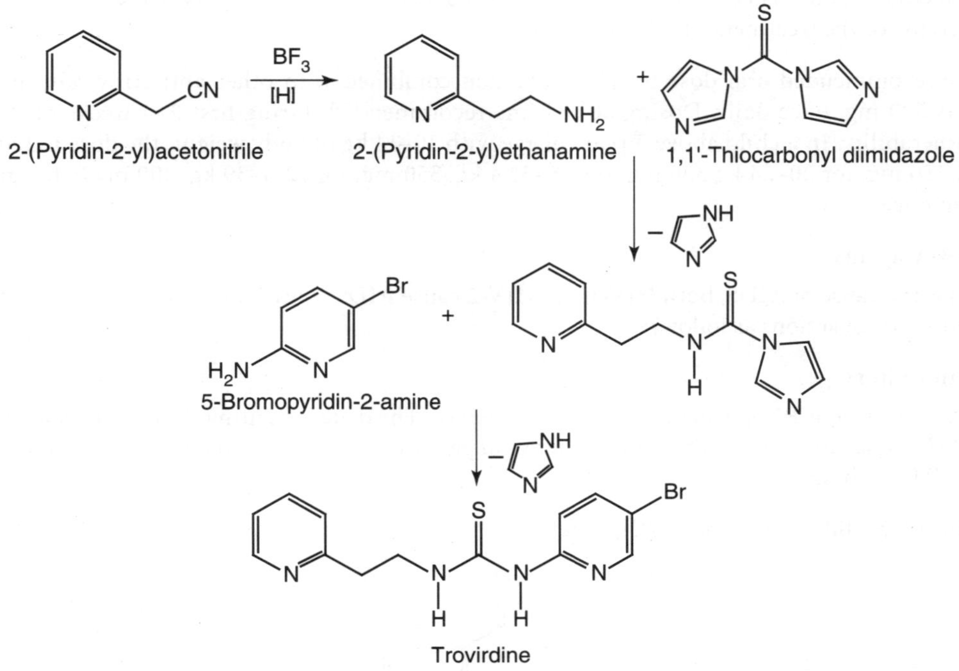

2-(Pyridin-2-yl)acetonitrile → (BF₃, [H]) → *2-(Pyridin-2-yl)ethanamine* + *1,1'-Thiocarbonyl diimidazole*

5-Bromopyridin-2-amine

Trovirdine

II. f. Benzoxazinones
Efavirenz (Efavir, Efferven, Evirenz)
Synthesis

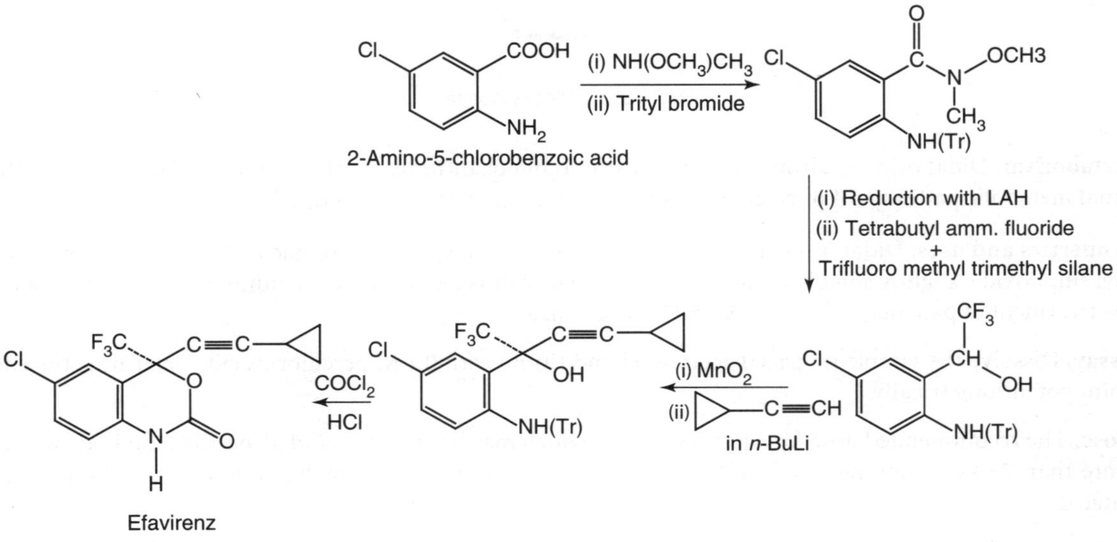

2-Amino-5-chlorobenzoic acid

(i) NH(OCH₃)CH₃
(ii) Trityl bromide

(i) Reduction with LAH
(ii) Tetrabutyl amm. fluoride
    +
Trifluoro methyl trimethyl silane

(i) MnO₂
(ii) cyclopropyl-C≡CH in n-BuLi

COCl₂, HCl

Efavirenz

Properties and uses: Efavirenz is a white to slightly pink crystalline powder, soluble in dilute hydrochloric acid and in ethanol, but insoluble in water. It is a non-nucleoside RT inhibitor used as a part of the combination therapy for the treatment of HIV infection.

Dose: The recommended oral dose for HIV infection combined with other antiretrovirals, in the case of adults is 600 mg, once daily. Dosing at bedtime recommended during first 2–4 weeks of therapy to improve tolerability. In a child above 3 years of age with 10–14 kg of body weight, the dose is 200 mg; for 15–19 kg, 250 mg; for 20–24 kg 300 mg; for 25–32.4 kg, 350 mg; for 32.5–39 kg, 400 mg ≥ 40 kg; 600 mg to be taken once a day.

III. Anti-HIV agents

HIV virus is the cause of AIDS, both HIV-1 and HIV-2 cause AIDS. Anti-HIV agents are classified according to their mode of actions as follows:

III a. RT inhibitors

Reverse transcription is RNA dependent DNA polymerase. The drug inhibiting RT interferes with the replication of HIV and stops the synthesis of further viral particle. They are classified into nucleoside and non-nucleoside RT inhibitors.

Didanosine (2′,3′-dideoxyinosine (DDI), Videx)

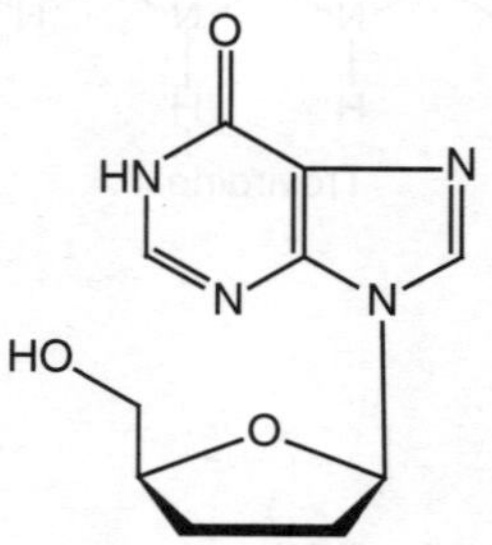

2′,3′ Dideoxyinosine

Metabolism: Didanosine is ultimately converted into hypoxanthine, xanthine, and uric acid through the usual metabolic pathways of purines. The latter is a nontoxic metabolic product.

Properties and uses: Didanosine is a white crystalline powder, sparingly soluble in water, soluble in dimethyl sulphoxide, slightly soluble in methanol and ethanol. It is a nucleoside RT inhibitor recommended for the treatment of patients with advanced HIV infections.

Assay: Dissolve the sample in glacial acetic acid and titrate with 0.1 M perchloric acid. Determine the end point potentiometrically.

Dose: The recommended dose for adults as tablets, which may be chewable and dispersible, for body weight more than 75 kg is 300 mg; for 50–74 kg body weight, 200 mg; for 35–49 kg body weight, 125 mg with antacids.

Synthesis

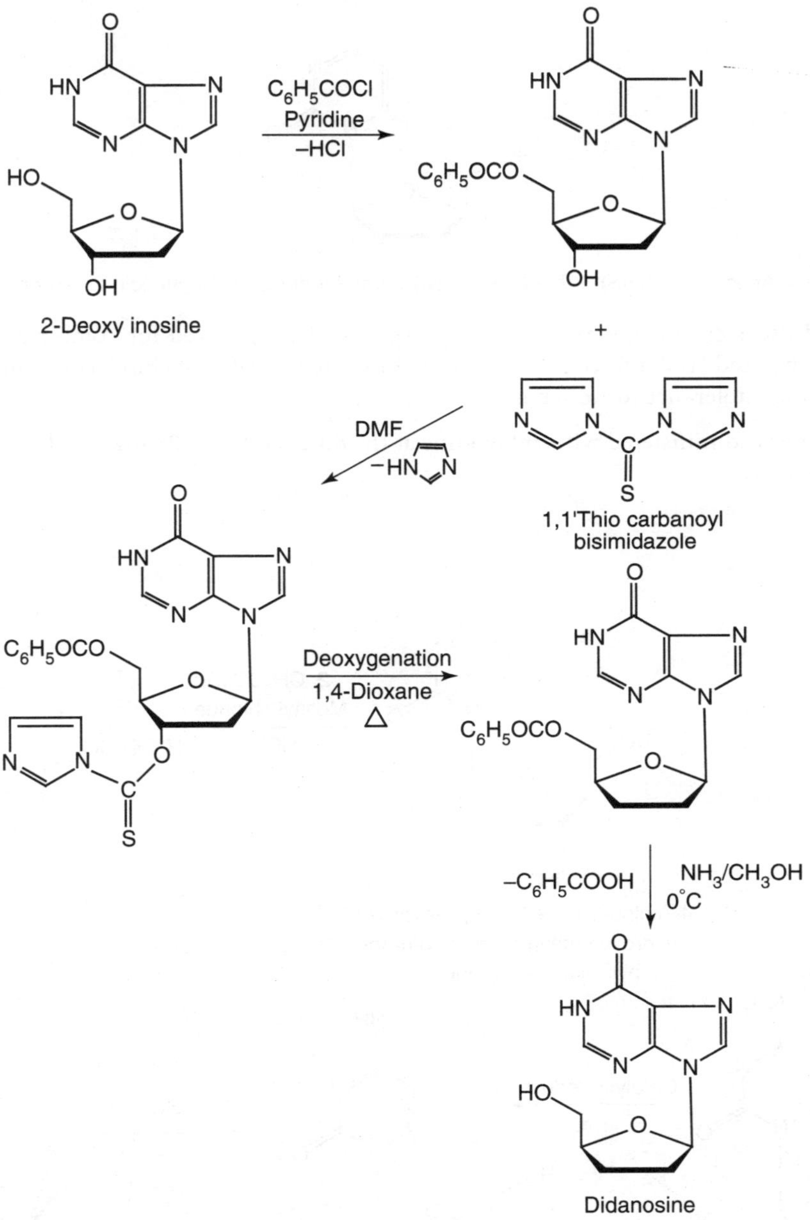

2-Deoxy inosine
C6H5COCl
Pyridine
–HCl
C6H5OCO
+
1,1'Thio carbanoyl
bisimidazole
DMF
–HN
Deoxygenation
1,4-Dioxane
△
–C6H5COOH
NH3/CH3OH
0°C
Didanosine

Zalcitabine (DDC, Hivid)

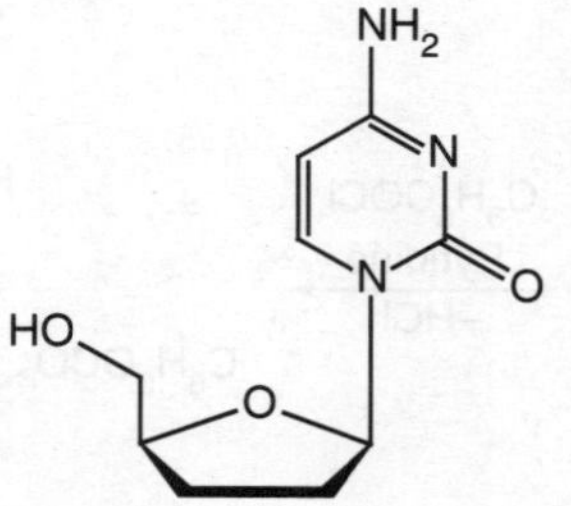

4-Amino-1-((2R,5S)-5-(hydroxymethyl)-tetrahydrofuran-2-yl)pyrimidin-2(1H)-one

Properties and uses: Zalcitabine exists as white crystals. It is approved for combination therapy with zidovudine in advanced HIV infection, who has demonstrated significant clinical or immunological deterioration, showing intolerance to zidovudine.

Dose: Zalcitabine is administered with zidovudine at the dose level of 2–25 mg of zalcitabine and 600 mg of zidovudine per day.

Synthesis
Route I.

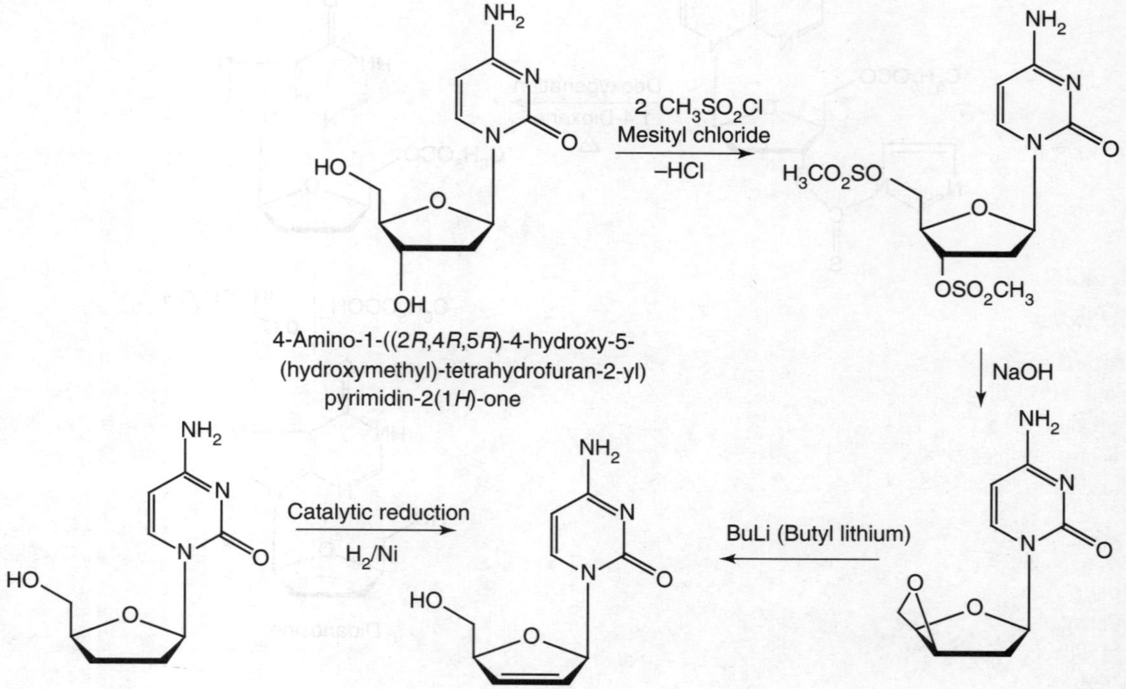

4-Amino-1-((2R,4R,5R)-4-hydroxy-5-(hydroxymethyl)-tetrahydrofuran-2-yl)pyrimidin-2(1H)-one

Zalcitabine

Route II.

[Reaction scheme: Starting cytidine derivative (with NHAc) → Zn/Cu couple, Reductive elimination with AcO-C(CH₃)₂-O- → intermediate dideoxy nucleoside with NHAc → Raney–Ni, H₂/Pd–C → **Zalcitabine** (with NH₂)]

Zidovudine (ZDV) [azido-deoxythymidine (AZT), Retrovir]

[Structure of Zidovudine shown with azide group N⁻=N⁺=N]

1-((2R,4R,5S)-4-azido-5-(hydroxymethyl)-tetrahydrofuran-2-yl)-5-methylpyrimidine-2,4(1H,3H)-dione

Metabolism: Most of the administered drug is converted to its inactive glucuronide metabolite and it is excreted unchanged through urine.

Properties and uses: ZDV is a white or brownish powder, sparingly soluble in water and soluble in anhydrous ethanol. It is a nucleoside RT inhibitor, having activity against HIV, and hence, it is used for the treatment of AIDS and AIDS-related complex (ARC). It increases the survival and improves the quality of life of patients with complications, such as severe weight loss, fever, and pneumocytosis. As it crosses the blood brain barrier, it has favourable effect on the neurological symptoms of AIDS.

Assay: It is assayed by adopting liquid chromatography technique.

Dose: The recommended dose for adults in the case of oral asymptomatic HIV-infection initially is 100 mg every 4 h, while awake (500 mg a day), after 1 month, the dose may be reduced to 100 mg every 4 h. For intravenous infusion, the dose is 1–2 mg/kg infused over 1 h for every 4 h around the clock (6 times a day).

Synthesis

[Scheme: 2'Deoxythymidine → (with (C₆H₅)₃CCl, Pyridine, –HCl) → 5'-O-trityl intermediate → (Mesityl chloride, –HCl) → 3'-OSO₂CH₃ mesylate → (LiN₃ (Lithium azide), DMF; N₂, 100°C; 3 h) → 3'-azido-5'-O-trityl thymidine → (HBr, Detritylation) → Zidovudine]

Lamivudine (Lamda, Rolam, Lamvir)

4-Amino-1-((2S,5R)-2-(hydroxymethyl)-1,3-oxathiolan-5-yl)pyrimidin-2(1H)-one

Synthesis

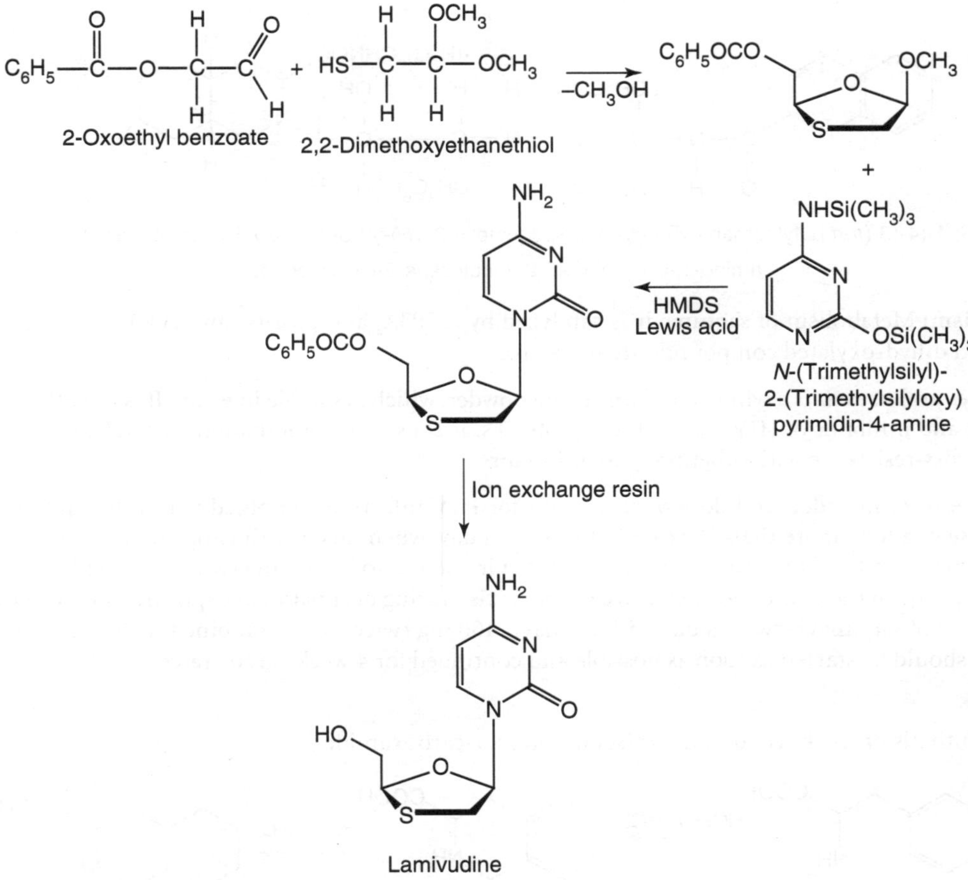

[Scheme: 2-Oxoethyl benzoate + 2,2-Dimethoxyethanethiol → (−CH₃OH) → intermediate (C₆H₅OCO-substituted oxathiolane with OCH₃) + N-(Trimethylsilyl)-2-(Trimethylsilyloxy)pyrimidin-4-amine → (HMDS, Lewis acid) → protected nucleoside → (Ion exchange resin) → Lamivudine]

Properties and uses: Lamivudine is a white powder, soluble in water, sparingly soluble in methanol and slightly soluble in ethanol. It is a nucleoside RT inhibitor, used in combination with ZDV for the treatment of diseases caused by HIV infection.

Assay: It is assayed by adopting liquid chromatography technique.

Dose: The recommended dose for chronic hepatitis B in the case of adults is 100 mg once daily. For a child more than 2 years, the dose is 3 mg/kg once daily, maximum is 100 mg per day for HIV infection. The recommended dose for concomitant HIV and hepatits B infection, in the case of adults is 150 mg twice a day or 300 mg once daily, in combination with other antiretrovirals. In the case of a child, 3 months–12 years, the dose is 4 mg/kg twice a day, maximum dose is 300 mg per day.

III. b. HIV protease inhibitors

i. Saquinavir (Saquin)

N-((S)-1-(4-(3-(*tert*-butylcarbamoyl)-octahydroisoquinolin-2(1H)-yl)-3-hydroxy-1-phenylbutan-2-ylamino)-4-amino-1,4-dioxobutan-2-yl)quinoline-2-carboxamide

Metabolism: Metabolism of saquinavir is catalyzed by $CYP3A_4$ and possibly by $CYP3A_5$. The metabolites mono and dihydroxylated compounds are not active.

Properties and uses: It is a white to off-white fine powder, which is soluble in water. It is a synthetic peptide analogue and inhibitor of HIV-1 and HIV-2 proteases. It is used in combination with RT inhibitors, but it has less cross-resistance with other protease inhibitors.

Dose: The recommended oral dose of saquinavir for HIV infection combined with other antiretrovirals, in the case of adults more than 16 years is 1 g twice a day, when taken with ritonavir 100 mg, it is twice a day. Alternatively, the administered dose of saquinavir could also be 400 mg twice a day with ritonavir 400 mg twice a day. In the case of postexposure prophylaxis, during occupational exposure to HIV, the dose for adults is 1 g of saquinavir twice a day with ritonavir 100 mg twice a day, combined with other antiretrovirals, and should be started as soon as possible and continued for 4 weeks, if tolerated.

Synthesis

Step I. Synthesis of *N-t*-butyl-decahydroisoquinoline-3-carboxamide (A)

2-Amino-3-phenyl propanoic acid → (HCHO/HCl) → 1,2,3,4-Tetrahydroisoquinoline-3-carboxylic acid → (H_2/Rh–C) → Decahydroisoquinoline-3-carboxylic acid

(i) $C_6H_5CH_2OCOCl$ (N-protection)
(ii) DCC(COOH-activation)
(iii) $H_2NC(CH_3)_3$
(iv) H_2/Pd(*N*-deprotection)

N-Tert-Butyl-decahydroisoquinoline-3-carboxamide (**A**)

Step II. Condensation of (**A**) and (**B**)

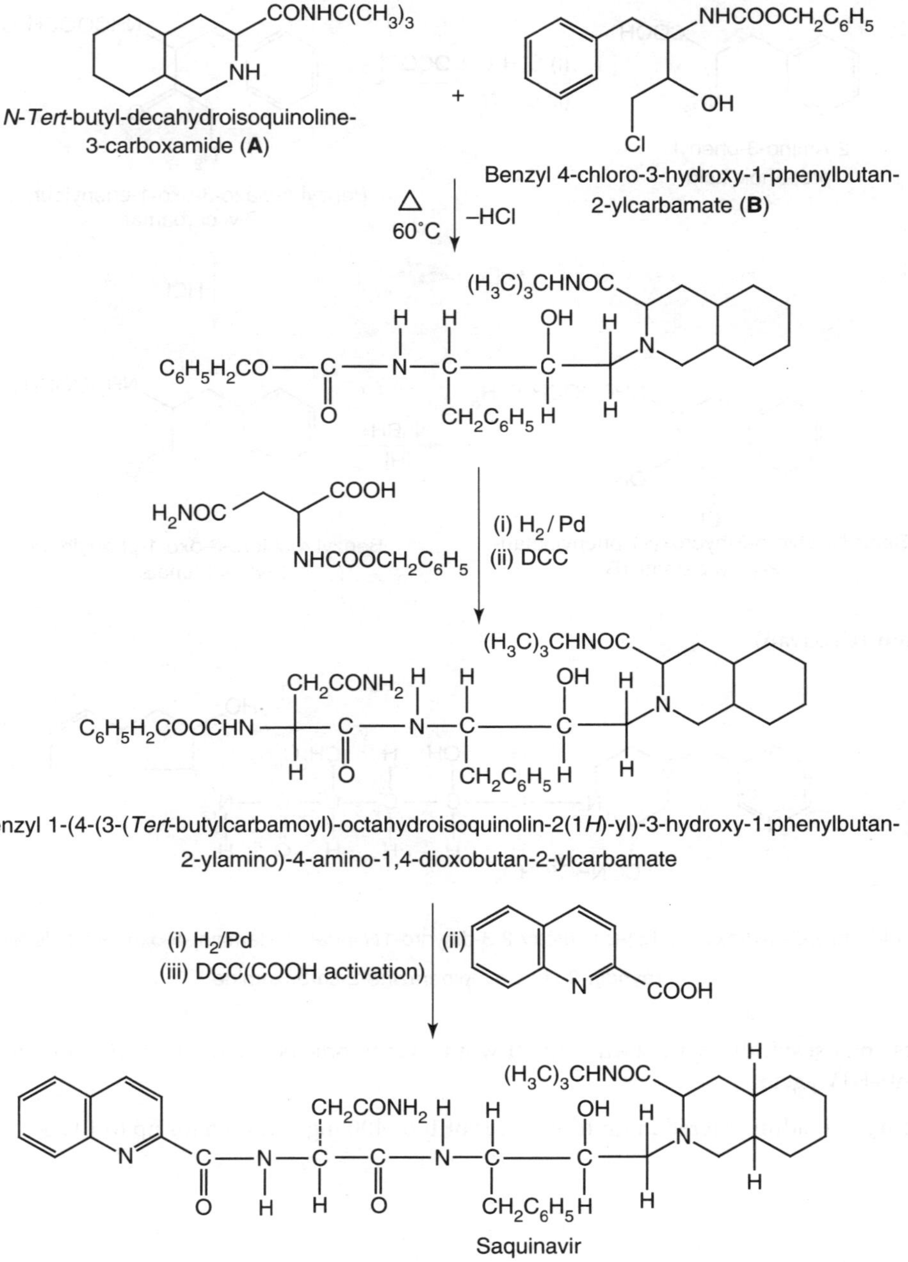
CONHC(CH3)3
NH
N-Tert-butyl-decahydroisoquinoline-3-carboxamide (A)
+
NHCOOCH2C6H5
OH
Cl
Benzyl 4-chloro-3-hydroxy-1-phenylbutan-2-ylcarbamate (B)
Δ 60°C
–HCl
(H3C)3CHNOC
C6H5H2CO
CH2C6H5
H2NOC
COOH
NHCOOCH2C6H5
(i) H2 / Pd
(ii) DCC
CH2CONH2
C6H5H2COOCHN
Benzyl 1-(4-(3-(Tert-butylcarbamoyl)-octahydroisoquinolin-2(1H)-yl)-3-hydroxy-1-phenylbutan-2-ylamino)-4-amino-1,4-dioxobutan-2-ylcarbamate
(i) H2/Pd
(iii) DCC(COOH activation)
(ii)
Saquinavir

Step III. Synthesis of Benzyl 4-chloro-3-hydroxy-1-phenylbutan-2-yl carbamate (**B**)

ii. Indinavir (Crixivan)

(S)-1-(4-benzyl-2-hydroxy-5-((1S)-2-hydroxy-2,3-dihydro-1H-inden-1-ylamino)-5-oxopentyl)-N-tert-butyl-4-(pyridin-3-ylmethyl)piperazine-2-carboxamide

Properties and uses: Indinavir is a white to off-white hygroscopic powder, soluble in water or in methanol. Used as anti-HIV agent.

Dose: Indinavir is administered in multiple doses of 100–400 mg every 6 h for up to 10 days.

Synthesis

Step I: Synthesis of an intermediate (A)

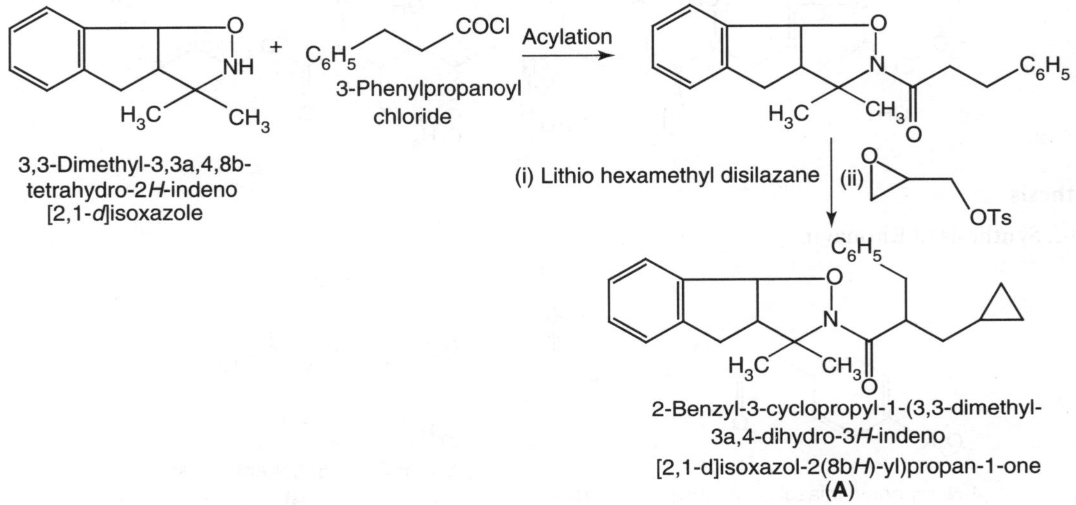
O
NH
H3C
CH3
+
C6H5
COCl
Acylation
3-Phenylpropanoyl
chloride
3,3-Dimethyl-3,3a,4,8b-
tetrahydro-2H-indeno
[2,1-d]isoxazole
O
N
C6H5
H3C
CH3
O
(i) Lithio hexamethyl disilazane
(ii)
O
OTs
C6H5
O
N
H3C
CH3
O
2-Benzyl-3-cyclopropyl-1-(3,3-dimethyl-
3a,4-dihydro-3H-indeno
[2,1-d]isoxazol-2(8bH)-yl)propan-1-one
(A)

Step II:

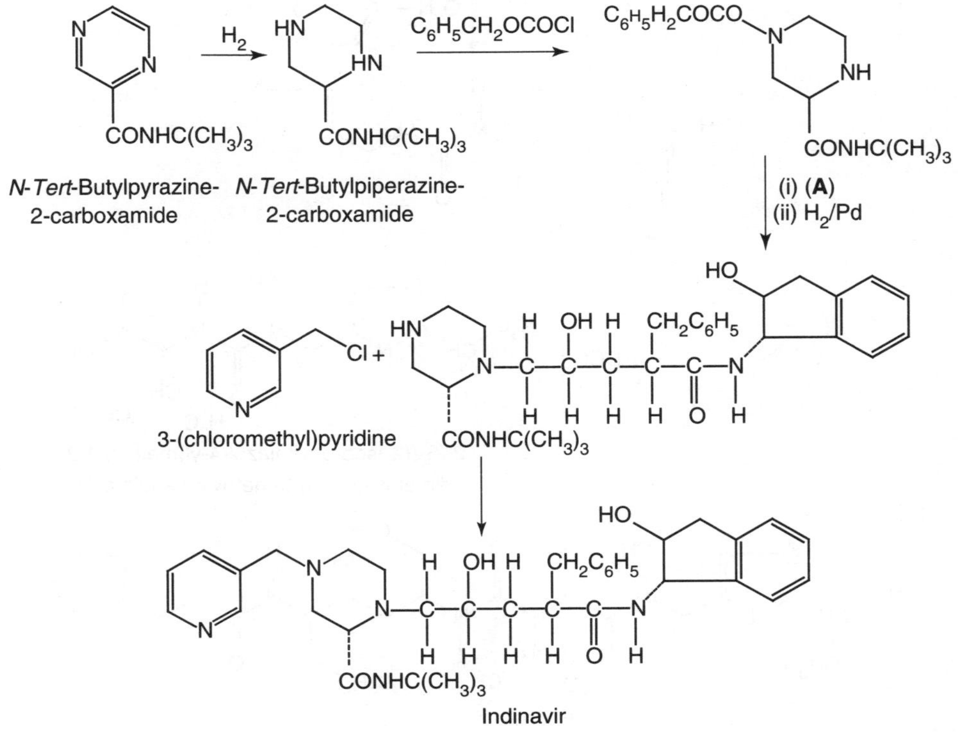
N
N
CONHC(CH3)3
H2
HN
HN
CONHC(CH3)3
C6H5CH2OCOCl
C6H5H2COCO
N
NH
CONHC(CH3)3
N-Tert-Butylpyrazine-
2-carboxamide
N-Tert-Butylpiperazine-
2-carboxamide
(i) (A)
(ii) H2/Pd
HO
N
Cl +
HN
N
H OH H CH2C6H5
C C C C C N
H H H H O H
3-(chloromethyl)pyridine
CONHC(CH3)3
HO
N
N
N
H OH H CH2C6H5
C C C C C N
H H H H O H
CONHC(CH3)3
Indinavir

iii. Ritonavir (Empetus, Ritomax, Ritovir)

Synthesis

Step-I. Synthesis of Ritonavir

4-Nitrophenyl thiazol-5-ylmethyl carbonate

2,5-Diamino-1,6-diphenylhexan-3-ol
(A)

2-(3-((2-Isopropylthiazol-4-yl)methyl)-1,3-dimethylureido)-3-methylbutanoic acid

Ritonavir

Step-II: Synthesis of (A)

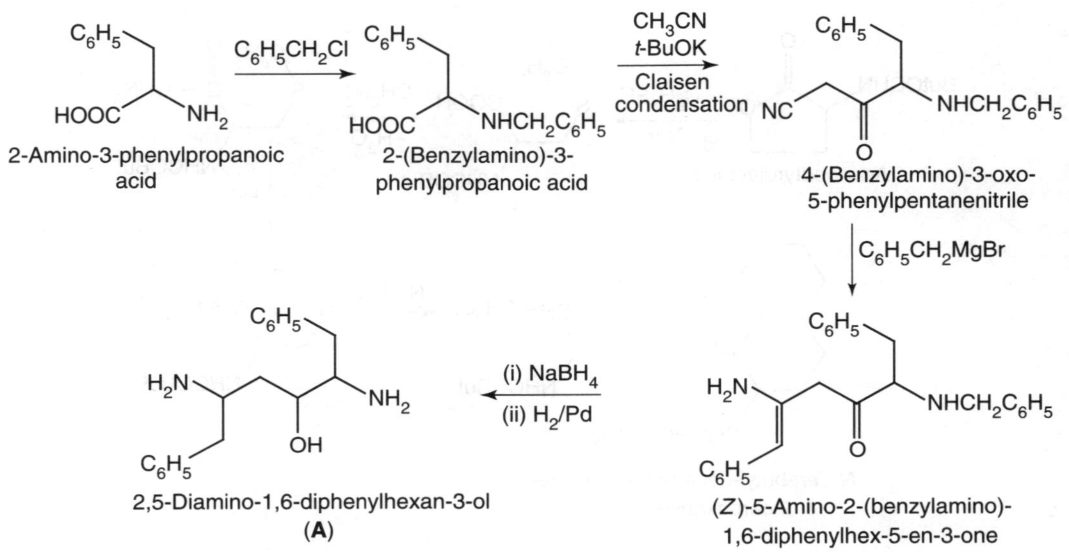

[Scheme: 2-Amino-3-phenylpropanoic acid → (via C₆H₅CH₂Cl) → 2-(Benzylamino)-3-phenylpropanoic acid → (via CH₃CN, *t*-BuOK, Claisen condensation) → 4-(Benzylamino)-3-oxo-5-phenylpentanenitrile → (via C₆H₅CH₂MgBr) → (Z)-5-Amino-2-(benzylamino)-1,6-diphenylhex-5-en-3-one → (i) NaBH₄ (ii) H₂/Pd → 2,5-Diamino-1,6-diphenylhexan-3-ol (**A**)]

Metabolism: Ritonavir is metabolized by CYP3A4; the metabolites are isolated from urine. They are isopropylthiazole oxidation products.

Properties and uses: Ritonavir is white to light tan powder with a bitter metallic taste. It is soluble in methanol and in isopropyl alcohol, but insoluble in water.

Dose: The recommended oral dose for HIV infection combined with other antiretroviral, in the case of adults, initially is 300 mg twice a day for the day one. The dose may be increased gradually by 100 mg twice a day and over a period of up to 14 days to 600 mg twice a day. In the case of a child more than 2 years, the recommended dose is 250 mg/m² twice a day. Increase the dose by 50 mg/m² twice a day, at 2–3 day intervals, up to 400 mg/m² twice a day. Maximum dose is 600 mg twice a day. As a pharmacokinetic enhancer, in the case of adults, to enhance the efficacy of other protease inhibitors the dose is 100–200 mg once or twice a day.

iv. Nelfinavir (Emnel, Nelvir, Retronel)

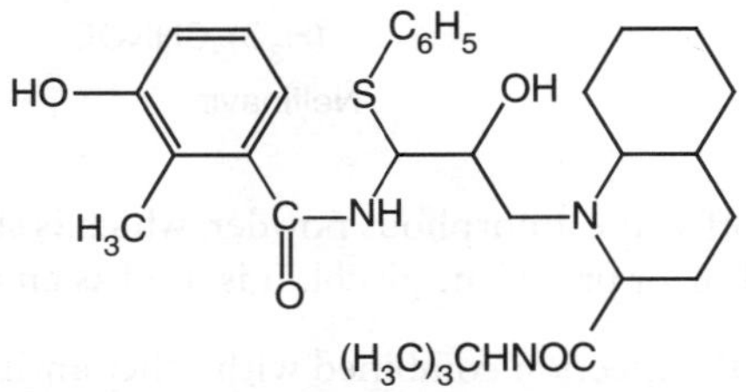

N-Tert-Butyl-1-(2-hydroxy-3-(3-hydroxy-2-methylbenzamido)-3-(phenylthio)propyl)-1,2,3,4-tetrahydroquinoline-2-carboxamide

Synthesis

[Scheme: Synthesis of Nelfinavir starting from Aminobutyrolactone, via reaction with C₆H₅SH/NaH, then COOH intermediate (NHCOBut), CH₂N₂/−H₂O to give diazoketone, HCl to give chloroketone, NaBH₄ reduction to chlorohydrin, coupling with N-Tert-butyl-decahydroquinoline-2-carboxamide, (i) H₂/Pd, (ii) acylation with 3-hydroxy-2-methylbenzoic acid derivative to give Nelfinavir.]

Properties and uses: It is a white to off-white amorphous powder, which is slightly soluble in water, soluble in methanol, ethanol, isopropyl alcohol, or propylene glycol. It is used as an anti-HIV agent.

Dose: The recommended dose for HIV infection combined with other antiretrovirals in the case of adults is 1.25 g twice a day or 0.75 g thrice a day. In the case of a child: For 2–13 years is 45–55 mg/kg twice a day or 25–35 mg/kg thrice a day. Maximum dose for a child is 0.75 g thrice a day.

SAR of Adamantane Amines

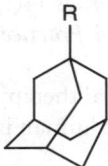

- α–methyl derivative of adamantane produced Rimantidine.
- α–methyl–1–adamantane methylamine is flumadine.
- N-Alkyl and N,N-dialkyl derivatives of adamantadine exhibit antiviral activity similar to that of adamantadine HCl.
- Except glycyl derivatives, N–acyl derivatives shows decreased antiviral action and tromantadine possesses efficacy against clinical *Herpes labialis* and *H. gentalis*.
- Replacement of the amino group with OH, SH, CN, or halogen produced inactive compounds.
- Optical isomers and the racemic mixtures of rimantadine are equally active.
- *Influenza* A_2 virus, is more susceptible to adamantanespiro–5–pyrrolidine derivative.

PROBABLE QUESTIONS

1. Enumerate a few DNA virus and RNA virus and mention the diseases produced by them. Classify the antiviral agents with suitable examples.
2. How will you synthesize the following:
   (a) Amantadine HCl (b) Methisazone
3. Give the names of three important drugs that specifically interfere with viral nucleic acid replication. Discuss the synthesis of one such drug selected.
4. What are protease inhibitors? Mention a few examples and write the synthesis of indinavir.
5. Classify the antiviral drugs on the basis of their mode of action. Draw the structure, chemical name, and uses of at least one potent drug form each category.
6. Write the structure, chemical name, and uses of two important antiviral drugs that affect translation on cell ribosomes. Outline the synthesis of any one of them.
7. Enumerate the drugs used in HIV infection and write the synthesis of any one of them.
8. Discuss the following in detail:
   (a) Important antiviral drugs (b) Mode of action of antiviral drugs.

SUGGESTED READINGS

1. Abraham DJ (ed). *Burger's Medicinal Chemistry and Drug Discovery* (6th edn). New Jersey: John Wiley, 2007.
2. *British Pharmacopoeia*, Medicines and Healthcare Products Regulatory Agency. London, 2008.
3. Bruntan LL, Lazo JS, and Parker KL. *Goodman and Gilman's: The Pharmacological Basis of Therapeutics* (11th edn). New York: McGraw Hill, 2006.

4. Cann AJ. *Principles of Molecular Virology* (3rd edn). New York: Academic Press, 2001.
5. Crumpacker CS. 'Molecular targets of antiviral therapy'. *N Engl J Med* 321: 163–72, 1989.
6. Faulds D and Brogden RN. 'Didanosine'. *Drugs* 44(1): 96–116, 1992.
7. Gennaro AR. *Remington: The Science and Practice of Pharmacy* (21st edn). New York: Lippincot Williams and Wilkins, 2006.
8. Havlir DN and Richman DD. 'Antiretroviral therapy'. *Curr Opin Infect Dis* 8: 66–73, 1995.
9. Hirsch MS and D'Aquilla RT. 'Therapy for human immunodeficiency virus infection'. *N Engl J Med* 328: 1686–695, 1993.
10. *Indian Pharmacopoeia*. Ministry of Health and Family Welfare. New Delhi, 1996.
11. Knipe DM and Howley PM (ed). *Fundamental Virology* (4th edn). New York: Lippincott Williams and Wilkins, 2001.
12. Lemke TL and William DA. *Foye's Principle of Medicinal Chemistry* (6th edn). New York: Lippincott Williams and Wilkins, 2008.
13. Lednicer D and Mitscher LA. *The Organic Chemistry of Drug Synthesis*. New York: John Wiley, 1995.
14. Mansuri MM and Martin JC. 'Antiviral agents'. In *Annual Reports in Medicinal Chemistry*, Bristol JA (ed), pp. 133–40. San Diego, USA: Academic Press, 1991.
15. Reines EE and Gross PA. 'Antiviral agents'. *Med Clin North Am* 72: 691, 1988.
16. Sommadosi JP. 'Nucleoside analogs'. *Clin Infect Dis* 16: 57–515, 1993.
17. Wagner EK and Hewlett MJ (eds). *Basic Virology*. Malden, MA: Blackwell, 1999.
18. Zoon KC. *Human Interferons: Structure and Function*, pp. 1–12. London: Interferon Academic, 1987.

Chapter 8

Antiamoebic Agents

INTRODUCTION

Amoebiasis affects about 10% of the world's population, causing invasive diseases in about 50 million people and death in about 1,00,000 of these annually. This infection is, especially, common in lower socio-economic groups and institutionalized individuals living under crowded and poor hygienic conditions. Two morphologically identical, but genetically and biochemically distinct, species of *Entamoeba* (*E. histolitica* and *E. dispar*) are the causative organisms. Human beings are the only host for this organisms. Ingested amoebic cysts from contaminated food or water survive and form acid gastric contents and transform them into trophozoites that usually cause colitis which is either acute or chronic (dysentery). In some cases, they target the brain and the liver producing abscesses and systemic diseases.

This parasitic disease is one of the major causes of illness and death in many countries. World Health Organization (WHO) has classified this disease as follows:

1. Asymptomatic
2. Symptomatic
    a. Intestinal Amoebiasis
        i. Dysentery
        ii. Nondysenteric colitis
        iii. Amoeboma
        iv. Amoebic appendicitis.
    b. Extraintestinal amoebiasis
        i. Hepatic acute nonsupporative
        ii. Liver abscesses
3. Cutaneous involvement of other organs

Lung, brain, and spleen without the obvious liver involvement are some examples under this category. Antiamoebic agents are drugs used to treat amoebiasis. The potential drug should be active within the bowel lumen, in the bowel wall, and particularly in the liver. Worldwide, nearly 480 million people are infected with *E. histolytica*, of whom 10% develope clinical disease. The infection is transmitted exclusively by the faecal—oral route; human beings are the only known hosts.

CLASSIFICATION OF AMOEBICIDES

I. Luminal amoebicides: Diloxanide furoate.
It is active only against intestinal forms of amoeba.

II. Systemic amoebicides: Dihydroemetin, Choroquine.
These agents have been employed primarily to treat severe amoebic dysentery or hepatic abscesses.

III. Mixed amoebicides: Metronidazole, tinidazole, and ornidazole.
These agents are active against both intestinal and systemic forms of amoeba.

SYNTHESIS AND DRUG PROFILE

I. Luminal amoebicdes

i. Diloxanide Furoate (Furamide)

4-(2, 2-Dichloro-*N*-methylacetamido)phenyl furan-2-carboxylate

Synthesis

Metabolism: The diloxanide furoate is administered orally and is hydrolyzed in the gut to give diloxanide.

Diloxanide furoate —GIT→ [furan-2-carboxylic acid] —OH + HO—[phenyl]—N(CH₃)—C(=O)—CHCl₂

Dioxanide

Properties and uses: Diloxanide furoate is a white crystalline powder, very slightly soluble in water, slightly soluble in ethanol and ether. It is dichloro acetamide derivative that is nontoxic, mainly used in the treatment of chronic amoebiasis. It is less effective in the treatment of acute intestinal amoebiasis.

Assay: Dissolve the sample in anhydrous pyridine and titrate against 0.1 M tetrabutylammonium hydroxide. Determine the end point potentiometrically.

Dose: The recommended oral dose is 500 mg three times daily for 10 days (Diloxanide furoate 250 mg + Tinidazole 300 mg) two tablets daily. Diloxanide furoate 250 mg + Metronidazole 250 mg two tablets thrice daily for 10 days.

Dosage forms: Diloxanide tablets B.P.

III. Mixed amoebicdes

1. Metronidazole (Flagyl, Metrogyl)

2-(2-Methyl-5-nitro-1H-imidazol-1-yl)ethanol

Synthesis

Glyoxal (OHC–CHO) + 2NH₃ + CH₃CHO —Cyclization→ 2-methylimidazole

—HNO₃/H₂SO₄→ 2-methyl-5-nitroimidazole

—ClCH₂CH₂OH, NaOH→ Metronidazole

Mode of action: The reactive intermediate formed in the parasital reduction of the 5-nitro group of metronidazole covalently binds to the DNA of the parasite and triggers the lethal effects. Potential reactive intermediates include the nitroxide, nitroso, hydroxylamine, and amine.

Metabolism: In the liver, metabolism of metronidazole leads to two major metabolites, hydroxylation of the 2-methyl group to 2-hydroxymethyl metronidazole and oxidation to metronidazole acetic acid (MAA).

Properties and uses: Metronidazole is a white or yellowish crystalline powder, slightly soluble in water, acetone, alcohol, and methylene chloride. It is used in the treatment of intestinal and hepatic amoebiasis.
Assay: Dissolve the sample in anhydrous acetic acid and titrate with 0.1 M perchloric acid. Determine the end point potentiometrically.

Dose: For amoebiasis, the administered dose is 750 mg orally three times a day for 5–10 days. For trichomoniasis, the prescribed dose is 250 mg orally three times a day for 7 days. For giardiasis, the prescribed dose is 250 mg orally three times daily for 5–7 days.

Dosage forms: Metronidazole gel B.P., Metronidazole intravenous infusion B.P., Metronidazole suppositories B.P., Metronidazole tablets B.P.

2. **Tinidazole** (Fasigyn)

1-(2-(Ethylsulfonyl)ethyl)-2-methyl-5-nitro-1H-imidazole

Mode of action: Tinidazole's mechanism of action is similar to that of metronidazole. It is used in the treatment of intestinal and hepatic amoebiasis with a potential greater efficacy than metronidazole.

Metabolism: Tinidazole is metabolized by hydroxylation at the 2-methyl group and catalyzed by CYP3A4 to form inactive compound.

Synthesis

$$C_2H_5SCH_2CH_2OH \xrightarrow{\text{Peracid}} C_2H_5SO_2CH_2CH_2OH \xrightarrow{\text{Tosyl chloride}} C_2H_5SO_2CH_2CH_2OTs$$

+ 2-Methyl-5-nitro imidazole

↓ −TsOH

Tinidazole

Properties and uses: Tinidazole is a white or pale yellow crystalline powder, practically insoluble in water, soluble in acetone and in methylene chloride, and sparingly soluble in methanol. Used as an antiprotozoal and antibacterial agent.

Assay: Dissolve the sample in anhydrous acetic acid and titrate with 0.1 M perchloric acid. Determine the end point potentiometrically.

Dose: For giardiasis, the administered dose is 2 mg as a single dose.

3. Ornidazole (Ornida, Dazolic, Onidaz)

1-Chloro-3-(2-methyl-5-nitro-1*H*-imidazol-1-yl)propan-2-ol

Synthesis:

2-Methyl-5-nitro-1*H*-imidazole + Epichlorhydrin $\xrightarrow{\text{NaH}}$ Ornidazole

Properties and uses: It has a longer duration of action than metronidazole and used as an antiprotozoal.

Dose: The administered dose for amoebic dysentery in the case of adults is 1.5 g as a single daily dose for 3 days. Alternatively, for patients, whose weight is more than 60 kg, the dose is 1 g two times a day for 3 days. In the case of a child, the administered dose is 40 mg/kg daily. For amoebiasis, the recommended dose for adults is 5 g two times a day for 5–10 days. And in the case of a children, the dose is 25 mg/kg as a single daily dose for 5–10 days.

For giardiasis, in the case of adults, the dose is 1–1.5 g as a single daily dose for 1–2 days. In the case of a child, the dose is 30–40 mg/kg daily. In the case of trichomoniasis, the dose for adults is 1.5 g as a single daily dose or 0.5 g two times a day for 5 days. Treat sexual partners concomitantly. In the case of child, the dose is 25 mg/kg as a single dose. In the case of intravenous administration, during severe amoebic dysentery and amoebic liver abscess the prescribed dose for adults initially is 0.5–1 g infusion followed by 0.5 g every 12 h for 3–6 days. For a child, the dose is 20–30 mg/kg body weight daily.

4. Nitazoxanide

2-((5-Nitrothiazol-2-yl)carbamoyl)phenyl acetate

Synthesis

5-Nitrothiazol-2-amine + 2-Acetoxybenzoic acid $\xrightarrow{-H_2O}$ Nitrazoxanide

Mode of action: Nitazoxanide is a member of the 5-nitro heterocylces and is a prodrug forming a short-lived redox active intermediate. It appears to be more selective than metronidazole.

Uses: Used as an antiprotozoal agent.

5. Nimorazole (Nitroimidazole)

Synthesis

Glyoxal + 2NH₃ + Formaldehyde $\xrightarrow{-3H_2O}$ Imidazole $\xrightarrow{HNO_3/H_2SO_4}$ 5-Nitro-imidazole $\xrightarrow[\text{(ii) ClH}_2\text{CH}_2\text{C}-\text{N}\bigcirc\text{O}]{\text{(i) NaOH}}$ Nimorazole

Properties and uses: It possesses antiamoebic activity, and hence, used against intestinal and hepatic amoebiasis.

PROBABLE QUESTIONS

1. Classify antiamoebic agents and write the synthesis of any three of them.
2. Write synthesis, metabolism, and uses of Diloxanide furoate, Metronidazole, and Tinidazole.

SUGGESTED READINGS

1. Abraham DJ (ed). *Burger's Medicinal Chemistry and Drug Discovery* (6th edn). New Jersey: John Wiley, 2007.
2. Archer S. 'The chemotherapy of schistosomiasis'. *Ann Rev Pharmacol Toxicol* 25: 485, 1985.
3. Bruntan LL, Lazo JS, and Parker KL. *Goodman and Gilman's: The Pharmacological Basis of Therapeutics* (11th edn). New York: McGraw Hill, 2006.
4. *British Pharmacopoeia*. Medicines and Healthcare Products Regulatory Agency. London, 2008.
5. Freeman CD, Klutman NE, and Lamp KC. 'Metronidazole: A therapeutic review and update'. *Drugs* 54: 679–708, 1997.
6. Gennaro AR. *Remington: The Science and Practice of Pharmacy* (21st edn). New York: Lippincot Williams and Wilkins, 2006.
7. Gutteridge WEE. 'New antiprotozoal agents'. *Int J Parasitol* 17: 121–29, 1987.
8. Harries J. 'Amoebiasis—a review'. *J R Soc Med* 75: 190–97, 1982.
9. *Indian Pharmacopoeia*. Ministry of Health and Family Welfare. New Delhi, 1996.
10. Lednicer D and Mitscher LA. *The Organic Chemistry of Drug Synthesis*. New York: John Wiley, 1995.
11. Lemke TL and William DA. *Foye's Principle of Medicinal Chemistry* (6th edn). New York: Lippincott Williams and Wilkins, 2008.

12. Mandel GL, Bennett JE, and Dolin R (eds). *Principles and Practices of Infectious Diseases*, Vol. I (4th edn). New York: Churchill-Livingstone, 1995.
13. Meshnick SR. 'The chemotherapy of African trypanosomiasis'. In *Parasitic Diseases*, Vol. 2, Mansfield JM (ed), pp.165–99. New York: Marcel Dekker, 1984.
14. Reynolds EF (ed). *Martindale the Extra Pharmacopoeia* (31st edn). London: The Pharmaceutical Press, 1997
15. Testa B (ed). *Advances in Drug Research*, Vol. 21. New York: Academic Press, 1991.
16. Wilson JD et al (ed). *Harrison's Principles of Internal Medicine* (12th edn), p. 772. New York: McGraw Hill, 1992.
17. Woolfe G. 'The chemotherapy of amoebiasis'. In *Progress in Drug Research*, Vol. 8, Jucker E (ed), pp. 11–52. Basel, Switzerland: Brikhauser Verlag, 1965.

Chapter 9

Antimalarials

INTRODUCTION

Antimalarial agents are drugs used for the treatment or prophylaxis of malaria. Malaria is caused by four species of *Plasmodium*, such as *Plasmodium falciparum, P. malariae, P. ovale*, and *P. vivax*. Three of which produces the mild forms of malaria by destroying red blood cells in peripheral capillaries and thus, causing anaemia. The bouts of fever correspond to the reproductive cycle of the parasite. However, the most dangerous is the *P. falciparum*. In this case, the infected red blood cells become sticky and form lumps in the capillaries of the deep organs of the body and cause microcirculatory arrest. This disease still affects about 200 millions people and causes at least 2 million deaths per year.

LIFE CYCLE OF PLASMODIUM

The different stages of the reproductive cycle (Fig. 9.1) of the malarial parasite and the drugs acting at different stages of this cycle are given below:

- Stage-I: No drug is effective in this stage.
- Stage-II: Primaquine and pyrimethamine can block at this stage.
- Stage-III: Primaquine can only prevent because fever occurs at this stage.
- Stage-IV: Chloroquine, amodiaquine, santoquine, proguanil.
- Stage-V: Primaquine only.

Two important phases of the parasite life cycle are the following:

1. Asexual cycle—occurs in the infected host.
2. Sexual cycle—occurs in the mosquito.

After the insect bite, the parasite forms rapidly. They leave the circulation and localize in the hepatocytes whereby they transform, multiply, and develop into tissue schizonts. The primary asymptomatic tissue stage lasts for 15 days and the tissue schizonts rupture, each releasing thousands of merozites. The released merozites invade more erythrocytes to continue the cycle's synchronous rupture of erythrocytes to continue the cycle. Synchronous rupture of erythrocytes and release of merozites into the circulation leads to

Chemotherapy

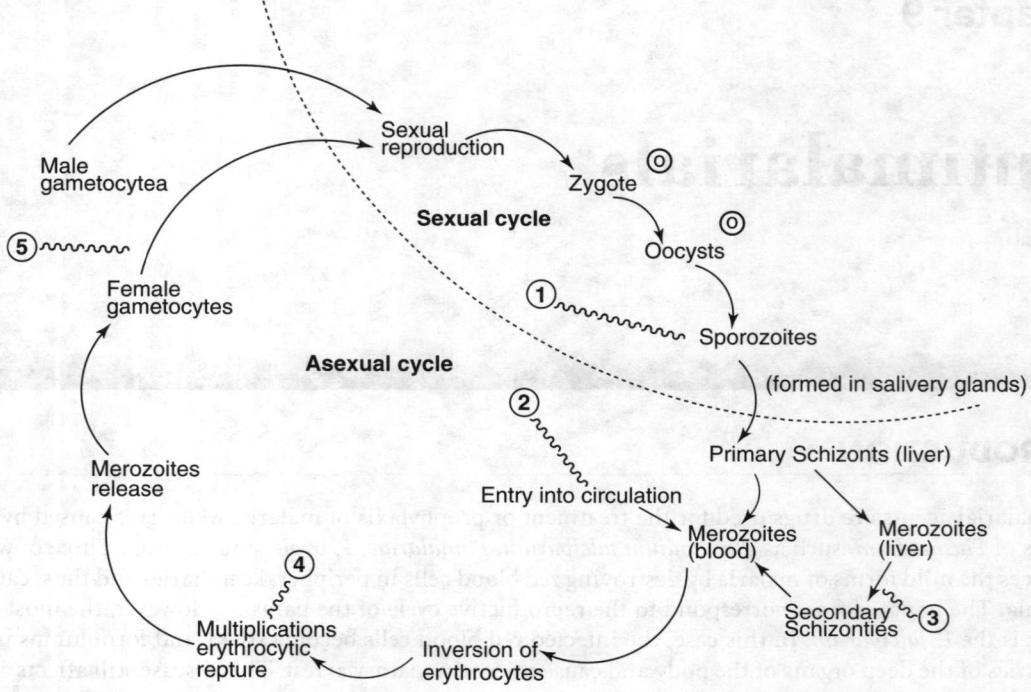

Figure 9.1 Life cycle of plasmodium.

febrile pattern attacks on day 1 and 3; hence, the designation is 'tertian malaria'. Some erythrocyte parasites differentiate into several forms known as gametophytes. After infecting human blood, female mosquito ingests them. Then the exflagellation of male gametocyte is followed by the male gametogenesis and the fertilization of the female gametocytes in the insect's guts. The resulting zygote, which develops as an oocyte in the gut wall, eventually gives rise to infective sporozoite, which invades the salivary glands of the mosquito. The insect then can infect another human by taking a blood meal.

CLASSIFICATION

I. Cinchona alkaloids

Name	R
Quinine	–OCH$_3$ (–) isomer
Quinidine	–OCH$_3$ (+) isomer (used as antiarrhythmic)
Cinchonine	–H (+) isomer
Cinchonidine	–H (–) isomer

II. 7-Chloro-4-Amino Quinolines

[Structure: 7-chloro-4-amino quinoline with NHR at position 4, R^1 at position 3, Cl at position 7]

Name	R	R^1
Cholorquine	–CH(CH$_3$)(CH$_2$)$_3$–N(C$_2$H$_5$)$_2$	–H
Amodiaquine	[phenyl ring with –CH$_2$N(C$_2$H$_5$)$_2$ and –OH substituents]	–H
Hydroxychloroquine	–CH(CH$_3$)–(CH$_2$)$_3$–N(C$_2$H$_5$)((CH$_2$)$_2$OH)	–H
Sontoquine	–CH(CH$_3$)–(CH$_2$)$_3$–N(C$_2$H$_5$)$_2$	–CH$_3$
Amopyroquine	[phenyl ring with –CH$_2$–pyrrolidine and –OH substituents]	–H

III. 8-Amino Quinolines

[Structure: 6-methoxy-8-amino quinoline with H$_3$CO at position 6 and NH-R at position 8]

6-Methoxy-8-amino quinoline derivatives

Name	R
Primaquine	$-CH(CH_3)-(CH_2)_3-NH_2$
Pamaquine	$-CH(CH_3)-(CH_2)_3-N(C_2H_5)_2$
Pentaquine phosphate	$-(CH_2)_5-NH-CH(CH_3)_2$
Isopentaquine	$-CH(CH_3)-(CH_2)_3-NH-CH(CH_3)_2$
Quinocide HCl	$-(CH_2)_3-CH(CH_3)-N(C_2H_5)_2$

IV. Acridine derivatives (9-amino acridine derivatives)

Name	R
Quinacrine	$-CH(CH_3)-(CH_2)_3-N(C_2H_5)_2$
Acriquine	$-(CH_2)_4-N(C_2H_5)_2$

V. Antifolates
a. Biguanids

Name	R	R'
Proguanil	–Cl	–H
Chloro proguanil	–Cl	–Cl
Bromoguanil	–Br	–H
Nitroguanil	–NO$_2$	–H

b. Diamino pyrimidines

Pyrimethamine (Daraprim)

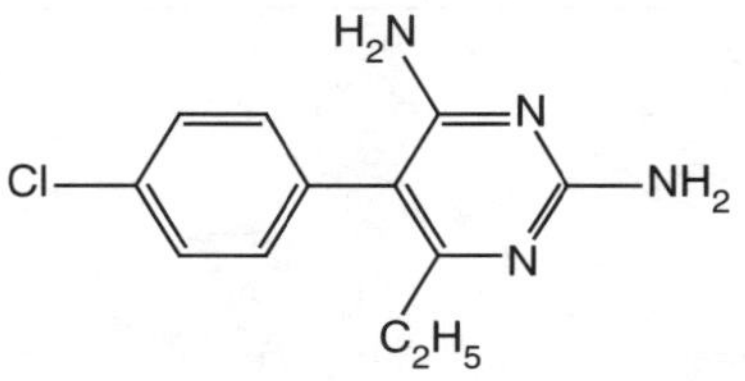

Trimethoprim

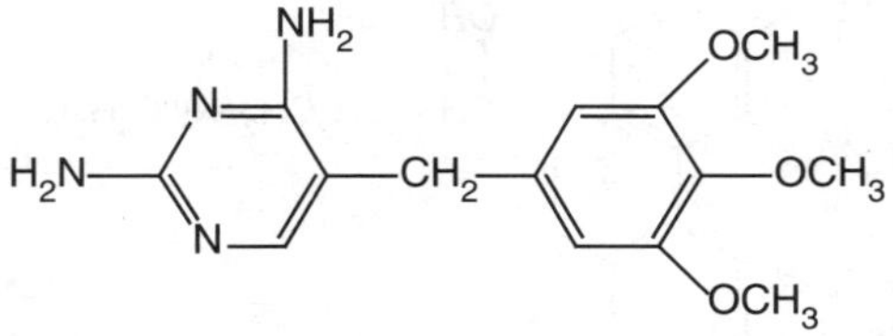

VI. Sulphonamides and Sulphones

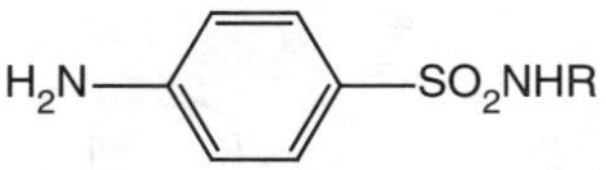

$H_2N-\text{C}_6H_4-SO_2NHR$

Name	R
Sulphadoxine	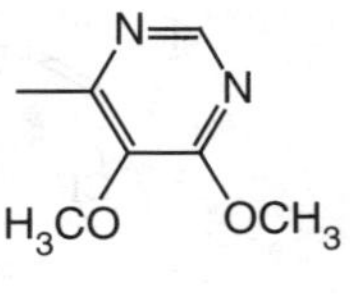 4-methyl-5,6-dimethoxypyrimidin-2-yl (methyl group, with H$_3$CO and OCH$_3$ substituents)
Sulphadiazine	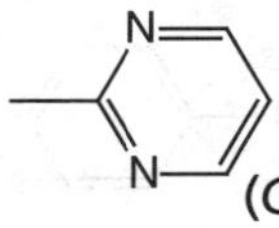 pyrimidin-2-yl

(*Continued*)

Name	R
(Continued)	
Sulphamethoxazole	3-methyl-5-methylisoxazole
Sulphalene	3-methyl-2-methoxypyrazine

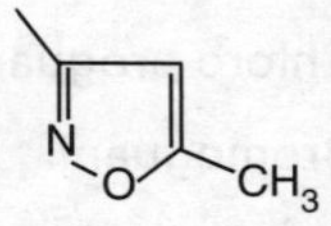

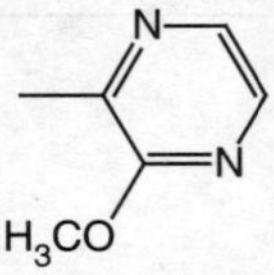

VII. Phenanthrine methanol

Halofentamine

VIII. Miscellaneous drugs

Halofantrine (Hafan)

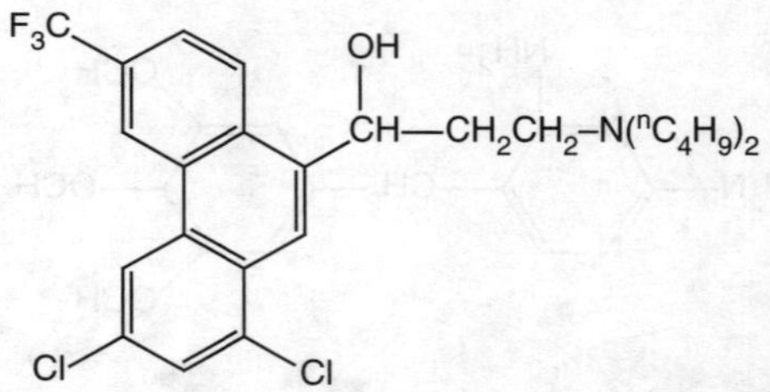

[Structure: phenanthrene with F_3C, two Cl substituents, and $CH(OH)-CH_2CH_2-N(^nC_4H_9)_2$ side chain]

Mefloquine

[Structure: quinoline with two CF_3 groups, HO–CH linked to piperidine ring]

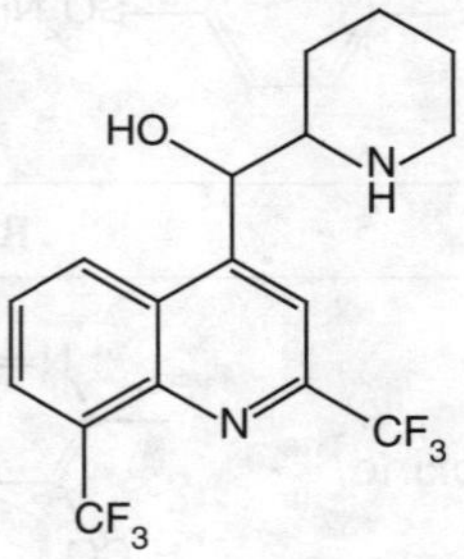

Dapsone

H_2N–C$_6$H$_4$–SO_2–C$_6$H$_4$–NH_2

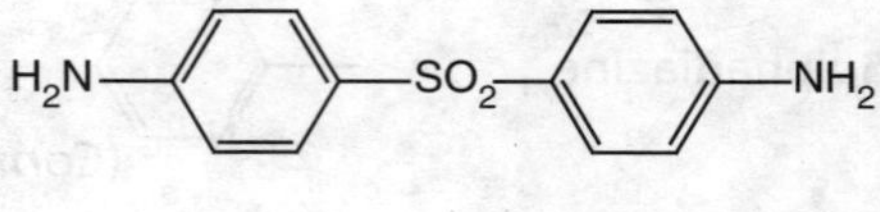

Artemether, Artemotil

R = CH$_3$; Artemether
R = C$_2$H$_5$; Artether

Artesunate

SYNTHESIS AND DRUG PROFILE

I. 4-Substituted Quinolines

Mode of Action: Three different mechanism of actions are suggested for these drugs:

DNA interaction: The mechanism of action for quinine is that the drug gets intercalated into the DNA of the parasite. It is based on the fact that the concentration required for the inhibition of nucleic acid synthesis is significantly higher than that necessary for the inhibition of the plasmodium parasite.

Ferriprotoporphyrin IX: The plasmodium parasite utilizes host haemoglobin as a source of amino acid. On digestion of the haemoglobin, the haem is released as ferriprotoporphyrins IX and it produces haemolysis of the erythrocyte parasites. Therefore, ferriprotoporphyrin that is released is converted into nontoxic products and they, in turn, to haemozoites by the polymerase enzyme. The steps involved in the conversion to haemozoites are inhibited by the chloroquine.

Weak base hypothesis: The 4-substituted quinolines have weak base and because of this pKa they are thought to accumulate in a location, which is acidic (parasite lysozome pH 4.8–5.2). As the extracellular fluid of the parasite is at pH 7.4, the weak base will move towards a more acidic pH of lysosome. Once the acid–base reaction occurs, elevating the pH in the lysozome, that in turn reduces the parasite's ability to digest haemoglobin, thus reducing the availability of amino acids.

Metabolism of Quinine: It is metabolized in the liver to 2-hydroxy derivative followed by additional hydroxylation on the quinoline ring with the 2,3-dihydroxy derivative, as the major metabolite. This metabolite has low activity and is rapidly excreted in urine.

Properties and uses: Quinine hydrochloride exists as fine, silky needles, often in clusters, colourless, soluble in water and in alcohol. It is used in the treatment of malaria.

Assay: Dissolve the sample in alcohol, add 0.01 M hydrochloric acid, and titrate with 0.1 M sodium hydroxide. Determine the end point potentiometrically.

Chloroquine (Nivaquin, Aralen, Lariago)

Synthesis

Step I. Synthesis of 4,7-dichloro quinoline

Step-II: Preparation of 1-diethyl amino-4-amino pentane

Step III. Condensation of the products of *Step I* and *Step II*

Metabolism: The drug is metabolized by *N*-dealkylation through CYP2D6, and CYP3A4 isoenzymes. It has been reported that the level of metabolism correlates closely with degree of resistance.

Properties and uses: Chloroquine exists as white or almost white crystalline powder, soluble in water and in methanol, very slightly soluble in ethanol. It is mainly used as an antimalarial. Chloroquine also has antihistaminic and antiinflammatory properties. It is used to treat hepatic amoebiasis, rheumatoid arthritis, discoid lupus erythematosus, cutanea tards, solar urticaria, and polymorphous light eruptions. Chloroquine and other 4-amino quinolines are not effective against exoerythrocytic parasites. It is an example for poor selective toxicity. Adverse reactions include retinopathy, haemolysis in patients with glucose-6-phosphate dehydrogenase deficiency (same mutation that confers resistance against malaria), muscular weakness, exacerbation of psoriasis and porphyria, and impaired liver function.

Assay: Dissolve the sample in anhydrous acetic acid and titrate with 0.1 M perchloric acid. Determine the end point potentiometrically.

Dose: The recommended dose as a prophylactic and a suppressive is 500 mg once per week. As a therapeutic the dose, initially, is 1 g followed by 500 mg in 6 h, and 500 mg on the 2nd and 3rd day.

Dosage forms: Chloroquine sulphate injection I.P., B.P., Chloroquine sulphate tablets I.P., B.P.

Amodiaquine HCl (Camoquin)

Synthesis

Properties and uses: It exists as yellow crystalline powder with a bitter taste, and is soluble in water. It is very similar to chloroquine and does not have any advantages over the other 4-amino quinoline drugs. It is used for suppressing *P. vivax* and *P. falciparum* infections being 3–4 times more active than quinine.

Dose: The recommended dose initially is 600 mg followed by 300 mg doses 6, 24, and 48 h later.

Hydroxy chloroquine (Plaquenil)

Synthesis

Step I. Preparation of side chain-N-ethyl-N-(2-hydroxyethyl)-4-amino pentylamine

Step II. Condensation of the product of *Step I* with 4,7-dichloro quinoline

Properties and uses: Hydroxychloroquine is a white or almost white crystalline powder, soluble in water, practically insoluble in ethanol and in ether. It is equivalent to the chloroquine, but it is less toxic and used in the place of chloroquine against normally sensitive strains. It is mainly used as an antimalarial. It is also used for the treatment of rheumatoid arthritis and lupus erythematoses.

Assay: Dissolve the sample in water, add 1 M sodium hydroxide, and extract with dichloromethane. Combine the dichloromethane extracts and evaporate. Add anhydrous acetic acid and titrate against 0.1 M perchloric acid, using oracet blue B solution as indicator.

Dose: In *P. falciparum* infections, the dose is 1.25 g in a single dose or in two divided doses at 6 h intervals; in rheumatoid arthritis, 400 mg daily; in lupus erythematosus, 200 to 400 mg 1 or 2 times daily.

Dosage forms: Hydroxychloroquine tablets B.P.

STRUCTURE–ACTIVITY RELATIONSHIP

- At C-4 position, the dialkylaminoalkyl side chain has 2-5 carbon atoms between the nitrogen atoms, particularly the 4-diethylaminomethyl butyl amino side chain that is optimal for activity, as in chloroquine and quinacrine.
- The substitution of a hydroxyl group on one of the ethyl groups on the tertiary amine (hydroxy quinoline), reduces toxicity.
- Incorporation of an aromatic ring in the side chain (e.g. amodiaquine) gives a compound with reduced toxicity and activity.
- The tertiary amine in the side chain is important.
- The introduction of an unsaturated bond in the side chain was not detrimental to activity.
- The 7-chloro group in the quinoline nucleus is optimal, the methyl group in position 3 reduces activity, and an additional methyl group in position 8 abolishes activity.
- The D-isomer of chloroquine is less toxic than its L-isomer.

II. 8-Amino quinolines

Mode of action: While the mechanism of action of the 8-amino quinolines is unknown, it is known that primaquine can generate reactive oxygen species via an autoxidation of the 8-amino quinoline group with the formation of radical anion. As a result, cell destructive oxidants, such as hydrogen peroxide, super oxide, and hydroxyl radical can be formed.

Primaquine (Primaquine Phosphate)

Synthesis

Step I. Preparation of 1-phthalimido-4-bromo pentane

1,4-Dibromo pentane + Potassium phthalimide $\xrightarrow{-KBr}$ 1-Phthalimido-4-bromo pentane

Step II. Synthesis of 8-amino-6-methoxy quinoline

p-Acetamido anisole $\xrightarrow{HNO_3 / H_2SO_4}$

$\xrightarrow{H_2O}$

Skraup's synthesis (H_2SO_4, Nitrobenzene) with glycerol (H_2C-OH, $HC-OH$, H_2C-OH)

$\xrightarrow{Sn / HCl}$ 8-Amino-6-methoxy quinoline

Step III. Condensation of product of *Step I* and *Step II*

[Reaction scheme: 8-Amino-6-methoxy quinoline + 1-Phthalimido-4-bromo pentane, −HBr, gives the N-substituted intermediate, which upon Hydrolysis (−Phthalic acid) gives Primaquine.]

Metabolism: Primaquine is totally metabolized by CYP3A4 with primary metabolites having carboxy primaquine. Trace amounts of *N*-acetyl primaquine, aromatic hydroxylated products, and conjugation metabolites are seen.

[Structures: Primaquine → Carboxy primaquine; N-acetyl primaquine]

Properties and uses: Primaquine is a crystalline powder, soluble in water, and practically insoluble in alcohol. In vitro and in vivo studies indicate that the stereochemistry at the asymmetric carbon is not important for antimalarial activity. These appears to be less toxicity with the levorotatory isomer, but this is dose–dependent, and may not be of much importance as the doses used to treat exoerythrocytic *P. vivax* malaria. It is extensively used for the radical cure of relapsing *vivax* malaria, but it is not normally employed either for arresting the severe attacks of the disease or for the suppressive therapy. It invariably kills gametocytes of all the species, or inhibits their growth and development in the mosquito. It fails to produce any significant effect on other erythrocytic stages, and hence, it must not be employed alone for the treatment of malaria.

Assay: Dissolve the sample in anhydrous acetic acid and heat gently. Allow to cool and titrate with 0.1 M perchloric acid. Determine the end point potentiometrically.

Dose: The recommended dose for administration is 17.5–26.3 mg (10–15 mg of base) once daily for 14 days.

Pamaquine

Synthesis

Properties and uses: It was the first 8-amino quinoline marketed, used as an antimalarial agent.

III. Acridine Derivatives

Quinacrine

Synthesis

Reaction scheme: 2,4-Dichloro benzoic acid (as acid chloride, COCl) + 4-Methoxy aniline $\xrightarrow{KOH}$ intermediate (Cl–C$_6$H$_3$(COOH)–NH–C$_6$H$_4$–OCH$_3$) $\xrightarrow{POCl_3,\ Cyclization}$ acridone intermediate ⇌ 9-hydroxy acridine (Cl, OCH$_3$ substituted) $\xrightarrow{POCl_3}$ 9-chloro-acridine (Quinacrine intermediate) $\xrightarrow{R,\ -HCl}$ **Quinacrine**

R = NH$_2$CH(CH$_3$)(CH$_2$)$_3$N(C$_2$H$_5$)$_2$

Mode of action: Quinacrine acts at many sites within the cell, including intercalation of DNA strands, succinic dehydrogenase, mitochondrial electron transport, and cholinesterase. It may be tumerogenic and mutagenic and has been used as a sclerosing agent. Because it is an acridine dye, quinacrine can cause yellow discolouration of the skin and urine.

Properties and uses: It acts as a schizontocidal and now it is not used as an antimalarial agent. It is used in the treatment of leishmaniasis and some tape worm infestations.

IV. a. Biguanides

Mode of action: Biguanides inhibit dihydrofolate reductase enzyme and interfere in the folic acid metabolism. This leads to inhibition of the nuclear division in malarial parasites.

Proguanil HCl (Paludrine)

Cl—C$_6$H$_4$—NH—C(=NH)—NH—C(=NH)—NH—CH(CH$_3$)$_2$ · HCl

Synthesis

Step I. Synthesis of *p*-chloro phenyl guanidine

1-Chloro-4-nitrobenzene →(Reduction)→ 4-Chloroaniline →(CNBr)→ (4-Chlorophenyl)cyanamide →(H)/NH$_3$→ *p*-Chlorophenyl guanidine

Step II. Synthesis of isopropyl cyanamide

Isobutyric acid →(SOCl$_2$)→ (CH$_3$)$_2$CH—COCl →(NH$_3$)→ (CH$_3$)$_2$CH—CONH$_2$ →(Decarbonylation)→ Isopropylamine →(CNBr)→ Isopropyl cyanamide

Step III. Condensation of the products of *Steps I and II*

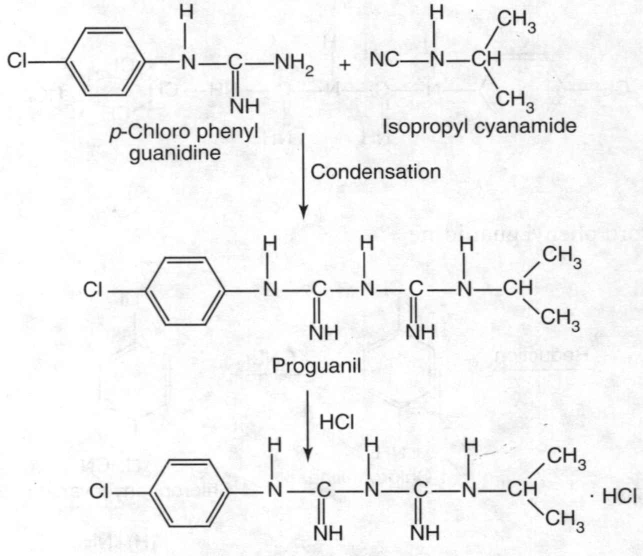

[Structures: p-Chloro phenyl guanidine + Isopropyl cyanamide → Condensation → Proguanil → HCl → Proguanil hydrochloride]

Metabolism: Proguanil is a prodrug, which is metabolized in the liver to diaminotriazine (cycloguanil) that acts as a dihydrofolate reductase inhibitor of *Plasmodium* species and inhibits DNA synthesis.

Properties and uses: Proguanil hydrochloride is a white crystalline powder, slightly soluble in water, sparingly soluble in ethanol, and practically insoluble in methylene chloride. It is used mainly for prophylactic treatment of malaria.

Assay: Suspend the sample in anhydrous acetic acid, shake and heat at 50°C for 5 min. Cool to room temperature, add acetic anhydride, and titrate with 0.1 M perchloric acid. Determine the end point potentiometrically.

Dose: The recommended dose as a prophylactic and a suppressant is 100 to 200 mg per day in nonimmune subjects; 300 mg/week or 200 mg twice/week in semi-immune subjects. In the case of acute *vivax* malaria, initial loading dose is 300 g–600 mg followed by 300 mg per day for 5–10 days. For the treatment of *falciparum* malaria, the dose is 300 mg two times daily for 5 days.

IV. b. Diaminopyrimidines

Mode of Action: It inhibits the reduction of folic acid and dihydrofolic acid to the active tetrahydrofolate coenzyme form.

Pyrimethamine (Daraprim)

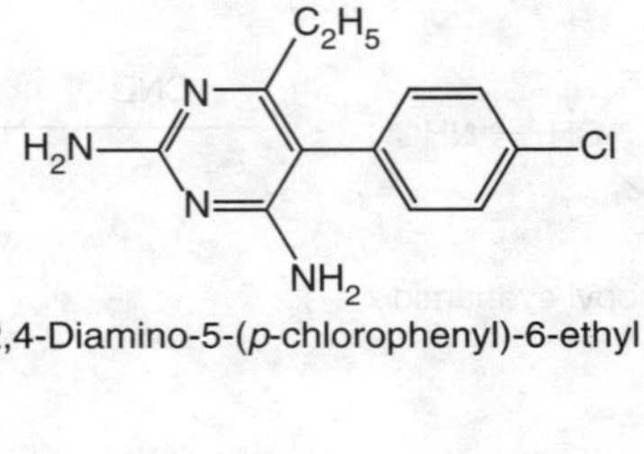

[Structure of pyrimethamine]

2,4-Diamino-5-(*p*-chlorophenyl)-6-ethyl pyrimidine

Synthesis

Properties and uses: Pyrimethamine exists as a white crystalline powder or colourless crystals, practically insoluble in water, and slightly soluble in alcohol. Pyrimethamine inhibits the reduction of folic acid and dihydrofolic acid to the active tetrahydrofolate coenzyme form. It finds its extensive use as a suppressive prophylactic for the prevention of severe attacks due to *P. falciparum* and *P. vivax*. It is also used in the treatment of taxoplasmosis and as an immuno suppressive agent.

Assay: Dissolve the sample in anhydrous acetic acid by heating gently. Cool and titrate with 0.1 M perchloric acid. Determine the end point potentiometrically.

Dose: The administered dose as a suppressive is 25 mg once a week, as a therapeutic 50–75 mg once a day for two days when used alone, otherwise 25 mg.

Dosage forms: Pyrimethamine tablets I.P., B.P.

Trimethoprim (Proloprim)

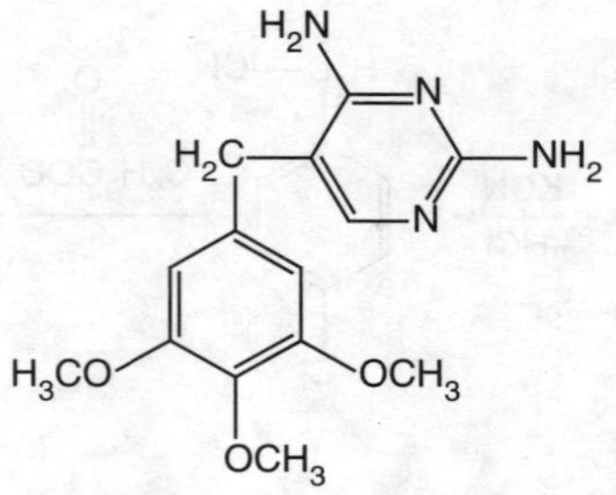

Synthesis

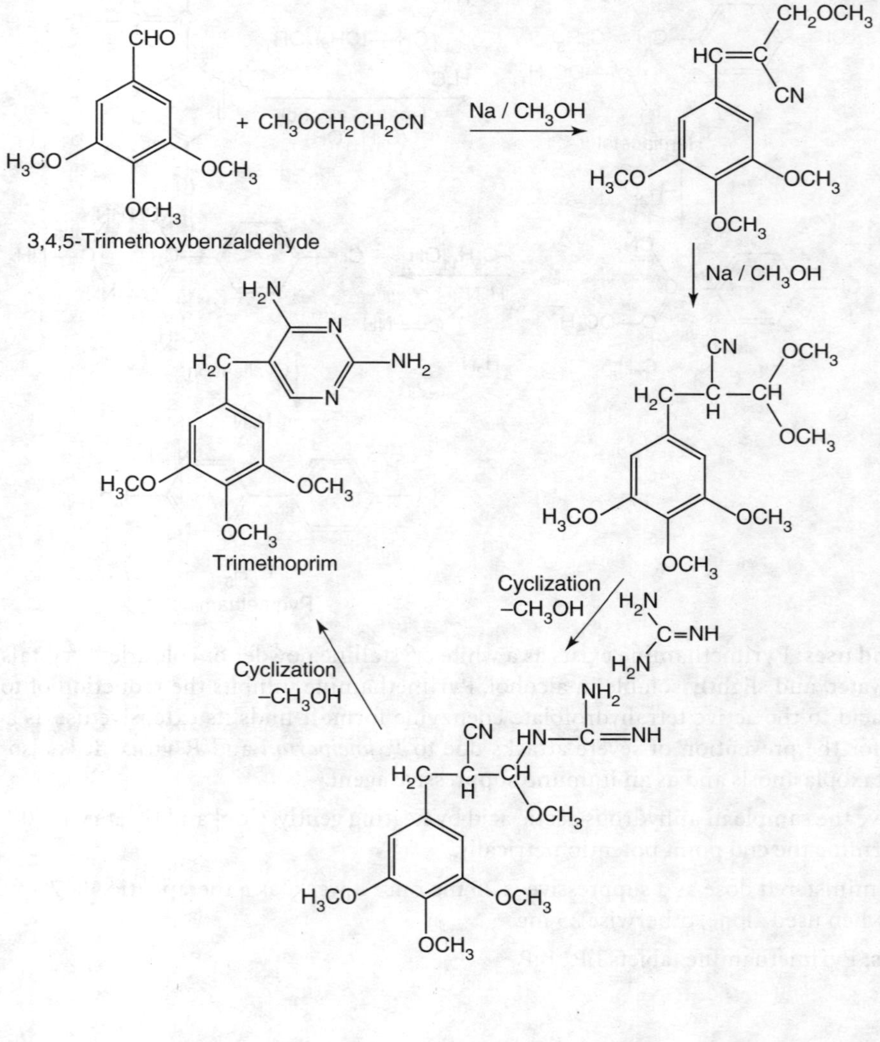

Properties and uses: Trimethoprim exists as a white or yellowish-white powder, very slightly soluble in water, and slightly soluble in ethanol. It is a potent inhibitor of dihydrofolate reductase. It has been employed in conjugation with sulphamethopyrazine in the treatment of chloroquine-resistant malaria. It has also been used in conjugation with sulphonamides in the treatment of bacterial infections. Trimethoprim is an antibacterial, effective against malarial parasite.

Assay: Dissolve the sample in anhydrous acetic acid and titrate with 0.1 M perchloric acid. Determine the end point potentiometrically.

Dose: The administered dose is 1.5 g with 1 g of sulphametopyrazine per day for 3 days.

Dosage forms: Co-trimoxazole intravenous infusion B.P., Co-trimoxazole oral suspension B.P., Paediatric co-trimoxazole oral suspension B.P., Co-trimoxazole tablets dispersible B.P., Co-trimoxazole tablets paediatric B.P., Co-trimoxazole tablets B.P., Trimethoprim oral suspension B.P., Trimethoprim tablets B.P.

V. Sulphones and sulphonamides

Mode of action: They only act against the erythrocytic stages of malaria parasite. The sulphadoxine interferes with the parasites ability to synthesize folic acid. Sulphonamides block the incorporation of *p*-amino benzoicacid (PABA) to form dihydropteroic acid. PABA is the central part of the folate structure. Sulphonamides exhibit significant toxicity because humans do not synthesize the vitamin folic acid. There are severe to fatal occurrences of erythema multiform, Stevens-Johnson syndrome, toxic epidermal necrolysis, and serum sickness syndromes attributed to the sulphadoxine.

VI. Micellaneous

Halofantrine

Metabolism: The drug is metabolized by *N*-dealkylation to desbutyl halofantrine by CYP3A4. The metabolites appear to be several folds more active than the parent drug.

Halofantrine

Desbutyl halofantrine

Synthesis

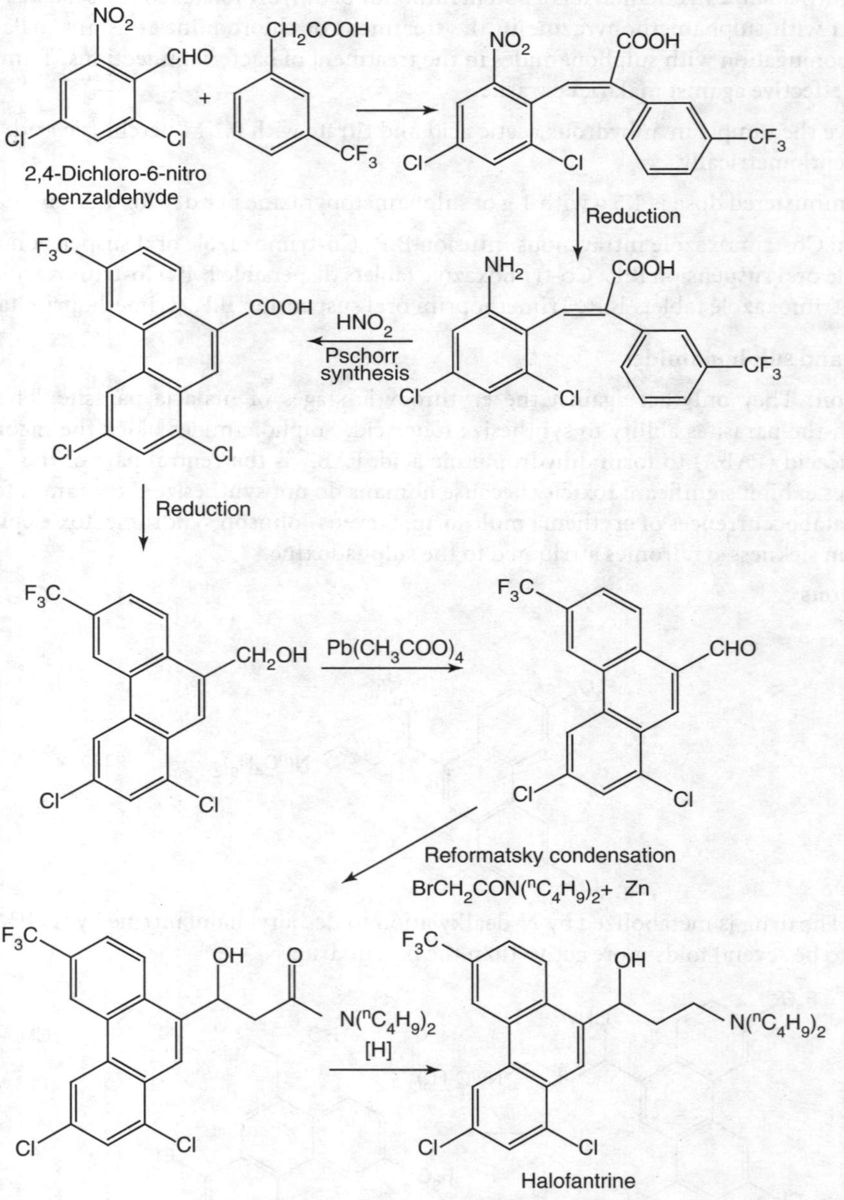

[Scheme: 2,4-Dichloro-6-nitrobenzaldehyde + CH₂COOH-C₆H₄-CF₃ → nitro-stilbene intermediate → Reduction → amino intermediate → HNO₂ / Pschorr synthesis → phenanthrene-COOH → Reduction → CH₂OH → Pb(CH₃COO)₄ → CHO → Reformatsky condensation with BrCH₂CON(^{n}C₄H₉)₂ + Zn → β-hydroxy amide → [H] → Halofantrine]

Properties and uses: Halofantrine is a white or almost white powder, practically insoluble in water, soluble in methanol, and sparingly soluble in alcohol. Structurally, halofentrine differs from all other antimalarial drugs and belongs to the latest generation of antimalarials. It is a good example of a drug design that incorporates bioisosteric principles evidenced by the tri-fluoro methyl moiety. It is schizonticidal and has no effect on the sporozoite, gametocyte, or hepatic stages. It is effective in the treatment and prophylaxis of chloroquine and multidrug resistant *P. falciparum*.

Assay: It is as assayed by adopting Liquid chromatography technique.

Artemether (Larither, Paluther) **and Artether**

Synthesis

R = CH$_3$; Artemether
R = C$_2$H$_5$; Artether

Dose: The administered dose for acute uncomplicated *falciparum* malaria in the case of adults is 80 mg daily to be taken with lumefantrine 480 mg daily. Doses to be taken at diagnosis and repeated after 8, 24, 36, 48, and 60 h. Total doses are six. For a child, the daily dose based on the body weight is as follows: 5–14 kg: 20 mg ; 15–24 kg: 40 mg with lumefantrine 240 mg; 25–34 kg; 60 mg with lumefantrine 360 mg and more than 34 kg; 80 mg with lumefantrine 480 mg. Doses to be taken at diagnosis and repeated after 8, 24, 36, 48, and 60 h and the total doses are 6.

Artesunate (Asunate, Ultera, Falcigo)

[Structure of Artesunate showing the sesquiterpene lactone with endoperoxide bridge and OCOCH₂CH₂COOH substituent]

Synthesis

[Dihydroartemisinin with OH group] + HOOCCH₂CH₂COOH →(DCC)→ Artesunate

Dose: The dose in the case of *falciparum* malaria for adults is 2.4 mg/kg via IM or IV administration to be repeated after 12 h and 24 h later; then, once daily thereafter. For a child, the dose is 2.4 mg/kg via IM or IV administration and to be repeated after 12 h and 24 h later; then, once daily thereafter.

Mefloquine

[Structure of Mefloquine: quinoline with two CF₃ groups, hydroxyl, and piperidine substituent]

Metabolism of mefloquine: It is metabolized through CYP3A4 oxidation to its major inactive metabolite called carboxy mefloquine and rest of the amount is excreted unchanged in urine.

Mefloquine → [Metabolite: quinoline with COOH, two CF₃ groups]

Metabolite

Properties and uses: Mefloquine hydrochloride is a white or slightly yellow crystalline powder, very slightly soluble in water, soluble in methanol and in alcohol. It is used as an antimalarial agent.

Assay: Dissolve the sample in anhydrous formic acid, add acetic anhydride and titrate with 0.1 M perchloric acid. Determine the end-point potentiometrically.

PROBABLE QUESTIONS

1. What are the casual organisms responsible for malaria? How do the antimalarials affect the life cycle of mosquito? Explain.
2. Write the mode of action, synthesis, and metabolism of any one of the 4-amino quinoline derivatives.
3. Discuss the synthesis of one important antimalarial drug belonging to the class:
   (a) Diaminopyrimidines (b) Sulphones.
4. Write the SAR of 4-amino quinolines.
5. Classify the synthetic antimalarials based on their basic chemical nucleus. Provide examples of at least one of the two compounds from each class.
6. Modifications of the side-chain at C-4 position on the 4-amino-7-chloroquinoline nucleus results in the following drugs:
   (a) Chloroquine phosphate (b) Amodiaquine hydrochloride (c) Santoquin
7. Outline the synthesis of proguanil hydrochloride from *p*-chlorophenyl guanidine and iso-propyl cyanamide. Write their structure, synthesis, and the dosage forms available.
8. Name the three important antimalarials derived from 8-amino-6-methoxy quinoline nucleus, their structure, chemical name, uses, and the synthesis of any one drug.
9. Elaborate the synthesis of mepacrine hydrochloride, the uses, and the dosage forms available.
10. Proguanil hydrochloride is the wonder drug for malaria that gets metabolized to its active form cycloguanil in vivo. Explain its biotransformation.

SUGGESTED READINGS

1. Abraham DJ (ed). *Medicinal Chemistry and Drug Discovery* (6th edn). New Jersey: John Wiley, 2007.
2. *British Pharmacopoeia*, Medicines and Healthcare Products Regulatory Agency. London, 2008.
3. Bruce-Chwatt LJ (ed). *Chemotherapy of Malaria*, Rev (2nd edn). Geneva: WHO, 1986.
4. Bruntan LL, Lazo JS, and Parker KL. *Goodman and Gilman's: The Pharmacological of Therapeutics* (11th edn). New York: McGraw Hill, 2006.
5. Butler AR and Wu Yu-Lin. 'Artemisinin (Qinghaosu). A new type of antimalarial drug'. *Chem Soc Rev* 85–90, 1992.
6. Cabantchuik ZI. 'Iron chelators as antimalarials: The biochemical basis of selective cytotoxicity'. *Parasitol Today* 11: 74–78, 1995.
7. Cooper WC. *Summary of Antimalarial Drugs*, Report No. 64. U.S. Public Health Service, 1949.
8. Findlay GM. *Recent Advances in Chemotherapy* (2nd edn), Vol. 2. Philadelphia: Blakiston, 1951.

9. Gennaro AR. *Remington: Science and Practice of Pharmacy* (21st edn). New York: Lippincot Williams and Wilkins, 2006.
10. Honingsbaum M. *The Fever Trail: In Search for the Cure for Malaria*. New York: Farrar, Straus, and Girous, 2001.
11. Hsuch KO and Tung P. 'Co-ordinating group for research on the structure of Quing Hau Sau: A new type of sesquiterpene lactone'. *Drugs of the Future* 22(3): 142, 1977.
12. *Indian Pharmacopoeia* Ministry of Health and Family Welfare. New Delhi, 1996.
13. Kremsner PG and Graninger W. 'Clindamycin in the treatment of experimental and human malaria'. *Rev Contemp Pharmacother* 26(3): 275–79, 1992.
14. Lednicer D and Mitscher LA. *The Organic Chemistry of Drug Synthesis*. New York: John Wiley, 1995.
15. Lemke TL and William DA. *Foye's Principle of Medicinal Chemistry* (6th ed). New York: Lippincott Williams and Wilkins, 2008.
16. Pratt WB. *Fundamentals of Chemotherapy*. London: Oxford University Press, 1973.
17. Panisko DM and Keystone JS. 'Treatment of malaria'. *Drugs* 39: 160, 1990.
18. Rozman RS and Canfield CJ. 'New experimental antimalarial drugs'. *Adv Pharmacol Chemother* 16: 1, 1979.
19. Reynolds EF (ed). *Martindale the Extra Pharmacopoeia* (31st edn). London: Pharmaceutical Press, 1997.
20. Stec EA. *The Chemotherapy of Protozoan Diseases*, Vols I–IV. Washington DC: Walter Reed Army Institute of Research, 1971.
21. Saxena AK and Saxena M. 'Advances in chemotherapy of malaria'. *Prog Drug Res* 30: 221, 1986.
22. Slater AFG and Cerani A. *Nature* 355: 167–69, 1992.
23. Thompson PE and Werbal LM. *Antimalarial Agents Chemistry and Pharmacology*. New York: Academic Press, 1972.

Chapter 10

Anthelmintics

INTRODUCTION

Anthelmintics are drugs used to treat parasitic infections due to worms. Worms that are pathogenic to human beings, namely, metazoa are conventionally classified into round worms (nematodes) and two types of flatworms, that is, flukes (trematodes) and tapeworms (cestodes). Anthelmintics act locally either to expel the worms from the gastrointestinal tract or systemically to eradicate the species and the developing forms of helmintics that invade the organs and tissues. This class of agents have added significance due to their wide prevalence in third-world countries and it is estimated over 2 billion people are affected. No cheaper medicines are available for this disease, even now, although the primitive Chinese and Egyptians have started treating this disease 3500 years ago.

CLASSIFICATION

The anthelmintic agents comprise of drugs of chemically diverse structures and their mechanism of action differs from one agent to another.

I. Benzimidazoles

These are versatile anthelmintic agents particularly effective against gastrointestinal nematodes. These are highly effective against *ascaris, enterobius, trichuris,* and hookworm infections as single or mixed infections.

S. No.	Drug	R
1	Albendazole	—S—CH$_2$CH$_2$CH$_3$
2	Mebendazole	—COC$_6$H$_5$
3	Flubendazole	—OC—C$_6$H$_4$—F
4	Cyclobendazole	—OC—cyclopropyl
5	Dribendazole	—SCH$_2$—cyclohexyl
6	Fenbendazole	—S—C$_6$H$_5$
7	Oxibendazole	—OCH$_2$CH$_2$CH$_3$
8	Parbendazole	—CH$_2$CH$_2$CH$_2$CH$_3$

II. Quinolines and isoquinolines
Oxamniquine

Praziquantel

III. Piperazine derivatives
Piperazine citrate

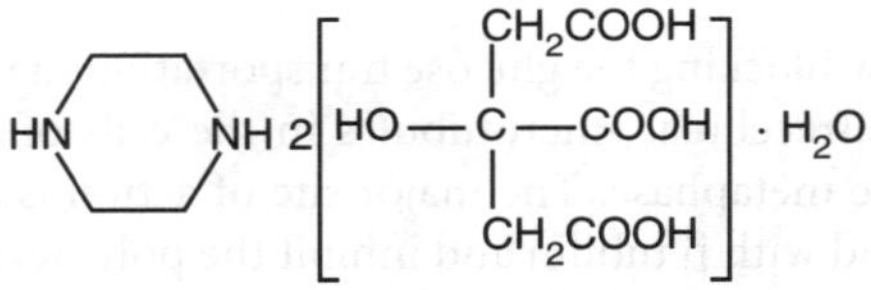

$$HN\diagup\hspace{-2pt}\diagdown NH \cdot 2\left[\begin{array}{c}CH_2COOH\\HO-C-COOH\\CH_2COOH\end{array}\right]\cdot H_2O$$

Diethyl carbmazine

$$H_3C-N\diagup\hspace{-2pt}\diagdown N-CON(C_2H_5)_2 \quad \left[\begin{array}{c}CH_2COOH\\HO-C-COOH\\CH_2COOH\end{array}\right]$$

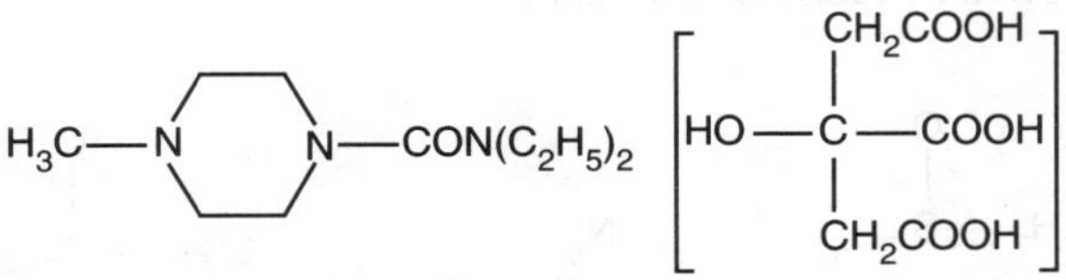

IV. Vinyl pyrimidines
Pyrantel pamoate

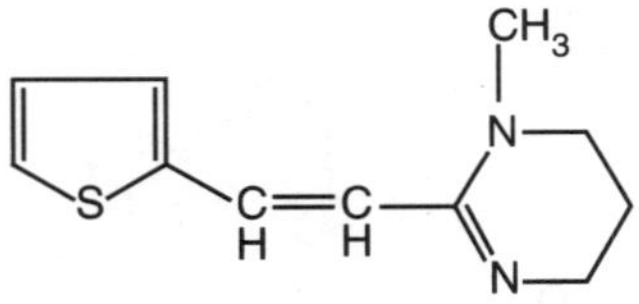

Oxantel

V. Amides
Niclosamide

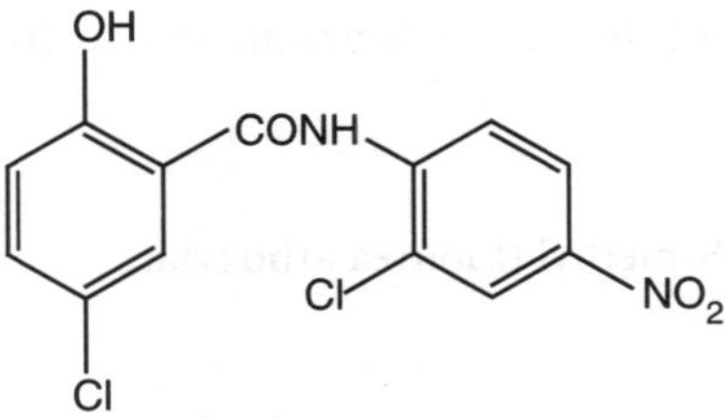

VI. Natural products: Avermectins
VII. Organo phosphorus: Metrifonate
VIII. Imidazothiazoles: Levamisole
IX. Nitro derivatives: Niridazole.

SYNTHESIS AND DRUG PROFILE

I. Benzimidazoles

Mode of action: These drugs act by blocking the glucose transportation in the parasites and lead to the depletion of glycogen storage of the intracellular microtubules in the cells of the worms, thereby arresting the nematodes and cell division in the metaphase. The major site of action is microtubular protein β tubulin of the parasite. These drugs are bound with β tubulin and inhibit the polymerization.

Metabolism: The parent compound is rapidly and almost completely metabolized by oxidative and hydrolytic processes.. The phase I oxidative reaction is commonly carried out by the cytochrome P450 catalyzed reaction, which may be followed by phase II conjugation.

Albendazole ⟶ Albendazole sulphoxide (active) ⟶

Mebendazole (Vermox)

Methyl-5-benzoly-2-benzimidazole carbamate

Synthesis

Step I. Synthesis of an intermediate-S-methyl thiourea arboxylate

S-methyl thio urea sulphate . H_2SO_4 + ClCOOCH$_3$ (Methyl chloro formate) $\xrightarrow{\text{NaOH} \atop PH_8}$ Methyl-S-methyl thiourea carboxylate

Step II. Synthesis of Mebendazole

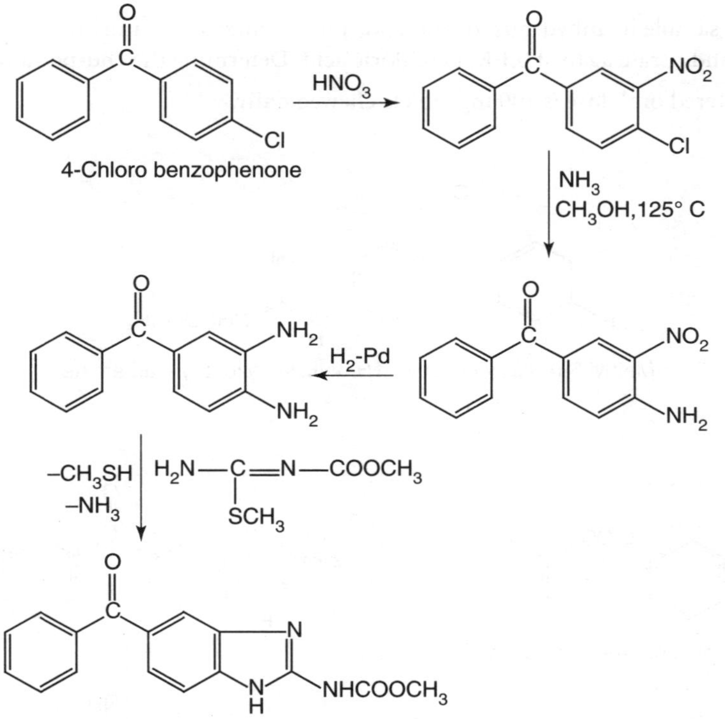

[Scheme: 4-Chloro benzophenone → (HNO₃) → nitro-chloro benzophenone → (NH₃, CH₃OH, 125° C) → nitro-amino benzophenone → (H₂-Pd) → diamino benzophenone → (H₂N—C(SCH₃)=N—COOCH₃, −CH₃SH, −NH₃) → Mebendazole]

Mebendazole

Metabolism: Mebendazole is metabolized by the reduction of the 5-carbonyl group to a secondary alcohol, which greatly increases the water solubility of this compound and thereby potentiates the excretion through urine. Secondary alcohol and amine are readily conjugated.

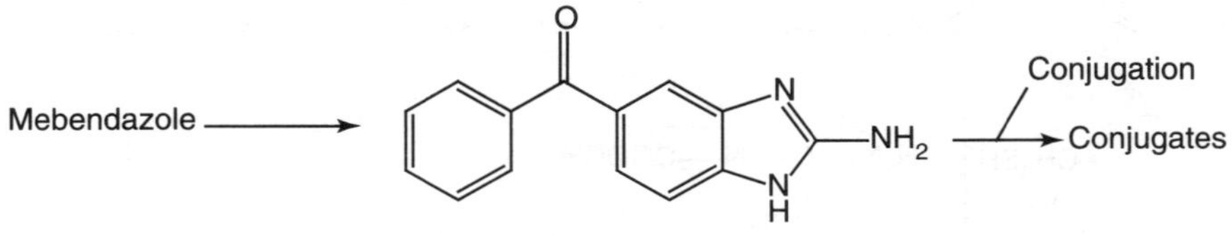

Mebendazole → Amino metabolite (2-amino benzimidazole with benzoyl group) → Conjugation → Conjugates

Mebandazole → Hydroxy metabolite (secondary alcohol with —N—C(=O)—OCH₃) → Conjugation → Conjugates

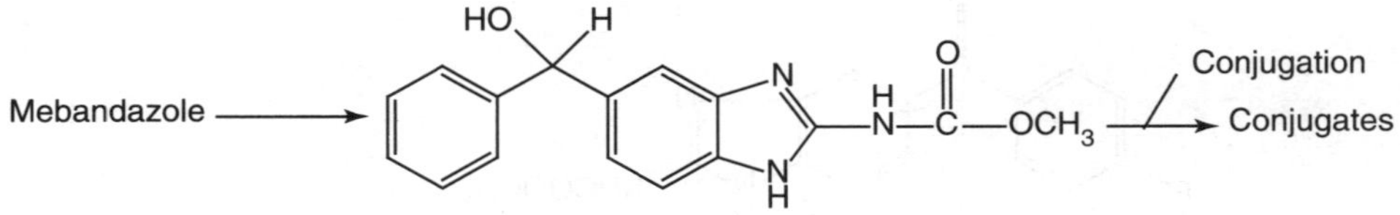

Properties and uses: Mebendazole is a white powder, practically insoluble in water, in alcohol, and in methylene chloride. It is used as an anthelmintic agent.

Assay: Dissolve the sample in anhydrous formic acid, add the mixture of anhydrous acetic acid and methyl ethyl ketone (1:7), and titrate against 0.1 M perchloric acid. Determine the end-point potentiometrically.

Dose: The administered oral dose is 100 mg tablets chewed daily.

Flubendazole

Methyl 5-(4-fluorobenzoyl)-1H-benzimidazol-2-yl-carbamate

Synthesis

Fluorobenzene + 4-Chloro-3-nitrobenzoyl chloride

Flubendazole

Properties and uses: Flubendazole is a white powder, practically insoluble in water, in alcohol, and in methylene chloride. It is used as an anthelmintic agent.

Assay: Dissolve the sample in anhydrous formic acid, add the mixture of anhydrous acetic acid and methyl ethyl ketone (1:7), and titrate against 0.1 M perchloric acid. Determine the end point potentiometrically.

Albendazole (Valbazen, Bentex, Zental)

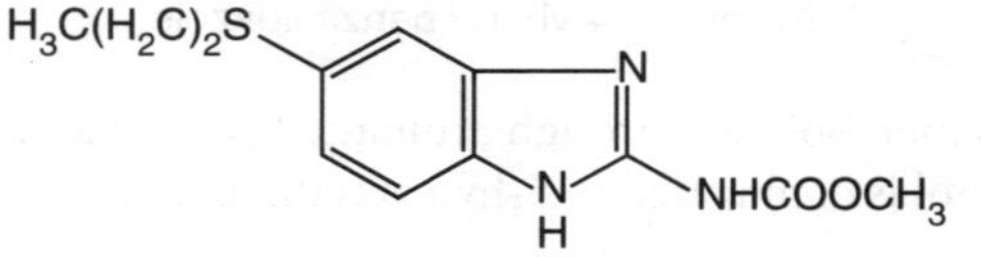

Methyl 5-(propylthio)-1*H*-benzoimidazol-2-yl-carbamate

Synthesis

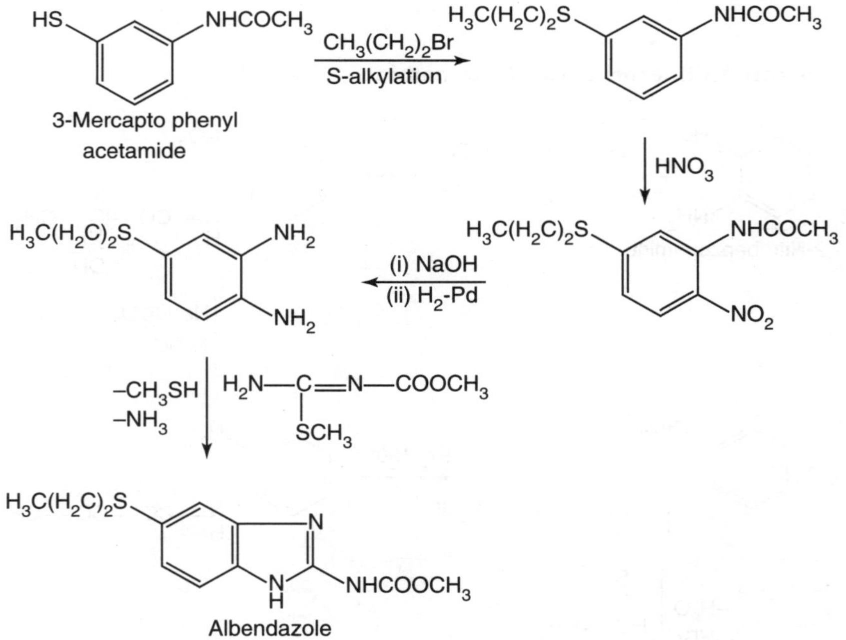

3-Mercapto phenyl acetamide

Albendazole

Properties and uses: Albendazole is a white or faintly yellowish powder, practically insoluble in water and alcohol, soluble in anhydrous formic acid, very slightly soluble in methylene chloride. It is used as an anthelmintic agent.

Assay: Dissolve the sample in anhydrous formic acid, add anhydrous acetic acid, and titrate against 0.1 M perchloric acid. Determine the end point potentiometrically.

Dose: The dose for controlling cysticercus cellulose is 5 mg/kg thrice daily for 30 days.

Thiabendazole (Mintezol)

2-(Thiazol-4-yl)-1H-benzimidazole

Metabolism: Thiabendazole is metabolized through aromatic hydroxylation at the fifth position catalyzed by CYP1A2. The resulting phenol is conjugated to 5-hydroxythiabendazole glucuronide.

Thiabendazole ⟶ [5-hydroxythiabendazole] $\xrightarrow[\text{Conjugation}]{\text{Glucuronic acid}}$ Glucuronide conjugate

Synthesis

Route I. From: o-Nitro aniline (or) 2-Nitrobenzenamine

2-Nitrobenzenamine + H₃C—CH(OH)—COCl ⟶ o-O₂N-C₆H₄-NH-CO-CH(OH)-CH₃

$\xrightarrow{\text{Na}_2\text{Cr}_2\text{O}_7 / \text{H}_2\text{SO}_4}$ o-O₂N-C₆H₄-NH-CO-CO-CH₃

$\xrightarrow{\text{Br}_2 / 180°\text{C}}$ o-O₂N-C₆H₄-NH-CO-CO-CH₂Br

$\xrightarrow[-\text{HBr}]{-\text{H}_2\text{O}, \; \text{HC(=S)-NH}_2 \; (\text{Thioformamide})}$ [2-nitrophenyl thiazole amide]

$\xrightarrow[\text{-H}_2\text{O}]{\text{(i) Zn/HCl} \quad \text{(ii) Cyclization}}$ Thiabendazole

Route II. From: Thiazolo nitrile

Thiazolonitrile → (C₆H₅NH₂ / AlCl₃) → intermediate → (NaOCl) → N-chloro intermediate → (KOH) → **Thiabendazole**

Properties and uses: It is a white, odourless, and tasteless powder, insoluble in water, slightly soluble in acetone, chloroform, or ether. It is used as a anthelminthic.

Dose: The dose orally is 25 mg/kg twice daily to a maximum of 3 g after meals. The dose for chewable tablets is 500 mg and oral suspension is 500 mg/5ml.

II. Quinoline and isoquinolines

Praziquantel (PZQ, Biltricide)

2-(Cyclohexanecarbonyl)-2,3,6,7-tetrahydro-1*H*-pyrazino[2,1-*a*]isoquinolin-4(11b*H*)-one

Metabolism: In serum, the major metabolites are 4-hydroxycyclohexyl carboxylate, but in the urine, 50%–60% of the initial PZQ exist as dihydroxylated products. Hydroxylation reactions are catalyzed by CYP2B6 and CYP3A4.

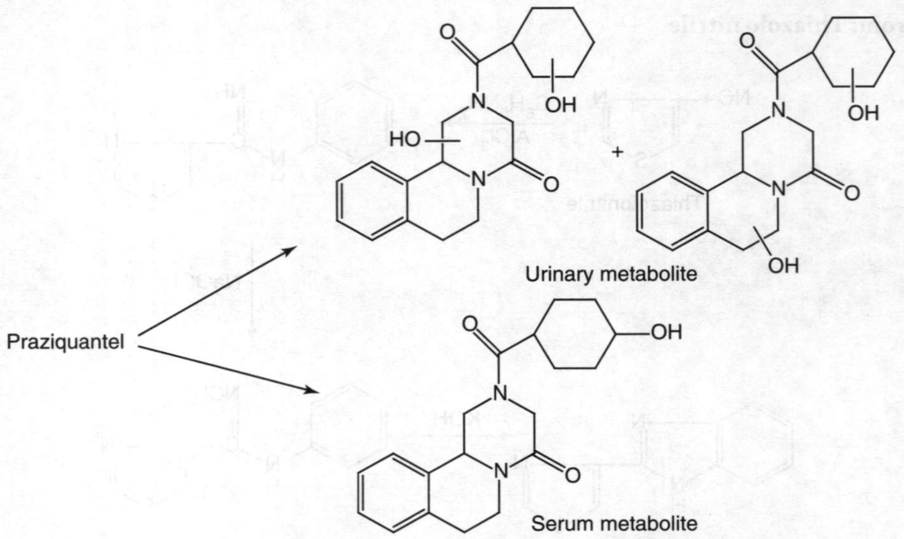
Praziquantel
HO
OH
N
O
+
OH
OH
Urinary metabolite
OH
Serum metabolite

Synthesis

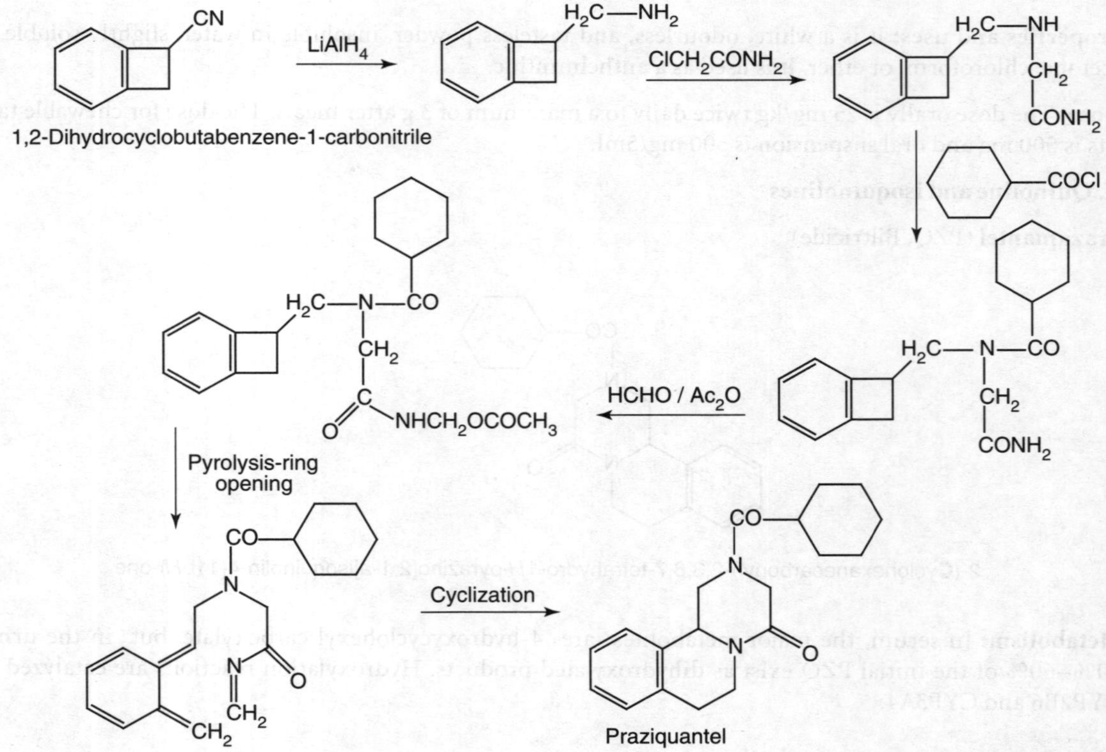
CN
LiAlH4
1,2-Dihydrocyclobutabenzene-1-carbonitrile
H2C—NH2
ClCH2CONH2
H2C—NH
CH2
CONH2
COCl
H2C—N—CO
CH2
CONH2
HCHO / Ac2O
H2C—N—CO
CH2
NHCH2OCOCH3
Pyrolysis-ring opening
CO
N
CH2
Cyclization
Praziquantel

Properties and uses: PZQ is a white crystalline powder, very slightly soluble in water, soluble in alcohol, and in methylene chloride. It is used for the treatment of schistosomiasis and liver fluke infections. It causes legumental damage to the worms, which activates the host defence mechanisms and results in the destruction of the worms.

Assay: It is assayed by adopting liquid chromatography technique.

Dose: The oral dose is 600 mg tablet two to three times a day.

Oxamniquine (Vansil)

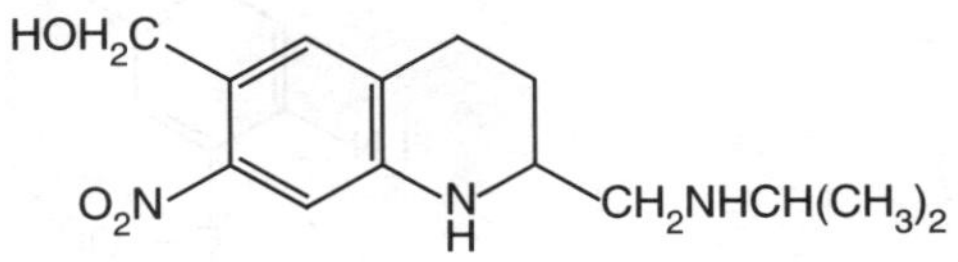

(2-((Isopropylamino)methyl)-7-nitro-1,2,3,4-tetrahydroquinolin-6-yl)methanol

Synthesis

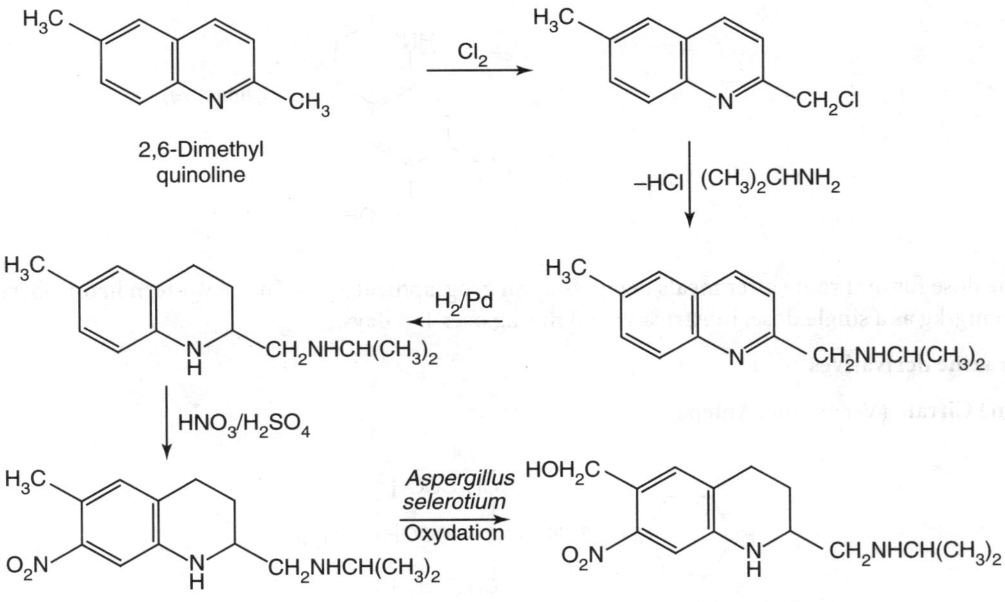

2,6-Dimethyl quinoline

Oxamniquine

Mode of action: *Schistosoma mansoni* is highly susceptible to oxamniquine. Adenosine-5′-triphosphate (ATP)-dependent enzymatic activation of the drug in susceptible schistosomes forms unstable phosphate esters, which disassociate to yield a chemically reactive carbocation this intermediate alkylates the DNA.

Metabolism: It is metabolized by oxidative reaction and it gives inactive metabolites of acid and alcohol derivatives.

Oxamniquine → Metabolic inactivation → (inactive) + (inactive)

Dose: The dose for oral route after meals depends upon geographical areas. In the western hemisphere, the dose is 15 mg/kg as a single dose, in Africa 15–60 mg/kg over 1–3 days.

III. Piperazine derivatives

Piperazine Citrate (Vermizine, Antepar)

Mode of action: The drug is highly effective against both *Ascaris lumbricoides* and *Enterobius (oxyuris) vermicularis*. These drugs cause the hyperpolarization of the ascaris muscles by gamma-aminobutyric acid (GABA) agonistic action, opening Cl⁻ channels, which cause relaxation, depress responsiveness to the contractile action of acetylcholine, and produce the suppression of spontaneous spike potentials with peristalsis.

Synthesis

$$\text{1,2 Dichloroethane} + \text{Ethane-1,2-diamine} \xrightarrow{-2NH_3} \text{Piperazine} \xrightarrow{\text{Citric acid}} \text{Piperazine citrate}$$

Properties and uses: Piperazine citrate is a white granular powder, soluble in water, and practically insoluble in alcohol, used as an anthelminthic. It can cause gastrointestinal and allergic reactions. It is contraindicated in epileptic patients.

Assay: Dissolve the sample in a mixture of anhydrous formic acid, acetic anhydride (2:3), and titrate quickly against 0.1 M perchloric acid. Determine the end point potentiometrically.

Dose: The administered dose always orally in the case of *ascaris* is 3.5 g as single dose daily for two consecutive days. For *oxyuriasis* (thread worms) the dose is 2.5 g given for 7 days.

Dosage forms: Piperazine citrate syrup I.P., Piperazine citrate tablets I.P., Piperazine citrate elixir B.P.

Diethyl cabamazine citrate (Vanaide, Vellcome)

Mode of action: It selectively acts on the microflora, causes attraction, and therefore, is readily phagocytosed by the tissue fixed monocytes. It also has an effect on the muscular activity of the microflora and causes hyper-polarization to destroy the worms.

Metabolism: The metabolism of diethyl carbamazepine leads to the compounds of methyl piperazine and piperazine. Nearly, all of the metabolites appear in the urine.

Diethylcarbamazine → H₃C—N(piperazine)N—C(=O)—N(C₂H₅)₂ with N→O (50%)

+

H₃C—N(piperazine)N—C(=O)—N(C₂H₅)(H) (23%)

Properties and uses: Diethylcarbanazine citrate is a white crystalline slightly hygroscopic powder, very soluble in water, soluble in alcohol, and practically insoluble in acetone. It is the drug of choice for treating *filariasis* infections. In adequate dosage, it clears the blood rapidly of the microfilariae and appears to be curative. Antihistamines or corticosteroids may be needed to control the allergic reaction caused by the disintegration of microfilariae. It is active against microfilariea of *Loa loa*, but may cause encephalopathy.

Assay: Dissolve the sample in anhydrous acetic acid, add acetic anhydride, and titrate with 0.1 M perchloric acid using crystal violet as indicator, until a greenish-blue colour is obtained.

Dose: The dose in the case of oral route for *Brugia malayi*, *Loa loa*, and *Wuchereria bancrofti* is 2 mg/kg three times daily after meals for 10–30 days. For *Caecal volvulus*, the dose is 0.5 mg/kg once on the first day and twice on the second day and the adverse effects limit the use of this drug.

Dosage forms: Diethylcarbamazine tablets B.P.

Synthesis

H₃C—N(piperazine)NH + ClCON(C₂H₅)₂ →(−HCl) H₃C—N(piperazine)N—CON(C₂H₅)₂

N-methyl piperazine   Diethyl carbamoyl chloride

↓ Citric acid

H₃C—N(piperazine)N—CON(C₂H₅)₂ · [HO—C(CH₂COOH)(COOH)(CH₂COOH)]

Diethylcarbamazine citrate

IV. Vinyl pyrimidines

Pyrantel (Antiminth, Combantrin)

1-Methyl-2-(2-(thiophen-2-yl)vinyl)-1,4,5,6-tetrahydropyrimidine

Synthesis

Thiophene-2-carbaldehyde + $CNCH_2COOH$ (Cyano acetic acid) $\xrightarrow[\text{(ii) } -CO_2]{\text{(i) Knoevenagel reaction}}$ thiophene-CH=CH-CN

$\downarrow CH_3OH/HCl$

thiophene-CH=CH-C(=NH)-OCH$_3$

$\xrightarrow{H_2N-CH_2-CH_2-CH(NHCH_3)}$

$\xrightarrow[-CH_3OH]{-NH_3}$ **Pyrantel**

Mode of action: Pyrantel is a depolarizing neuromuscular blocking agent. It induces marked persistent activation of the nicotinic receptors, which result in spastic paralysis of the worm. It is an alternative to mebendazole in the treatment of ascariasis and enterobiasis.

Properties and uses: It is a pale yellow or yellow powder, practically insoluble in water and in methanol, soluble in dimethyl sulphoxide. It is also as investigational drug for the treatment of hookworms, moniliformis, and trichostrongylus infections.

Assay: To the sample add acetic anhydride and glacial acetic acid, heat and stir. Allow to cool and titrate with 0.1 M perchloric acid. Determine the end point potentiometrically.

Doses: The dose for oral suspension or liquid is 50 mg/ml. A single dose of 11 mg/kg for ascarasis and enterobiasis.

V. Amides

Niclosamide (Niclocide)

Synthesis

[Structure: 5-Chlorosalicylic acid + SOCl₂ → acid chloride; + 2-chloro-4-nitroaniline → Niclosamide]

5-Chloro salicylic acid

Niclosamide

Mode of action: Niclosamide is also a potent mollusicide, which is effective against *Biomphaloria glabrata*, the principle action of the drug may be to inhibit anaerobic phosphorylation of adenosine diphosphate (ADP) by the mitochondria of the parasite, an energy producing process.

Properties and uses: Niclosamide exists as yellowish fine crystals, practically insoluble in water, sparingly soluble in acetone, and slightly soluble in ethanol. It is used as an anthelmintic.

Assay: Dissolve the sample in a mixture of equal volumes of acetone and methanol and titrate with 0.1 M tetrabutylammonium hydroxide. Determine the end point potentiometrically.

Dose: The dose orally to be taken after meals is 2 g chewable tablets.

Dosage forms: Niclosamide tablets B.P.

VI. Natural products

Avermectins (Mectizan)

Avermectin B_1a R= $-C(CH_3)(H)(C_2H_5)$ 80
Avermectin B_1b R= $-CH(CH_3)_2$ 20

Ivermectin

Mode of action: Avermectins specifically open the chloride channels in the invertebrate system distinct from the GABA-gated and glutamate-gated chloride channels.

Metabolism: It is metabolized and it gives 3-O-demethyl-22,23-dihydroavermectin $B_{1\alpha}$ monosaccharide.

Properties and uses: Avermectins are macrocyclic lactones with broad antinematocidal activity. This class of compound was isolated from a fermentation broth of a soil actinomycetics (*Streptomycin avermitils*). The drug avermectin is now effectively being used to treat and control *onchocera volvulus*, the filarial infection responsible for liver blindness. Ivermectin is a mixture of B_1a and B_1b (80:20) and is prepared by catalytic reduction of ivermectin B_1 (Abamectin)

VII. Organophosphorus compounds

Metrifonate (Bilacil)

Dimethyl 2,2,2-trichloro-1-hydroxyethylphosphonate

Synthesis

Dimethyl phosphate + Trichloro acetaldehyde → Metrifonate

Mode of action: Metrifonate is metabolized and rearranged in vivo to dichlorvos, which inhibits acetyl cholinesterase.

Properties and uses: Metrifonate is a white crystalline powder, soluble in water, in acetone, and in alcohol, and very soluble in methylene chloride, used as an anthelmintic.

Assay: Dissolve the sample in alcohol, add ethanolamine, and allow to stand for 1 h at 20°C–22°C. Add chilled nitric acid maintaining the temperature of the mixture at 20°C–22°C and titrate with 0.1 M silver nitrate. Determine the end point potentiometrically.

Doses: The recommended dose is 7.5 to 10 mg/kg given orally three times at intervals of 2 weeks.

VIII. Midazothiazoles

Levamisole (Bizole, Vermisol)

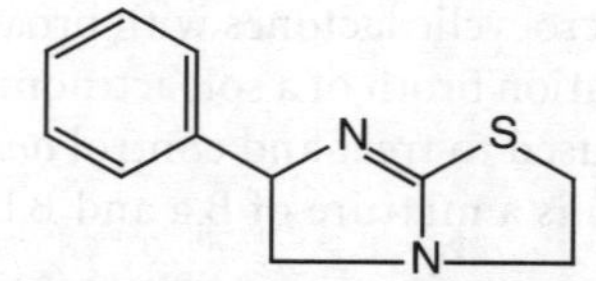

6-Phenyl-2,3,5,6-tetrahydroimidazo[2,1-*b*]thiazole

Synthesis:

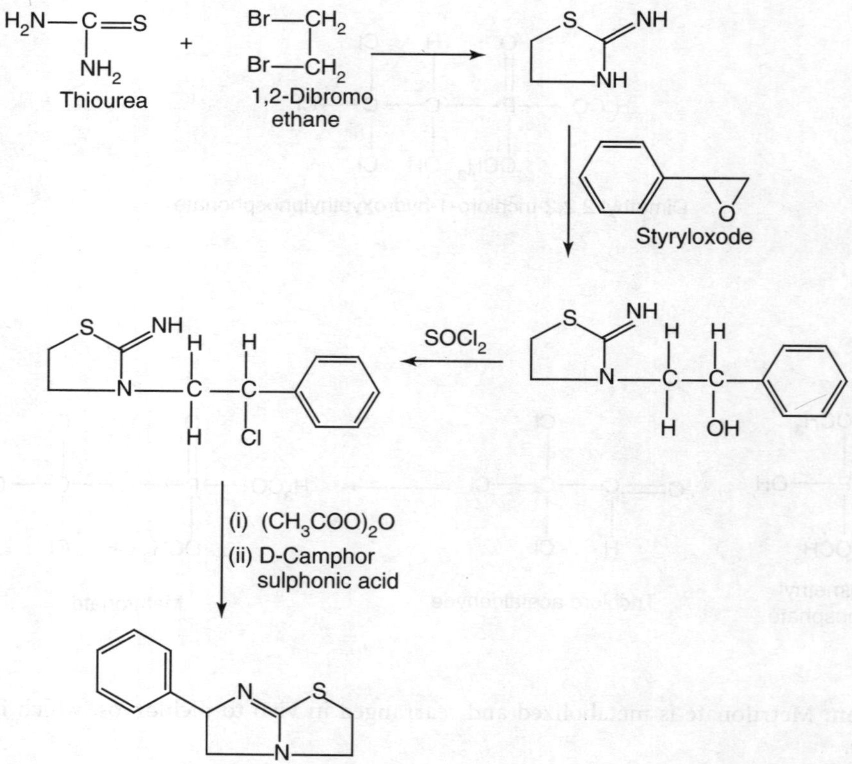

Thiourea + 1,2-Dibromoethane → (thiazoline imine intermediate)

+ Styryloxode →

(hydroxy intermediate) → SOCl$_2$ → (chloro intermediate)

(i) (CH$_3$COO)$_2$O
(ii) D-Camphor sulphonic acid

→ Levamisole

Mode of action: It stimulates the ganglion in the worms, causes tonic paralysis, which results in the expulsion of live worms. These also interfere with the carbohydrate metabolism by inhibiting fumarate reductase.

Dose: The administered dose is 15 mg as a single dose, repeated after 1 month to prevent recurrence.

IX. Nitro derivatives
Niridazole (Ambilhar)

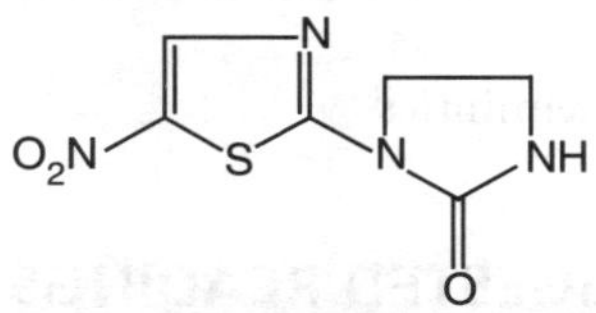

1-(5-Nitrothiazol-2-yl)imidazolidin-2-one

Synthesis

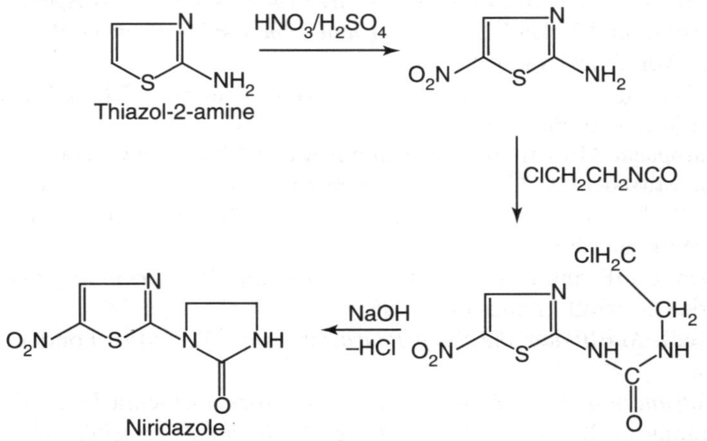

Thiazol-2-amine

Niridazole

Uses: Niridazole is used as an anthelmintic agent.

Dose: The recommended daily dose by oral route is 25 mg/kg daily in two divided doses.

PROBABLE QUESTIONS

1. Define anthelmintics and write the classification based on their chemical structure.
2. Write in detail about anthelmintics and provide suitable examples wherever necessary.
3. Outline the synthesis of the following drugs:
   (a) Albendazole (b) Thiabendazole.
4. How will you classify anthelmintics on the basis of chemical structures? Write the structure, chemical name, and uses of two examples from each category.
5. Describe the synthesis, mode of action, and uses of oxaminquine.
6. Write a short note on the following:
   (a) Pyrantel Pamoate (b) organophosphorus anthelmintic compounds.
7. What is avermectin? Describe its metabolism, mode of action, and uses.

8. Enumerate the various benzimidazoles derived from anthelmintics with their chemical structure, and write the synthesis, metabolism, and uses of mebendazole.
9. Mention an anthelmintic drug possessing quioline nucleus, describe its synthesis, metabolism and uses.
10. Write a note piperazine derived anthelmintics

SUGGESTED READINGS

1. Abraham DJ (ed). *Burger's Medicinal Chemistry and Drug Discovery* (6th edn). New jersey: John Wiley, 2007.
2. *British Pharmacopoeia*. Medicines and Healthcare Products Regulatory Agency. London, 2008.
3. Bruntan LL, Lazo JS, and Parker KL. *Goodman and Gilman's: The Pharmacological Basis of Therapeutics* (11th edn). New York: McGraw Hill, 2006.
4. Gennaro AR. *Remington: The Science and Practice of Pharmacy* (21st edn). New York: Lippincot Williams and Wilkins, 2006.
5. *Indian Pharmacopoeia*. Ministry of Health and Family Welfare. New Delhi, 1996.
6. Lednicer D and Mitscher LA. *The Organic Chemistry of Drug Synthesis*. New York: John Wiley 1995.
7. Lemke TL and William DA. *Foye's Principle of Medicinal Chemistry* (6th edn). New York: Lippincott Williams and Wilkins, 2008.
8. Mandel GL, Bennett JE, and Dolin R (eds). *Principles and Practices of Infectious Diseases*, Vol. I (4th edn). New York: Churchill-Livingstone, 1995.
9. Reynolds EF (ed). *Martindale the Extra Pharmacopoeia*. (31st edn). London: The Pharmaceutical Press, 1997.
10. Testa B (ed). *Advances in Drug Research*, Vol. 21. New York: Academic Press, 1991.
11. Wilson JD, Braunwald E, and Isselbacher KJ (eds). *Harrison's Principles of Internal Medicine* (12th edn), p. 772. New York: McGraw Hill, 1992.

Chapter 11

Antineoplastic Agents

INTRODUCTION

Antineoplastic agents are drugs used for the treatment of cancer, malignancy, tumour, carcinoma, sarcoma, leukaemia, or neoplasm (Greek neo = new, Plasm = formation). Neoplasm refers to a group of diseases caused by several agents, namely, chemical compounds and radiant energy. Cancer is characterized by an abnormal and uncontrolled, division of cells, which produces tumours and invades adjacent normal tissues. Often, cancer cells separate themselves from the primary tumour, and are carried by the lymphatic system to reach distant sites of the organs, where they divide and form secondary tumours (metastasis).

Cell Cycle Kinetics

Two key aspects of cellular life are the following:

1. DNA synthesis and mitosis to produce new cells.
2. Cell differentiation that produces specialized cells.

Limitations of Therapy

- Cancer cells very rapidly develop resistance to antineoplastic drugs.
- Differences between normal and neoplastic human cells are merely quantitative.
- Biochemical and morphological differences between normal and neoplastic cells are slight; therefore, antineoplastic agents are devoid of selective toxicity to tumour cells.
- Antineoplastic agents kill cells by first-order kinetics, that is, they kill a constant fraction of cells. However, some of the cancer cells elude killing and one of these cells may restabilize the tumour. It is extremely difficult to kill all the malignant cells.
- Most antineoplastic drugs are highly toxic to the patients.

Adverse Effects

The prominent adverse effects of antineoplastic drugs are exerted on rapidly proliferating normal tissues, in addition, to their chronic and cumulative toxicities.

- Bone marrow toxicity: Bleomycin, L-asparaginase.
- Hair follicle toxicity: Methotrexate, Vincristine, Cyclophosphamide, and Doxoroubicin.
- Hepatotoxicity: Azathiopurine, Mercaptopurine, and L-asparaginase.
- Skin rashes: Vinca alkaloids, Nitrosourea, Anthracyclins, and Mitomycin C.
- Pulmonary toxicity: Bleomycin, Methotrexate, and Busulfan.
- Cardiac toxicity: Doxorubicin, Daunorubicin, and Anthracyclins.
- Other toxicities: Intestinal epithelium, central nervous system (CNS) toxicity, nephrotoxicity, immuno-suppression, fever, anaphylaxis, cataracts, haemolytic anaemia, pancreatitis, pituitary insufficiency, adrenal insufficiency, coagulation problems, suppression of growth, and carcinogenicity.

CLASSIFICATION

Antineoplastic agents are classified as follows:

  I. Alkylating agents
 II. Antimetabolites
III. Antibiotics
 IV. Plant products
  V. Enzymes
 VI. Hormones
VII. Immuno therapy
VIII. Monoclonal antibodies
 IX. Radio-therapeutic agents
  X. Cyto-protective agents
 XI. Miscellaneous.

I. Alkylating agents

a. Nitrogen mustards

Mechlorethamine

Ifosamide

Cyclophosphamide

Melphalan

Uracil mustard

Chlorambucil

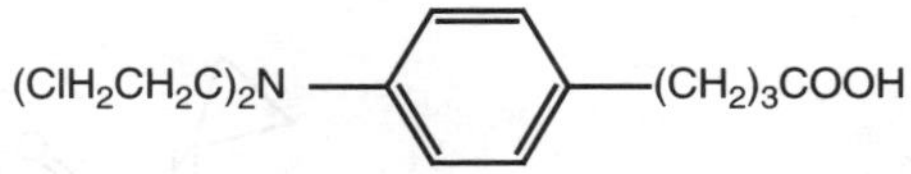

$(ClH_2CH_2C)_2N-\text{C}_6H_4-(CH_2)_3COOH$

Estramustine

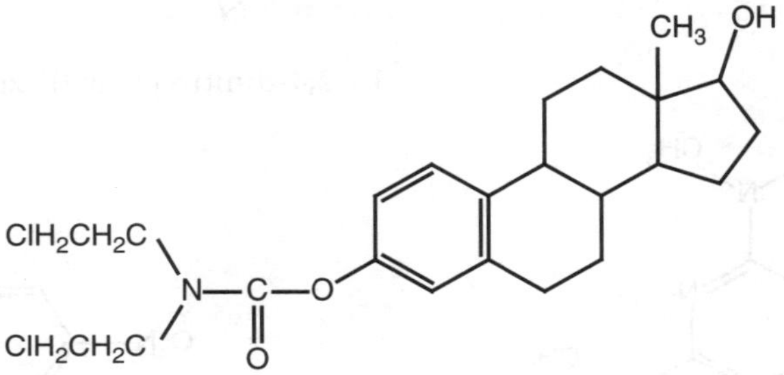

[Structure: estradiol with 3-O-carbamate bearing N(CH₂CH₂Cl)₂]

Chloroquine nitrogen mustard

b. Alkyl Sulphonate

Busulfan

$CH_3SO_2O(CH_2)_4OSO_2CH_3$

c. Nitrosoureas

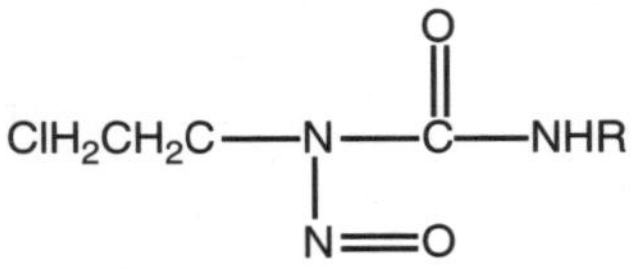

$ClH_2CH_2C-N(N=O)-C(=O)-NHR$

Name	R
Carmustine	—CH$_2$CH$_2$Cl
Lomustine	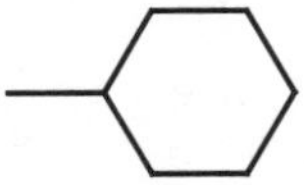 —cyclohexyl
Semustine	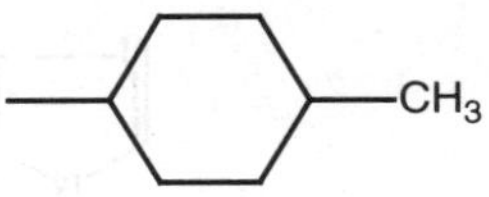 —(4-methylcyclohexyl)
Chlorozotocin	Glucose

d. Aziridines

Thiotepa

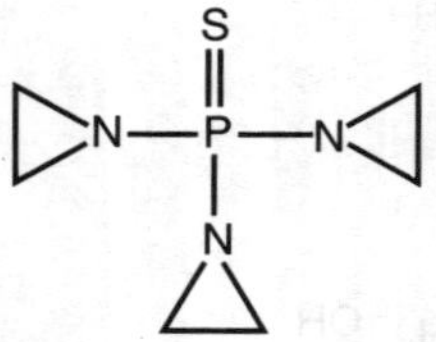

Benzo-tepa

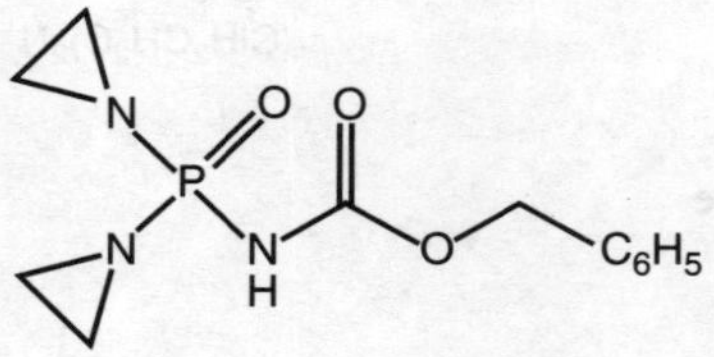

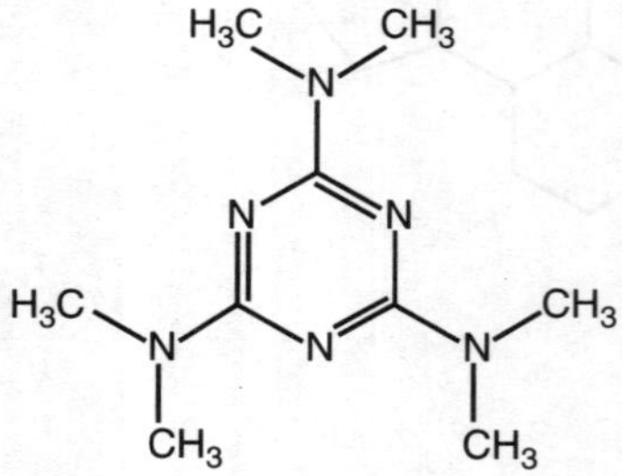

1,-(2,4-dinitro phenyl) aziridine

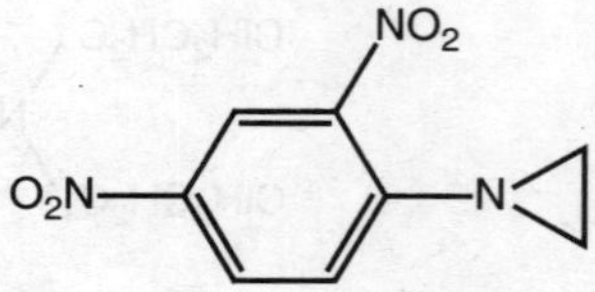

e. Altretamine

Triethylene melamine

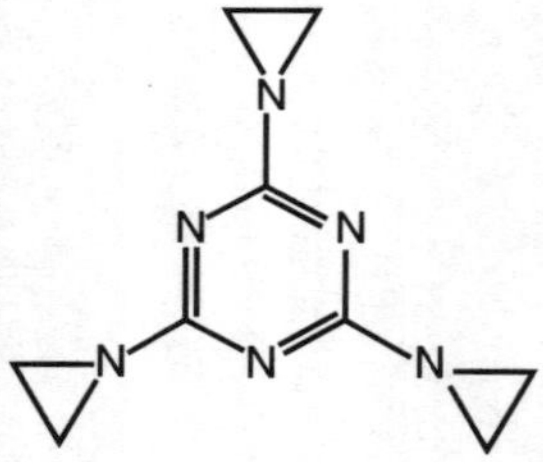

4 (1-aziridinyl)-2,6-dimethoxy triazine

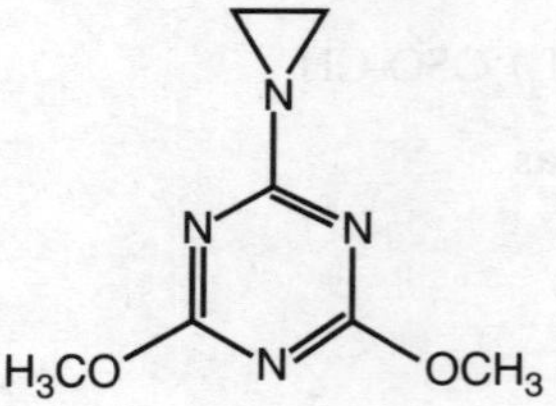

f. Methylhydrazines
Procarbazine

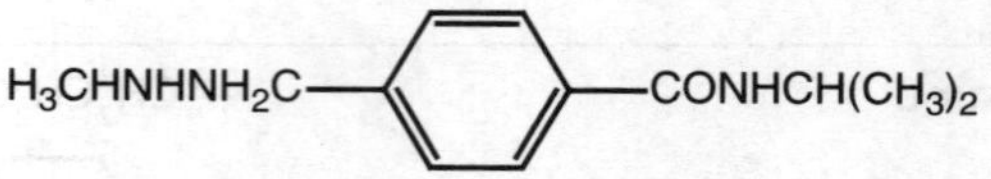

Dacarbazine

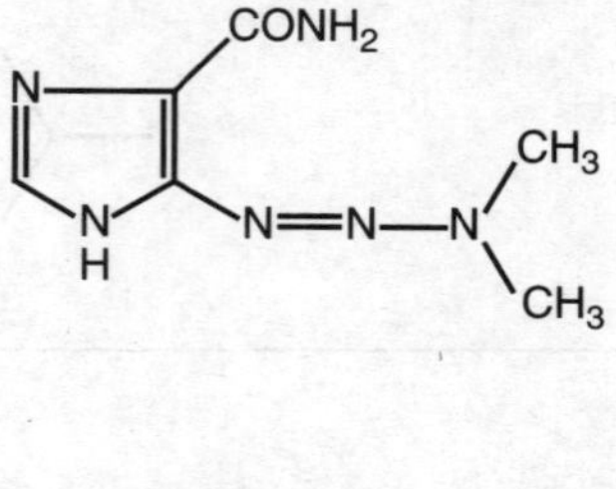

II. Antimetabolites

a. Pyrimdine analogues

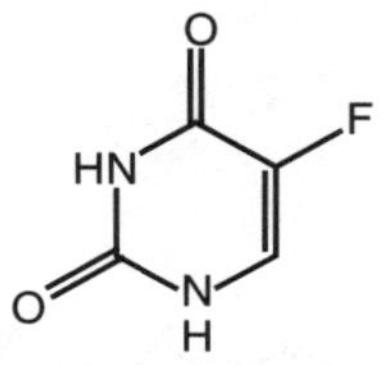

5-Flurouracil (5-FU)

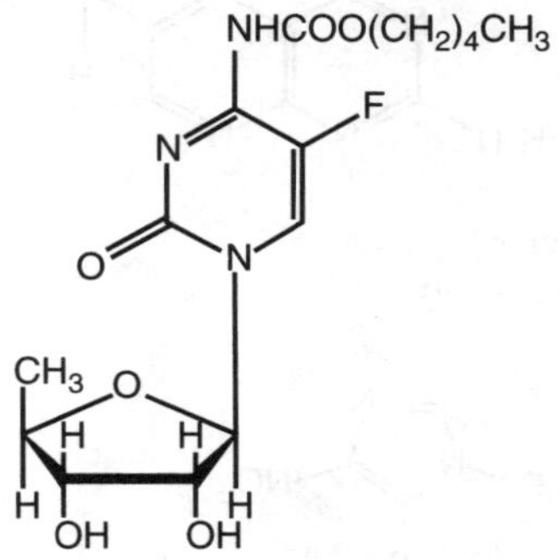

Capectitabine

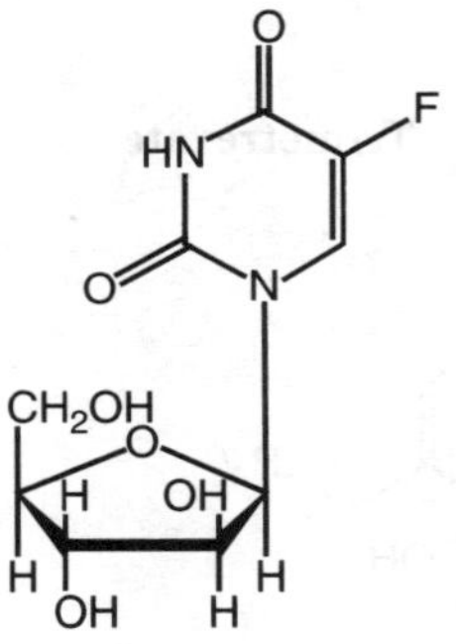

Floxuridine

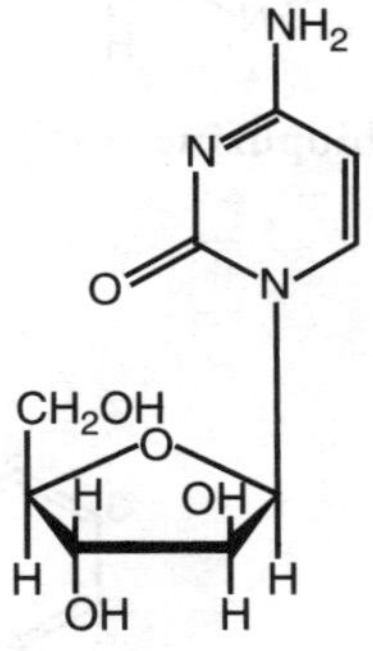

Cytarabine

b. Purine Analogues

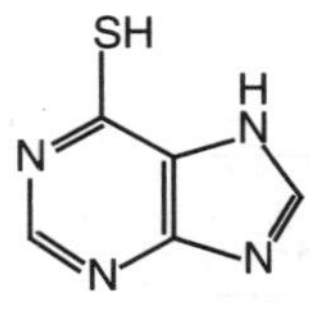

6-Mercaptopurine

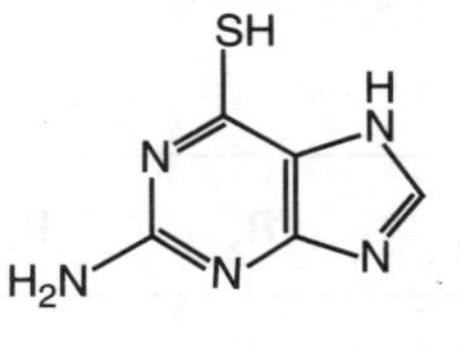

6-Thioguanine

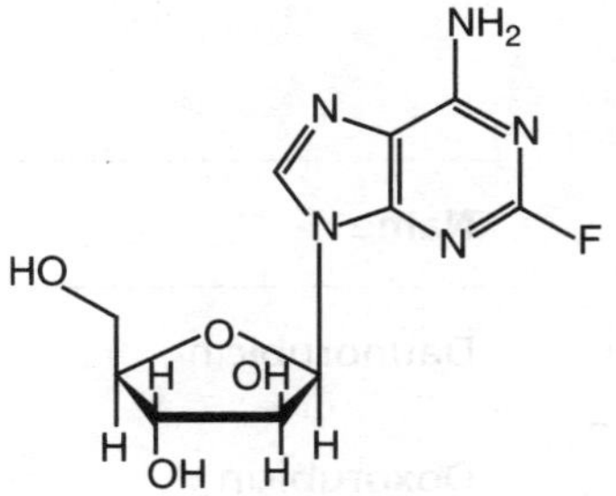

Fludarabine

c. Folic acid analogues

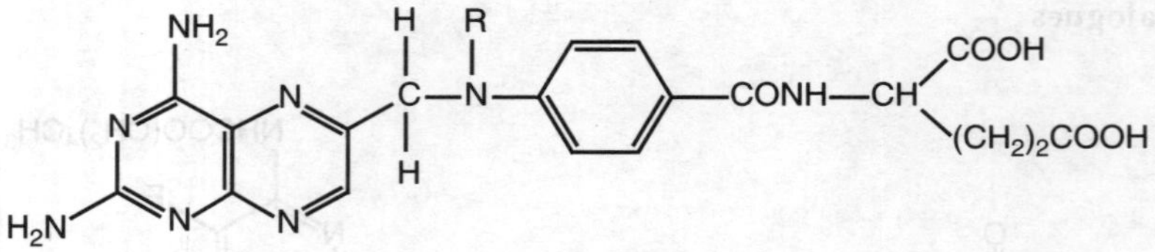

R = H (Aminopterin)
R = CH$_3$ (Methotrexate)

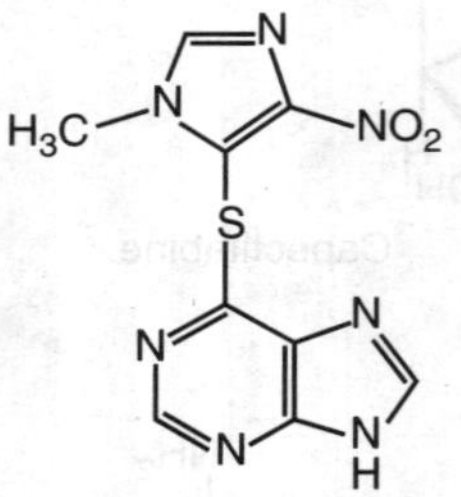

Azathiopurine

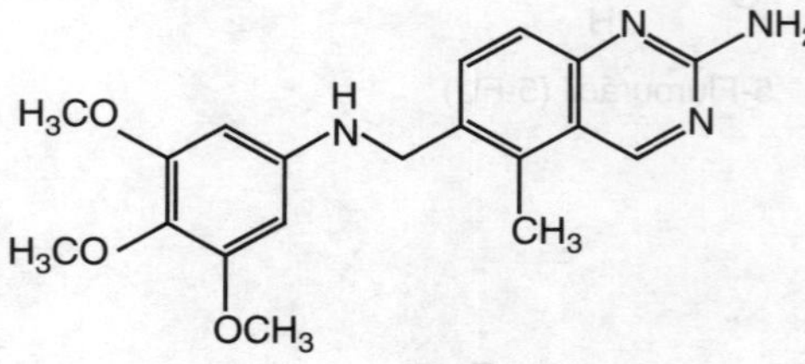

Trimetrexate

II. Antibiotics

a. Anthracyclines

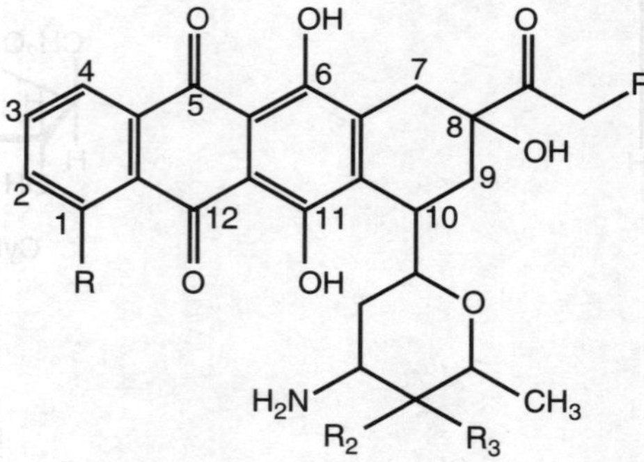

Name	R$_1$	R$_2$	R$_3$	R$_4$
Daunorubicin	–OCH$_3$	–H	–OH	–H
Doxorubicin	–OCH$_3$	–H	–OH	–OH

(Continued)

(Continued)

Name	R₁	R₂	R₃	R₄
Carminomycin	–OH	–H	–OH	–OH
Idarubicin	–H	–H	–OH	–H
Epirubicin	–OCH₃	–OH	–H	–OH

Valrubicin

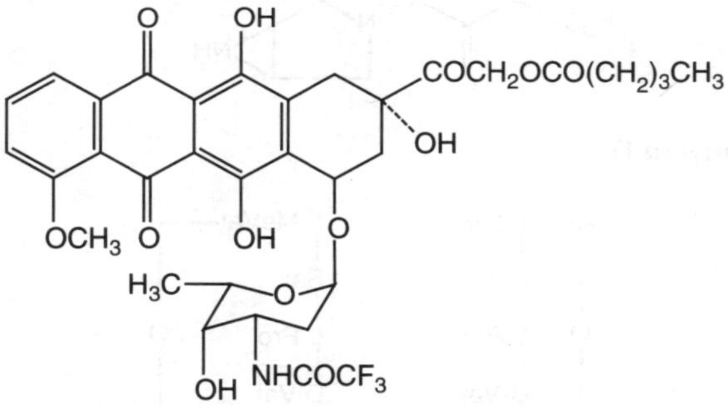

b. Bleomycins

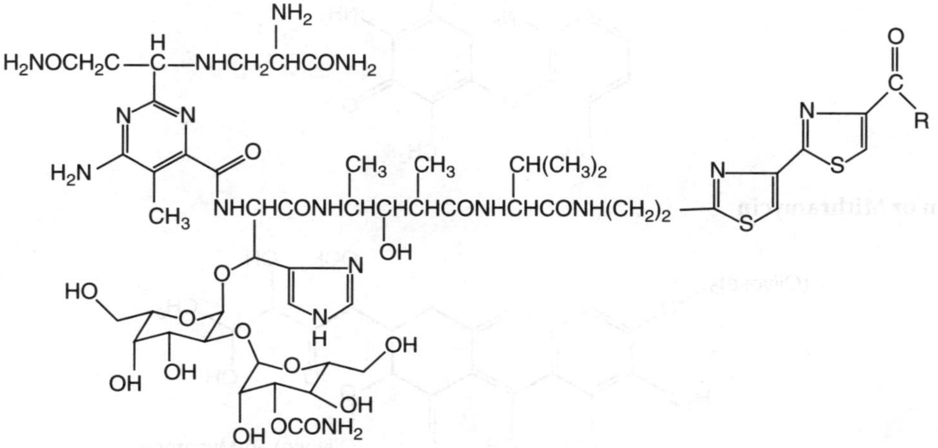

Bleomycinic acid R =	–OH
Bleomycin A$_2^-$ R =	–NH(CH$_2$)$_3\overset{\oplus}{S}$(CH$_3$)$_2$
Bleomycin B$_2^-$ R =	–NH(CH$_2$)$_4$NH–C(=NH)–NH$_2$

c. Mitomycins
Mitomycin C

Dactinomycin C or Actinomycin D

Plicamycin or Mithramycin

III. Plant products
a. Vinca alkaloids
Vinorelbine

Vincristine, Vinblastine

Vincristine R = CHO
Vinblastine R = CH$_3$

b. Camptothecin Derivatives

Name	R	R'
Camptothecin	–H	–H
Irinotecan	–C$_2$H$_5$	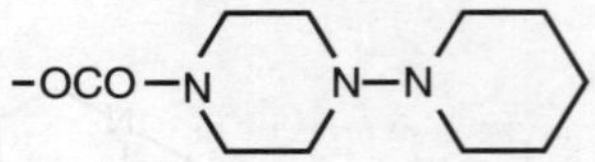 –OCO–N(piperazine)–N(piperidine)
Topotecan	–CH$_2$N(CH$_3$)$_2$	–OH

c. Epipodophyllo toxins

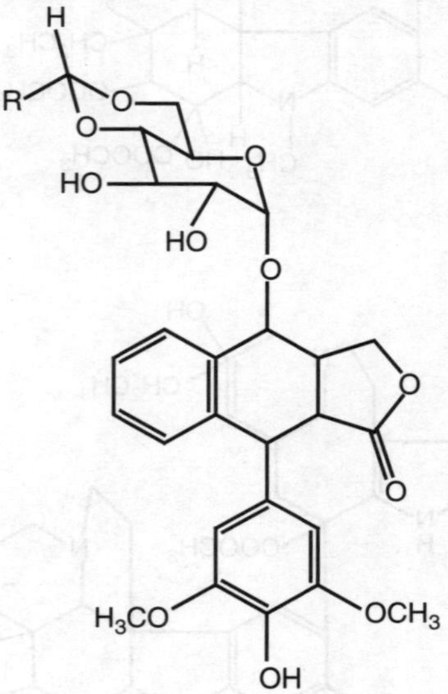

Etoposide   R = CH$_3$

Teniposide R = (2-thienyl)

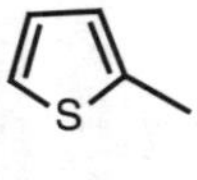

d. Taxol derivatives

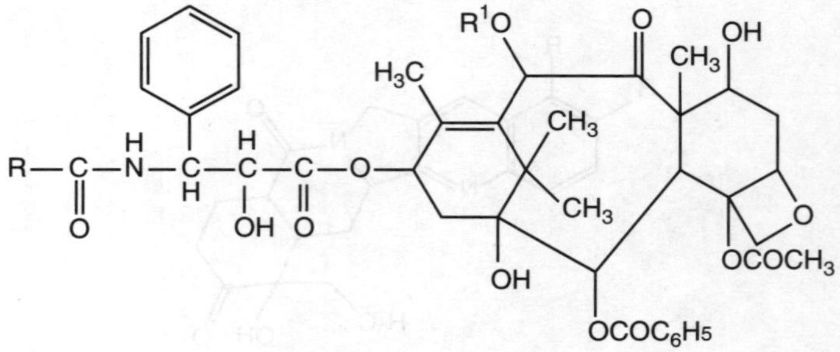

Name	R	R¹
Paclitaxel	—C₆H₅ (phenyl)	—COCH₃
Docetaxel	(CH₃)₃CO—	—H

IV. Enzymes
Examples—L-asparaginase, Pegaspargase

V. Hormones
a. Estorgenic derivatives

(i) 17-β-Estradiol R= H
(ii) Ethinyl estradiol R= —C≡CH

Diethylstilbosterol (nonsteroidal drug)

b. Progestine derivatives

Progesterone

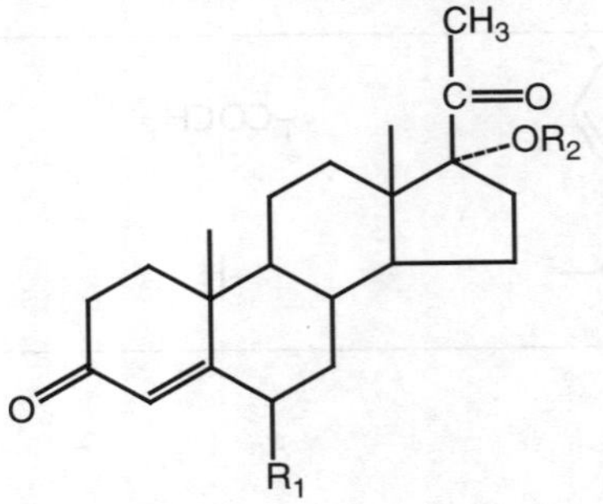

(i) Hydroxy progesterone caproate
   $R_1 = -H$, $R_2 = -COC_5H_{11}$
(ii) Medroxy progesterone acetate
   $R_1 = -CH_3$, $R_2 = -COCH_3$

Progestins
c. Testosterone derivatives
Testosterone

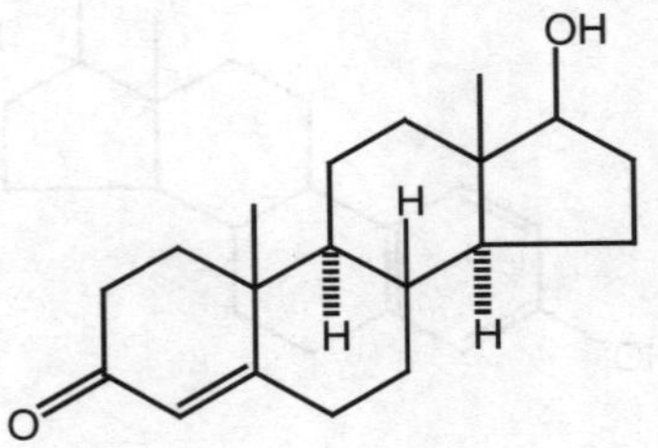

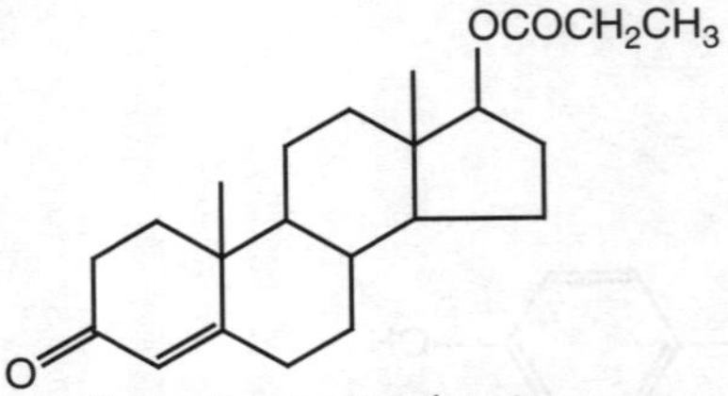

Testosterone propionate

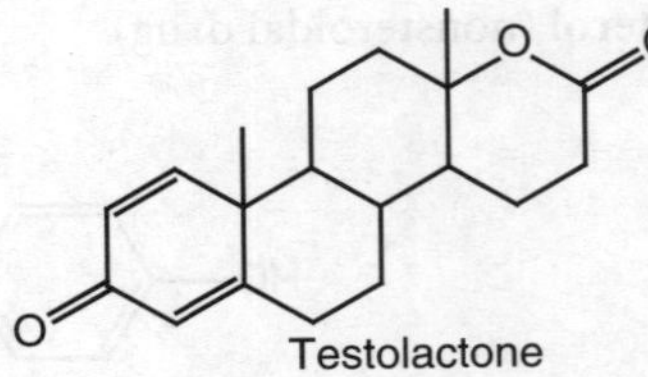

Testolactone

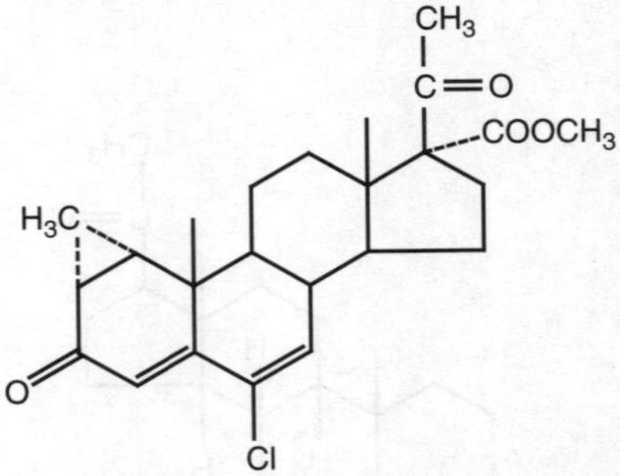

Cyproterone acetate

d. Steroidal anti-inflammatory agents

Prednisone

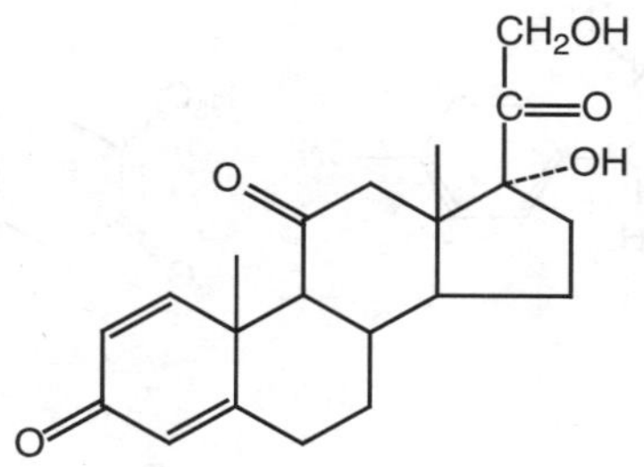

Flutamide (Nonsteroidal antiandrogen)

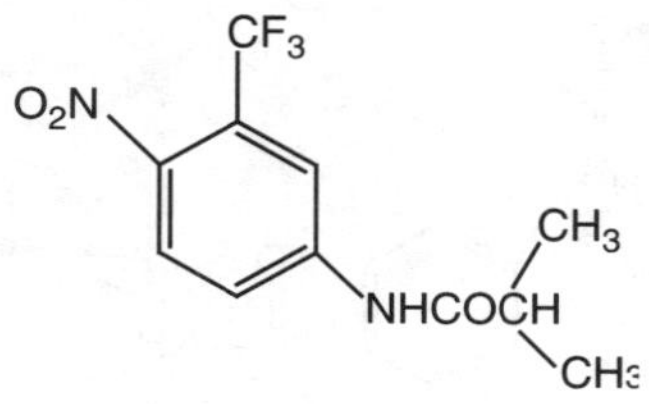

d. Miscellaneous agents

Mitotane

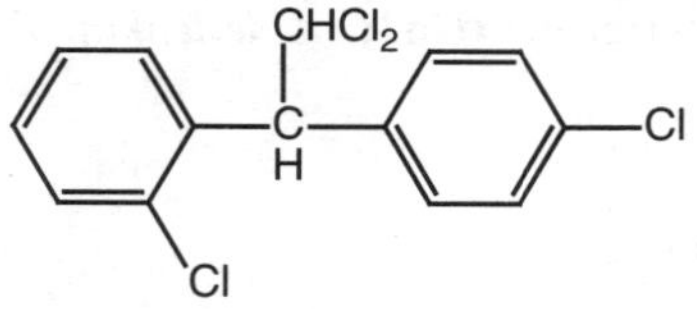

Tamoxifen

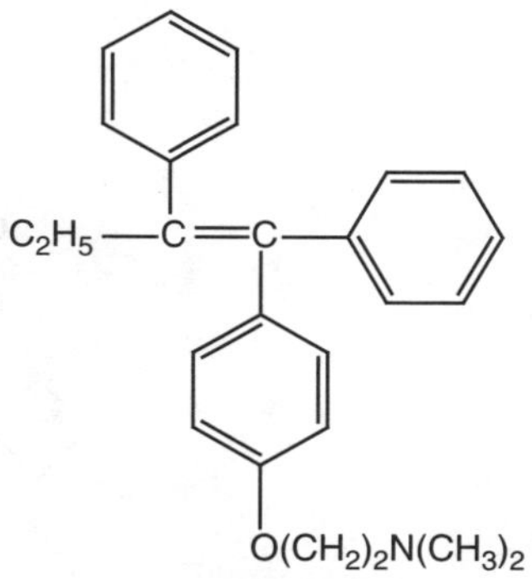

Letrozole

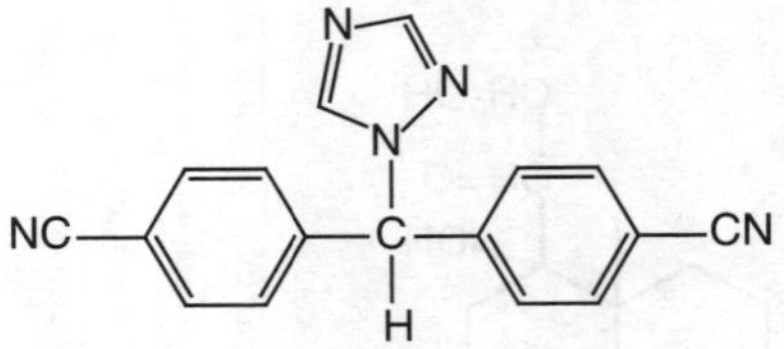

Dromostanolone

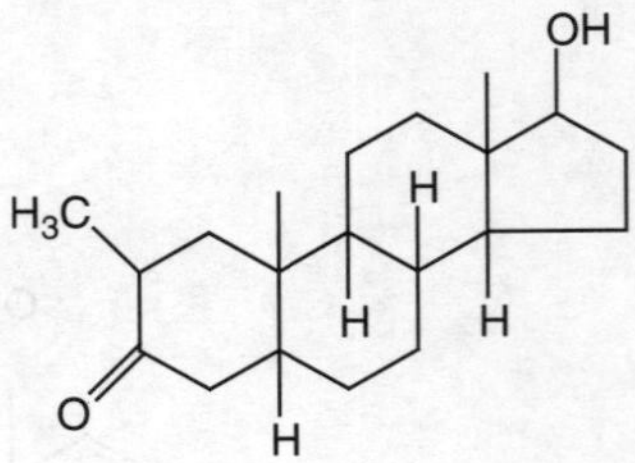

Pipobroman

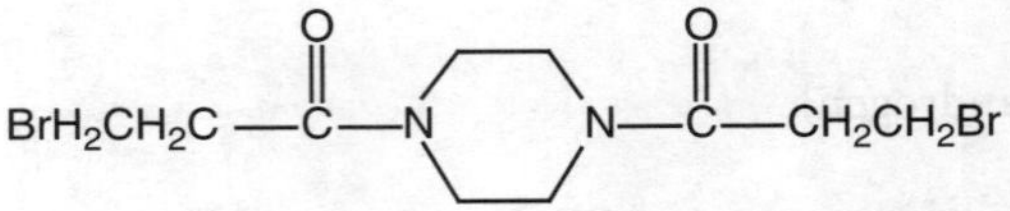

Aminoglutethimide

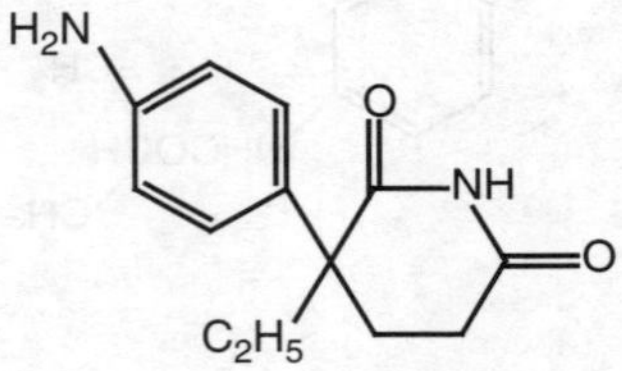

VI. Immuno therapay
Interferon α-2a; Interferon-2b; Interferon α-n3; *Aldesleukin*, Diftitox, *Denileukin*; and Bucillus calmette-Guerin (BCG).

VII. Monoclonal Antibodies
Rituximab, Gemtuzumab, Ozogamicin

VIII. Radio-therapeutic agents
Chromic phosphate P-32; Sodium phosphate P-32; Sodium iodide I-131; Strontium-89 chloride; Samarium Sm 153 lexidronam

IX. Cytoprotective agents
Mesna, Amifostine, Dexrazoxane

X. Miscellaneous

Cisplastin

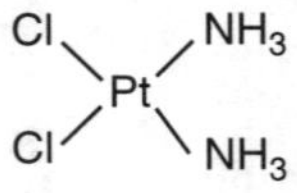

Carboplastin

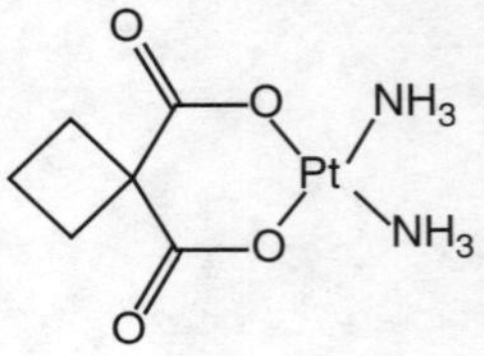

Hydroxy urea

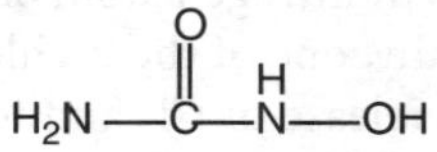

$H_2N-\overset{\overset{O}{\|}}{C}-\overset{H}{N}-OH$

Gallium nitrate

$Ga(NO_3)_3 \cdot 9H_2O$

Mitoxantrone

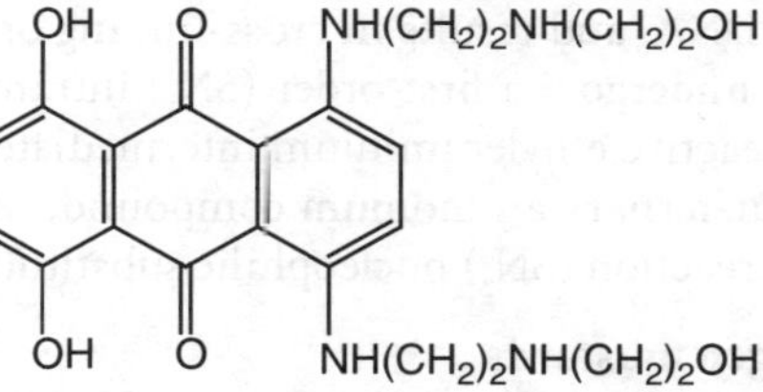

SYNTHESIS AND DRUG PROFILE

I. Alkylating agents

Step I: Intramoleular cyclization

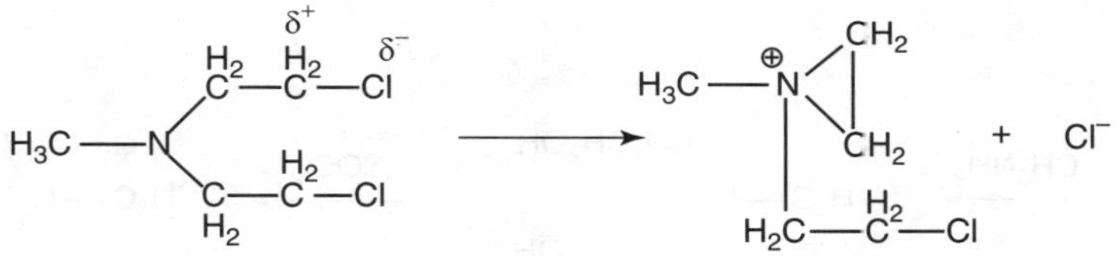

Step II: Nucleophilic attack of unstable aziridine

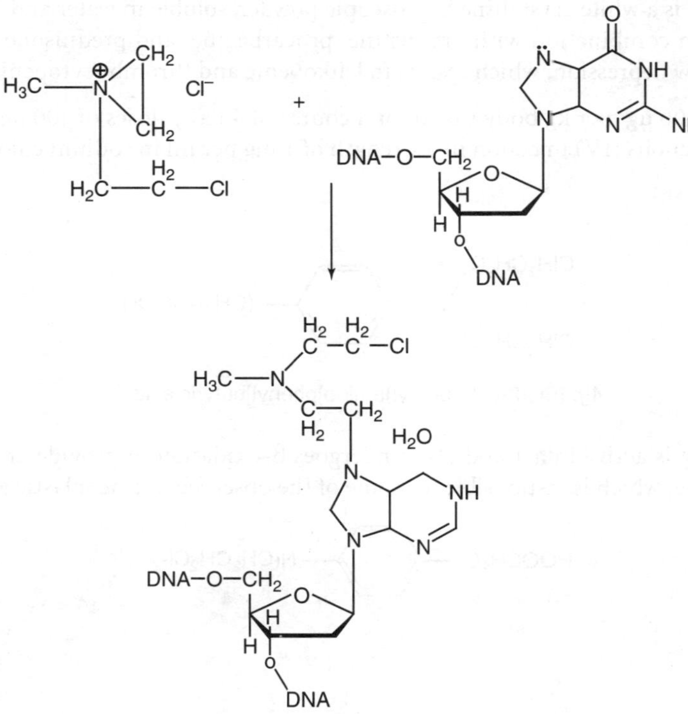

Mode of action: These compounds produce highly reactive carbonium ion intermediates that transfer alkyl group to cellular macromolecules by forming covalent bonds. It alkylates the 7th nitrogen atom of guanine residue in DNA, and results in cross-linking or abnormal base pairing. Initially, one of the 2-chloro ethyl side chain undergoes a first-order (SN_1) intramolecular cyclization with the release of Cl^- and formation of highly reactive ethyleniminium intermediate (Step I) By this reaction, tertiary amine is converted to an unstable quaternary ammonium compound, which react by forming carbonium ion. This precedes a second-order reaction (SN_2) nucleophilic substitution and alkylates the 7th N atom in guanine (Step II).

I. a. Nitrogen mustards

Mechlorethamine (Mustargen, Nitrogen mustard, Mustine)

$$H_3C-N(CH_2CH_2Cl)_2$$

2,2'-Dichloro-*N*-methyl diethylamine

Synthesis

$$2 \text{ Ethylene oxide} \xrightarrow{CH_3NH_2} H_3C-N(CH_2CH_2OH)_2 \xrightarrow{SOCl_2} H_3C-N(CH_2CH_2Cl)_2$$

Mechlorethamine

Properties and uses: It is a white crystalline hygroscopic powder, soluble in water and in alcohol. It is used in Hodgkin's disease in combination with vincristine, procarbazine, and prednisone. Most serious toxic reaction is bone marrow depression, which results in leukopenic and thrombocytopenia.

Dose: Single doses of 400 µg per kg body weight or a course of 4 daily doses of 100 µg per kg is normally administered by intravenous (IV) injection in a strength of 1 mg per ml in sodium chloride injection.

Chlorambucil (Leukaran)

$$(ClH_2CH_2C)_2N-C_6H_4-(CH_2)_3COOH$$

4[*p*-[Bis(2-chloroethyl)amino]phenyl]butyric acid

Metabolism: This drug is active intact and also undergoes β-oxidation to provide an active phenylacetic acid mustard metabolite, which is responsible for some of the observed antineoplastic activity.

$$HOOCH_2C-C_6H_4-N(CH_2CH_2Cl)_2$$

Synthesis

H_2N—⟨benzene⟩—$(CH_2)_3COOH$ + 2 ⟨ethylene oxide⟩

p-Amino phenyl butyric acid   Ethylene oxide

↓

$(HOH_2CH_2C)_2N$—⟨benzene⟩—$(CH_2)_3COOH$

↓ $SOCl_2$

$(ClH_2CH_2C)_2N$—⟨benzene⟩—$(CH_2)_3COOH$

Chlorambucil

Properties and uses: Chlorambucil is a white crystalline powder, practically insoluble in water, and soluble in acetone and alcohol. It is used in the treatment of chronic lymphocytic leukaemia, macroglobulinaemia, lymphosarcoma, and Hodgkin's disease.

Assay: Dissolve the sample in acetone, add water, and titrate with 0.1 M sodium hydroxide, using phenolphthalein as indicator.

Dose: Usual oral doses are 100–200 μg per kg body weight daily (usually 4–10 mg as a single daily dose) for 4–8 weeks.

Dosage forms: Chlorambucil tablets I.P., B.P.

Ifosfamide (Holoxan)

3-(2-Chloroethyl)-2-(2-chloroethyl)amino tetrahydro-2H-1,3,2-oxazaphosphorin-2-oxide

Properties and uses: Ifosfamide is a white crystalline hygroscopic powder, soluble in water and methylene chloride. It is used for testicular cancer, leukaemia, ovarian, and breast carcinoma.

Assay: It is assayed by adopting liquid chromatography technique.

Synthesis

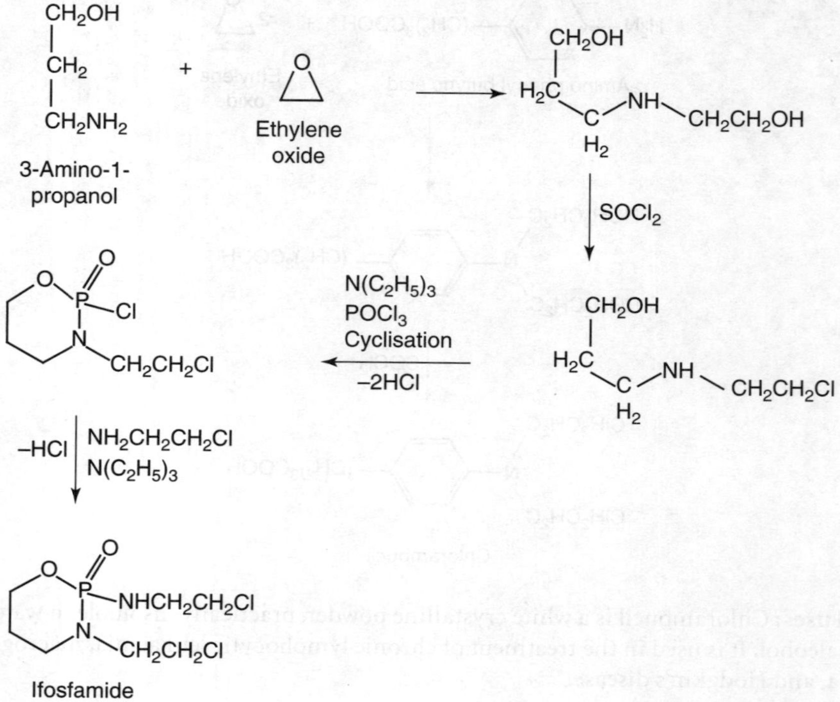

[Scheme: 3-Amino-1-propanol + Ethylene oxide → bis(hydroxyethyl) intermediate; SOCl₂ converts one OH to CH₂CH₂Cl; cyclisation with N(C₂H₅)₃ and POCl₃ (−2HCl) gives the cyclic phosphoramide chloride; reaction with NH₂CH₂CH₂Cl, N(C₂H₅)₃ (−HCl) yields Ifosfamide]

Ifosfamide

Dose: For the treatment of solid tumours of cervix, lungs, thymus, testes, and ovary; sarcoma; lymphoma of adults different licensed dosage regimens are available. Regimen 1: 8–12 g per m² divided over 3–5 days, repeat course every 2–4 weeks. Regimen 2: 6 g per m² divided over 5 days, repeat course every 3 weeks. Regimen 3: 5–6 g per m² (maximum, 10 g), given as a single 24 h infusion, repeat course every 3–4 weeks.

Cyclophosphamide (Cytoxan)

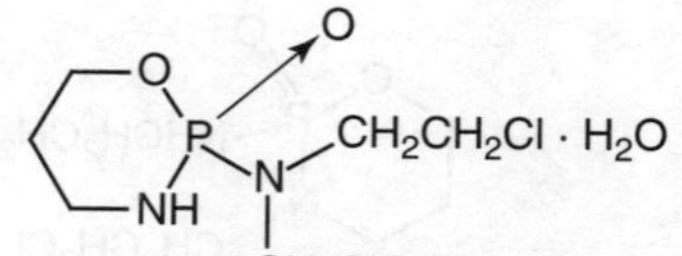

2-[Bis(2-chloroethyl)amino] tetrahydro-1, 3, 2-oxazaphosphorin-2-oxide monohydrate

Metabolism: The initial metabolic step is mediated primarily by CYP2B6 and involves hydroxylation of the oxazaphosphorine ring to generate a cabinolamine. CYP3A4 also catalyzes an inactivating N-dechloroethylation reaction, which yields nephrotoxic and neurotoxic chloroacetaldehyde.

Synthesis

Properties and uses: Cyclophosphamide is a white crystalline powder, soluble in water and alcohol. It is one among the widely used anticancer drugs and it is superior to many alkylating agents. It is active against multiple myeloma chronic lymphocytic leukaemias, acute leukaemia of children, Hodgkin's disease, breast, ovarian cancer, and lung cancer.

Assay: Dissolve the sample in sodium hydroxide solution in ethylene glycol, boil under reflux, and rinse with water, add 2-propanol, dilute nitric acid, 0.1 M silver nitrate, and ferric ammonium sulphate solution and titrate with 0.1 M ammonium thiocyanate.

474 Chemotherapy

Dose: Initial adult dose of 40–50 mg per kg given intravenously in divided doses over 2–5 days and for children 2–8 mg per kg daily through IV injection.

Dosage forms: Cyclophosphamide injection I.P., B.P., Cyclophosphamide tablets I.P., B.P.

Melphalan (Alkeran)

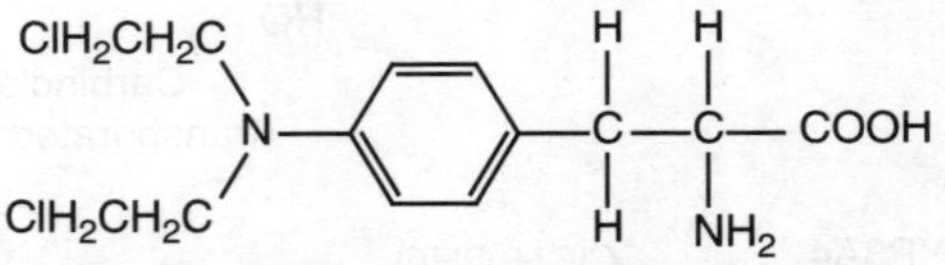

4-[Bis(2-chloroethyl)amino]-L-phenylalanine

Synthesis

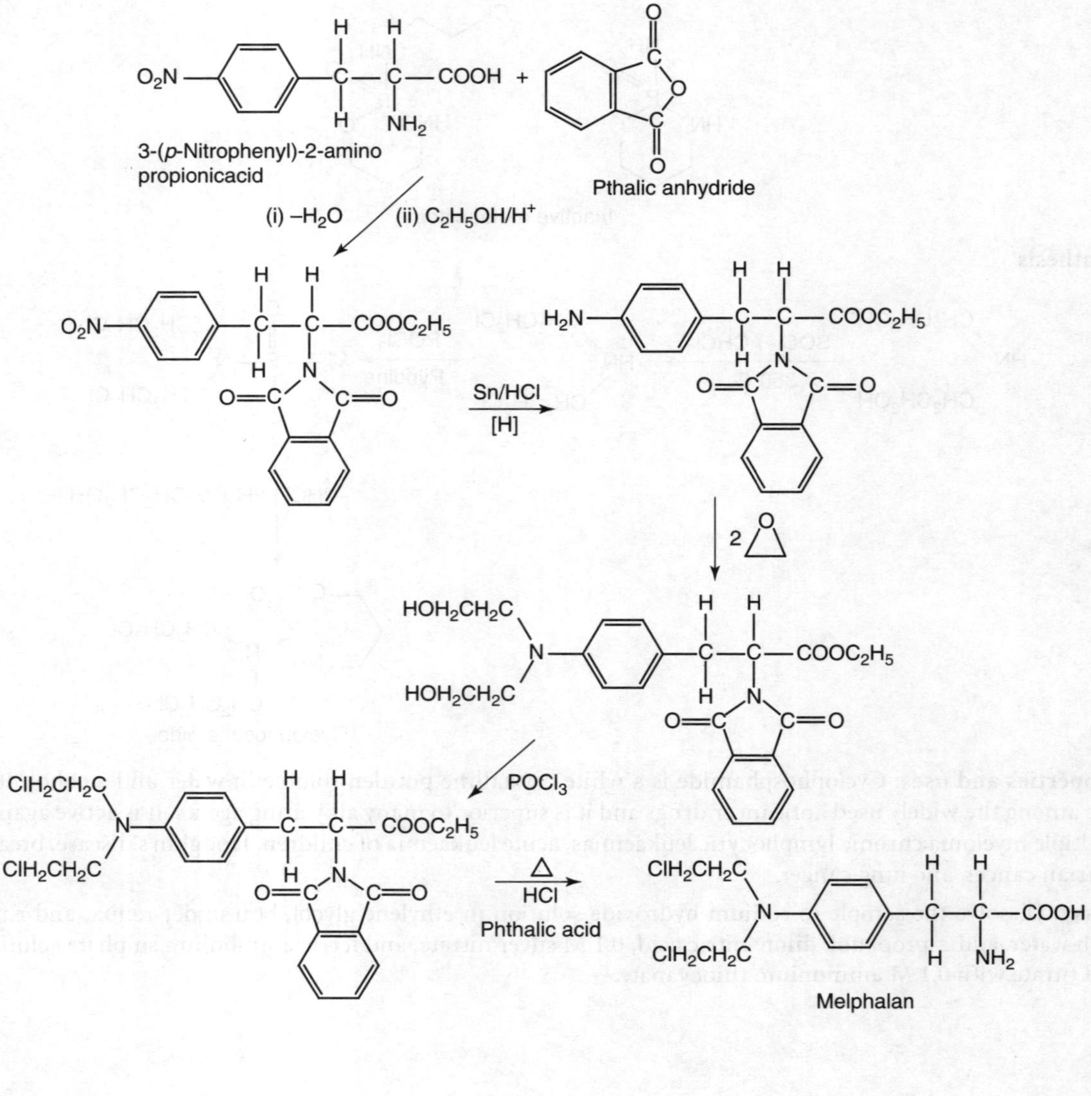

3-(p-Nitrophenyl)-2-amino propionic acid + Phthalic anhydride

(i) $-H_2O$ (ii) C_2H_5OH/H^+

Sn/HCl [H]

$2 \triangle$ (ethylene oxide)

$POCl_3$

Δ / HCl, Phthalic acid

Melphalan

Properties and uses: Melphalan is a white powder, practically insoluble in water and ether, slightly soluble in methanol and dissolves in dilute mineral acids. Melphalan is active against multiple myeloma, breast, testicular, and ovarian carcinoma.

Assay: To the sample add 20% w/v solution of potassium hydroxide, heat on a water bath, add water and nitric acid, cool, and titrate with 0.1 M silver nitrate. Determine the end point potentiometrically.

Dose: Dose orally is 150 µg per kg body weight daily for 4–7 days combined with prednisone 40–60 mg daily; 250 mg per kg daily for 4–5 days; or 6 mg daily by 2–3 weeks.

Dosage forms: Melphalan injection I.P., B.P., Melphalan tablets I.P., B.P.

Estramustine

Estradiol-3-bis-(2-chloroethyl)carbamate

Synthesis

Bis (2-chloroethyl) amine

Estradiol

Estramustine

Metabolism: The resonance-stabilized mustard-like antineoplastic agent utilizes an oestradiol carrier to deliver to the steroid dependent prostrate tissue selectively, and its use is limited to the palliative treatment of progressive prostrate cancer. In estramustine sodium phosphate, the essential 17 β-hydroxy group has been esterified with phosphoric acid, and the C-3 phenol has been carbamylated. The body still, however, transports the basic steroidal pharmacphore into the cells. The ionized sodium phosphate ester of the active 17 β-hydroxy group makes the compound water-soluble and to be able to distribute it in the blood. The ester is readily cleaved during absorption to provide the active 17 β-hydroxy group.

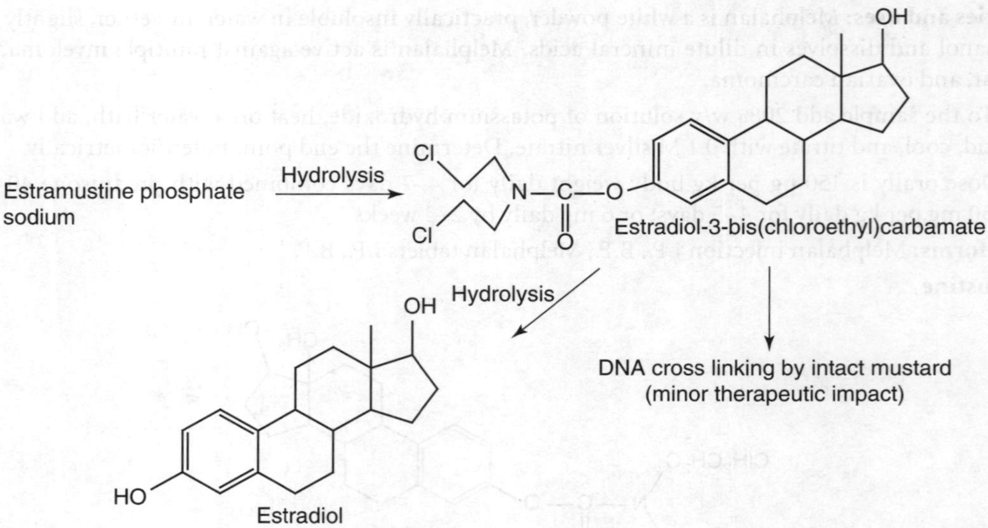

476 Chemotherapy

[Scheme: Estramustine phosphate sodium → (Hydrolysis) → Estradiol-3-bis(chloroethyl)carbamate → DNA cross linking by intact mustard (minor therapeutic impact); and (Hydrolysis) → Estradiol]

Properties and Uses: Estramustine sodium phosphate is a white powder, soluble in water and in methanol, and very slightly soluble in absolute ethanol. It is an alkylating agent, which is approved for metastatic/progressive cancer of the prostate, but is also active for advanced breast cancer. It causes nausea and vomiting, delayed bone-marrow depression, mild gynecomastia, thrombophlobitis, occasional myocardial infarction, hypertension, hypoglycaemia, and hepatotoxicity.

Assay: To the sample add 1M sodium hydroxide and boil under a reflux condenser. Cool and add 0.1 M silver nitrate and nitric acid dilute with water. Filter and titrate the excess of silver nitrate with 0.1 M ammonium thiocyanate using ammonium iron (III) sulphate as indicator.

Dosage forms: Estramustine phosphate capsules B.P.

Uracil Mustard

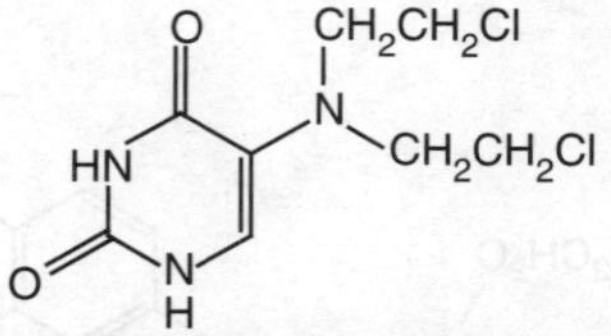

[Structure: 5-[Bis(2-chloro ethyl)amino] uracil]

Synthesis

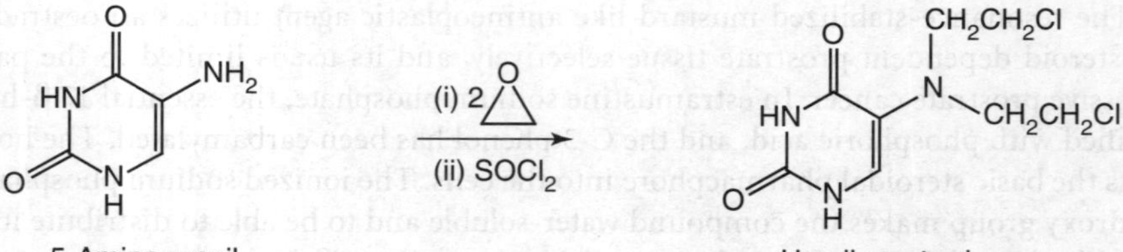

[Scheme: 5-Amino uracil → (i) 2 (epoxide) (ii) $SOCl_2$ → Uracil mustard]

Properties and uses: It is an off-white crystalline powder, odourless, and soluble in water or alcohol. It is used for the treatment of prostrate cancer.

I. b. Alkyl sulphones

Busulfan (mylearn)

$$CH_3SO_2O(CH_2)_4OSO_2CH_3$$
1,4-Bis(methanesulphonyloxy) butane

Synthesis

$$HO(CH_2)_4OH + 2CH_3SO_2Cl \xrightarrow[-2HCl]{Pyridine} CH_3SO_2O(CH_2)_4OSO_2CH_3$$

1,4-Butanediol   Busulfan

Metabolism: Busulfan undergoes sulphur stripping due to interaction with thiol compounds such as glutathione or cysteine and leads to loss of two equivalents of methosulphonic acid and formation of cyclic sulphonium intermediates, which is then converted into a metabolite 3-hydroxythiolane-1, 1-dioxide.

Properties and uses: Busulfan is a white crystalline powder, very slightly soluble in water and alcohol, soluble in acetone and acetonitrile. It is used in the treatment of chronic granulocytic leukaemia.

Assay: To the sample add water, boil under a reflux condenser, cool and titrate with 0.1 M sodium hydroxide using phenolphthalein as indicator until a pink colour is obtained.

Dose: For granulocytic leukaemia, the daily oral dose is 60 µg per kg body weight, up to a maximum single daily dose of 4 mg, and to be continued till the white cell count falls between 15,000 and 25,000 per mm^3

Dosage forms: Busulfan tablets I.P., B.P.

I.c. Nitrosourea
Carmustine

$$O=C\begin{cases}NHCH_2CH_2Cl\\NCH_2CH_2Cl\\|\\NO\end{cases}$$

N,N'-Bis(2-chloro ethyl)-N-nitroso urea

Properties and uses: Carmustine is a yellowish granular powder, very slightly soluble in water, very soluble in methylene chloride, and soluble in ethanol. It is used against brain tumours and leukaemia, which have metastasized to the brain, and these multiple states respond to a combination of carmustine and prednisone.

Synthesis

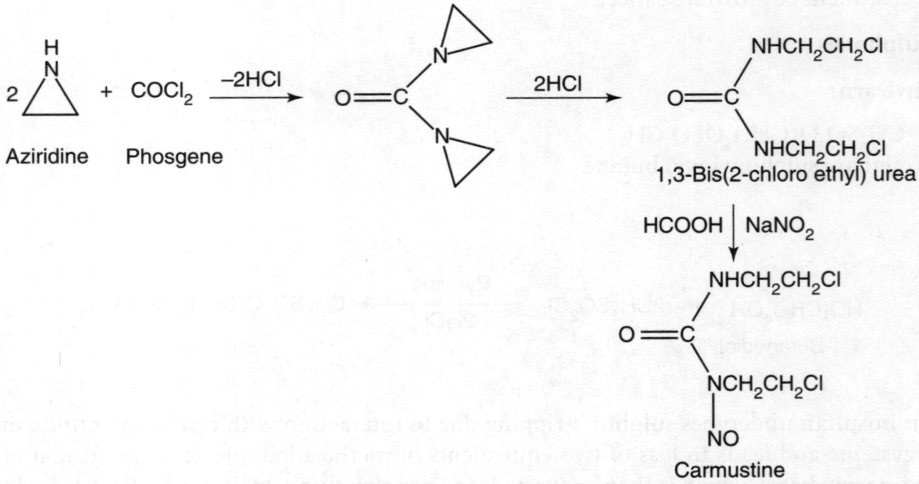

[Scheme: 2 Aziridine + COCl$_2$ (Phosgene) $\xrightarrow{-2HCl}$ 1,1'-carbonyldiaziridine $\xrightarrow{2HCl}$ 1,3-Bis(2-chloro ethyl) urea $\xrightarrow{HCOOH \mid NaNO_2}$ Carmustine]

Assay: Dissolve the sample in ethanol, dilute with water, and measure the absorbance at the maxima at 230 nm using ultraviolet spectrophotometer.

Lomustine and Semustine (Ceenu, Cinu)

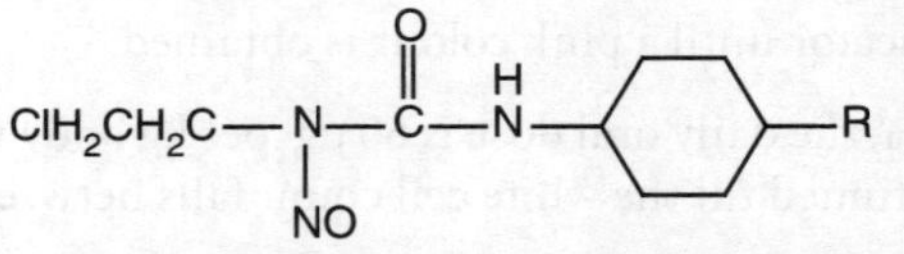

1-(2-Chloroethyl)-3-cyclohexyl-1-nitroso urea

Synthesis

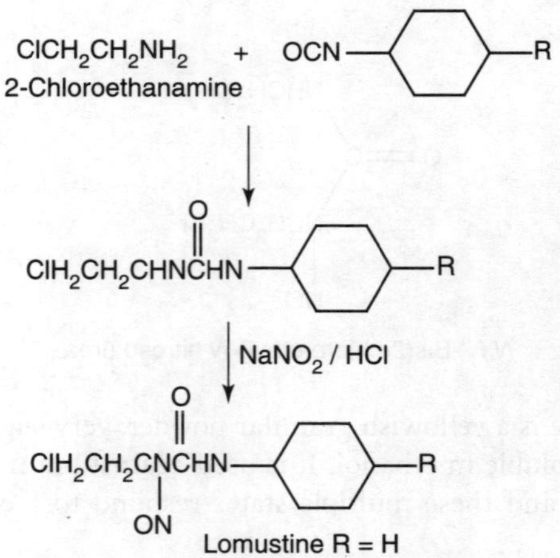

ClCH$_2$CH$_2$NH$_2$ (2-Chloroethanamine) + OCN—cyclohexyl—R

↓

ClH$_2$CH$_2$CHNCHN—cyclohexyl—R

↓ NaNO$_2$ / HCl

ClH$_2$CH$_2$CNCHN—cyclohexyl—R
       |
       NO

Lomustine R = H
Semustine R = CH$_3$

Properties and uses: Lomustine is a yellow crystalline powder, practically insoluble in water, soluble in acetone, methylene chloride, and alcohol. It is used against both primary and metastatic brain tumours and as secondary therapy in relapsed Hodgkin's disease.

Assay: Dissolve the sample in alcohol, add potassium hydroxide, and boil under a reflux condenser. Add water and nitric acid, cool and titrate with 0.1 M silver nitrate. Determine the end point potentiometrically. Perform a blank titration.

Dose: Usual dose is 130 mg/m^2 orally every 6 weeks.

Dosage forms: Lomustine capsules B.P.

I. d. Aziridines

Thiotepa

Tri-(1-aziridyl) phosphine sulphide

Synthesis

Trichlorophosphine sulphide + 3 Aziridine $\xrightarrow{-3HCl}$ Thiotepa

Metabolism: Thiotepa undergoes oxidative desulphuration forming an active cytotoxic metabolite known as Triethylene phosphoramide (TEPA). Aziridine metabolism occurs, with liberation of ethanolamine.

Properties and uses: Thiotepa exists as white crystalline flakes, freely soluble in water, chloroform, and ethanol. It is used as cytotoxic alkylating agent.

Assay: Transfer the sample to an iodine flask with the aid of 20% w/v solution of sodium thiosulphate and titrate immediately with 0.1 M hydrochloric acid, using methyl orange as indicator, until a faint red colour persists for 10 sec. Stopper the flask, allow to stand for 30 min, and titrate with 0.1 M sodium hydroxide using phenolphthalein as indicator. Subtract the volume of 0.1 M sodium hydroxide used from the volume of 0.1 M hydrochloric acid used.

Dosage forms: Thiotepa injection I.P., B.P.

Benzotepa

Benzyl di(aziridin-1-yl)phosphorylcarbamate

Synthesis

Ethylcarbamate → (POCl$_3$) → dichlorophosphoryl isocyanate → (C$_6$H$_5$CH$_2$OH) → intermediate → (2 Aziridine, −2 HCl) → Benzotepa

Altretamine

N^2,N^2,N^4,N^4,N^6,N^6-Hexamethyl-1,3,5-triazine-2,4,6-triamine

Synthesis

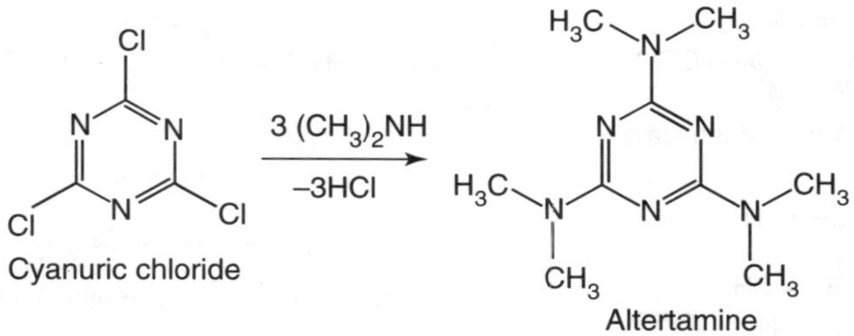

Cyanuric chloride + 3 (CH$_3$)$_2$NH $\xrightarrow{-3HCl}$ Altertamine

I.e. Methyl hydrazines
Procarbazine

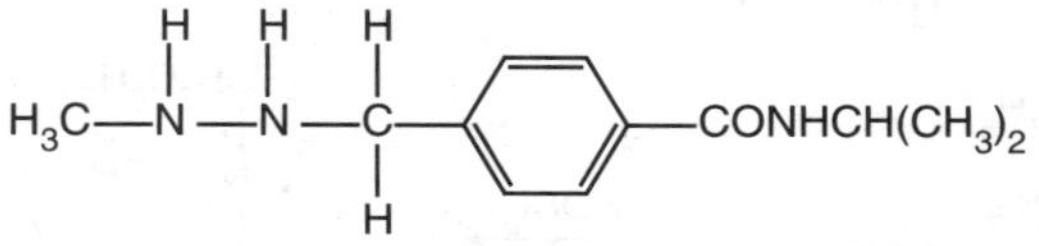

N-Isopropyl-2-(2-methyl hydrazine)-p-toluamide

Synthesis
Route-I. From: N-Isopropyl-p-methyl benzamide

N-Isopropyl-p-methyl benzamide + C$_2$H$_5$OOCN=NCOOC$_2$H$_5$ (Diethyl azodicarboxylate)

$\xrightarrow{-H_2}$

[intermediate with C$_2$H$_5$OOCHN—N and COOC$_2$H$_5$]

$\xrightarrow[-HI]{CH_3I}$

[N-methylated intermediate]

$\xrightarrow[NaOH/H_2O]{-2C_2H_5OH}$

[dicarboxylic acid intermediate with HOOCN and COOH]

$\xrightarrow[-2CO_2]{\Delta}$ Procarbazine

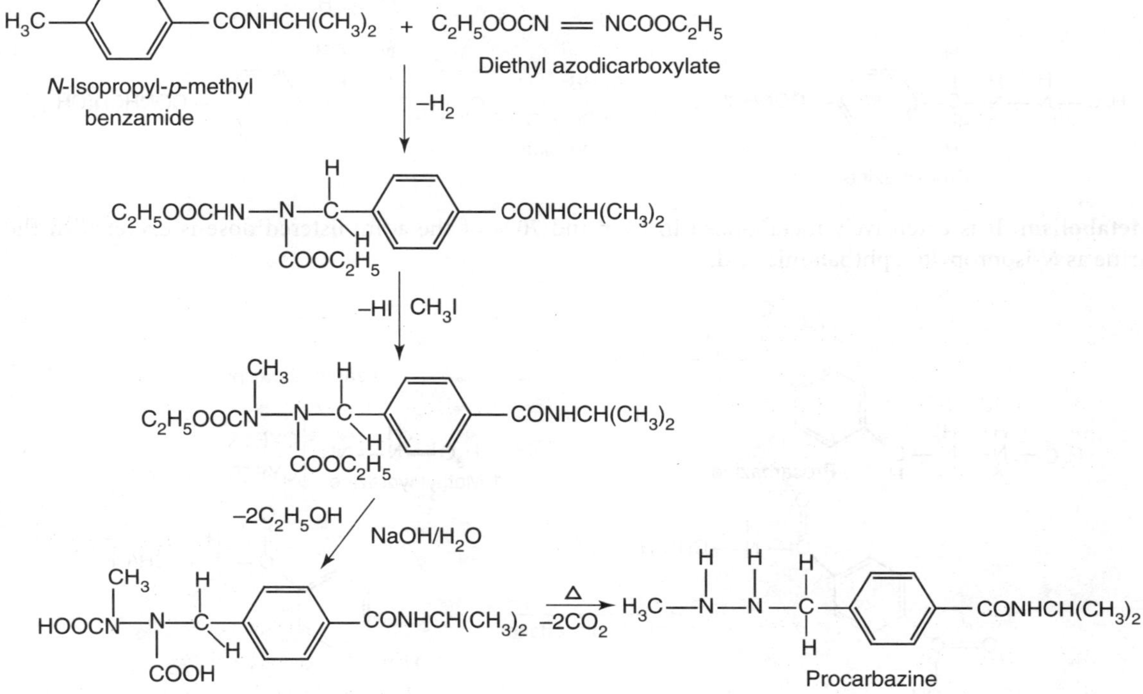

Route-II. From: Methyl-4-methylbenzoate

[Synthetic scheme: Methyl 4-methylbenzoate is treated with Br$_2$/UV (–HBr) to give 4-(bromomethyl)methyl benzoate along with N,N'-Bis(benzyl)-N-methyl hydrazine (CH$_2$C$_6$H$_5$–N(CH$_3$)–NHCH$_2$C$_6$H$_5$). These combine (–HBr) to give the benzyl-substituted intermediate bearing –COOCH$_3$. Hydrolysis with NaOH/H$_2$O (–CH$_3$OH) gives the corresponding –COOH; SOCl$_2$ converts it to –COCl; reaction with NH$_2$CH(CH$_3$)$_2$ (–HCl) gives the –CONHCH(CH$_3$)$_2$ amide; debenzylation with (i) HBr (ii) CH$_3$COOH furnishes Procarbazine: H$_3$C–NH–NH–CH$_2$–C$_6$H$_4$–CONHCH(CH$_3$)$_2$.]

Metabolism: It is extensively metabolized in liver and 70% of the administered dose is excreted in the urine as *N*-isopropylterephthalamic acid.

[Metabolism scheme: Procarbazine → Azaprocarbazine (oxidation of the CH$_2$ to C=O giving 4-(CH$_3$-N=N-CO-)C$_6$H$_4$-CONHCH(CH$_3$)$_2$); loss of 1-Methylhydrazine (H$_3$C–NH–NH$_2$) via CYP1A / CYP2B gives 4-formyl-N-isopropylbenzamide (OHC–C$_6$H$_4$–CONHCH(CH$_3$)$_2$); Aldehydeoxidase oxidation yields *N*-Isopropylterephthalamine acid (HOOC–C$_6$H$_4$–CONHCH(CH$_3$)$_2$) (major urinary product).]

Properties and uses: It exists as white to pale yellow crystalline powder with a slight odour and a bitter taste, soluble in water or alcohol, slightly soluble in chloroform, but insoluble in ether. Solutions are acid to litmus, stable in light, slowly oxidized in air, and stable at room temperature (in the presence of oxygen, oxidation is accelerated by increased temperature).

Decarbazine

5-(3,3-dimethyl-1-triazenyl)-1*H*-imidazole-4-carboxamide

Synthesis

5-Aminoimidazole-4-carboxamide → (NaNO$_2$ / HCl, Diazotisation) → 4-carboxamide-5-imidazole diazonium chloride

−CH$_3$Cl | (CH$_3$)$_3$N / CH$_3$OH

Decarbazine

Metabolism: Approximately 40% of the drug is excreted unchanged, but both the 5-amino imidazole-4-carboxamine and the carboxylic acid are seen in urine as metabolites.

Decarbazine → (CYP1A, CH$_2$O) → MTIC → AIC

MTIC = 3-Methyl-(triazen-1-yl) imidazole-4-carboxamide
AIC = 5-Amino Imidazole-4-carboxamide

Properties and uses: It is used as a cytotoxic agent, which is colourless to ivory coloured microcrystalline powder, soluble in water or alcohol.

II. Antimetabolites

Mode of action: These are analogues that resemble normal compounds of co-enzymes, which participate in the DNA synthesis and competitively inhibit the utilization of normal substrate or incorporates to make dysfunction.

II. a. Pyrimidine analogues

The structural modification of these metabolites may be on the pyrimidine ring.

5-Fluorouracil

5-Flouro-2,4-(1H,3H)pyrimidinedione

Synthesis

S-Ethyl isothiouranium bromide

Fluorouracil ← CFCl$_3$(inCFCl$_3$) Pressurebottle −78°C CF$_3$OF ← Trifluoromethyl hypofluorite

Mode of Action: It is converted into 5-flouro-2-deoxy uridine monophosphate, which inhibits thymidilate synthetase and blocks the conversion of deoxy uridic acid to deoxy thymidilic acid. For binding to thymidilate synthetase, this fluorinated pyrimidine prodrug must be converted to its deoxyribonucleotide. The active from of fluorouracil differs from the endogenous substrate only by the presence of the 5-flurogroup, which hold the key to the cytotoxic action of this drugs.

Metabolism: 20% of drug is excreted unchanged in urine and rest undergoes metabolism by polymorphic dihydro pyrimidine dehydrogenase to produce 5-fluoro 5, 6, dihydrouracil, which is converted to α-fluor-ouridopropionic acid by dihydropyrimidinase and to α-fluoro β-alanine by β-ureidopropionase.

Properties and uses: Fluorouracil is a white crystalline powder, sparingly soluble in water, and slightly soluble in alcohol. It is used topically in the treatment of pancancerous dermatoses, especially actinic keratosis, for which it is the treatment of choice, if the lesions are multiple, even if the lesions that are not clinically discernable respond. For this reason, the drug is applied to the entire affected area. Healing continues for 1 to 2 months after treatment. The drug does not affect nonkeratotic lesion. It is a secondary immuno-suppressive agent, and therefore, is not used in organ transplantation. It is the most active drug available for colorectal cancer. It is effective in the management of the breast, colon, pancreas, rectum, and stomach. It may have devastating bone marrow and gastrointestinal toxicity.

Assay: Dissolve the sample in dimethylformamide by gentle warming, cool and titrate with 0.1 M tetrabutylammonium hydroxide, using thymol blue as indicator.

Dosage forms: Fluorouracil injection I.P., B.P., Fluorouracil cream B.P.

Fluoxuridine

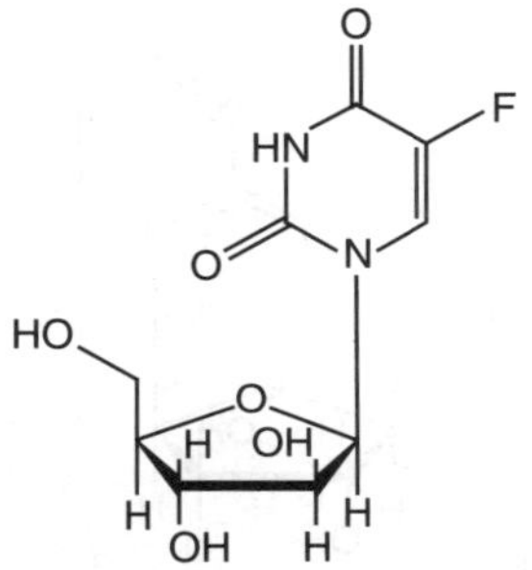

1-(2-Deoxy-D-ribofuranosyl)-5-flouorouracil

Synthesis

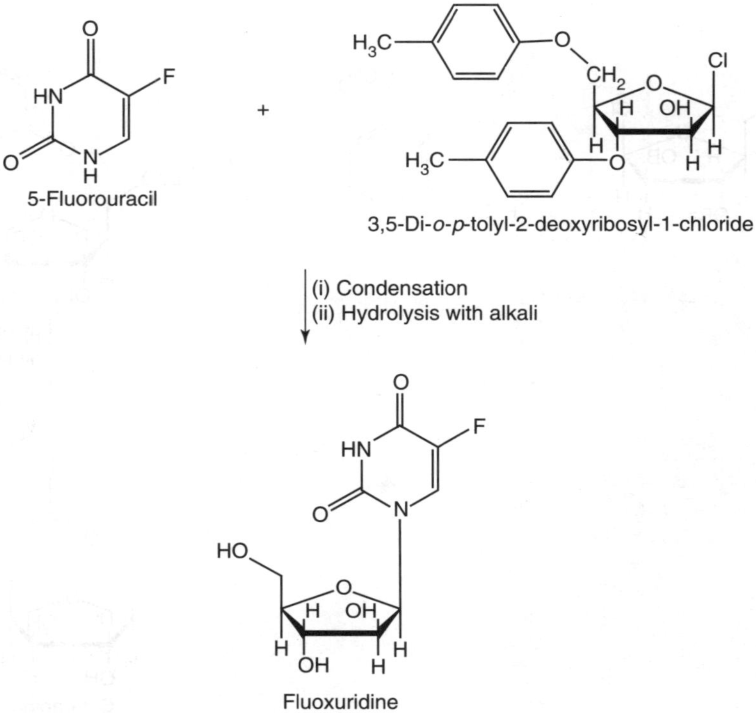

5-Fluorouracil + 3,5-Di-o-p-tolyl-2-deoxyribosyl-1-chloride

(i) Condensation
(ii) Hydrolysis with alkali

Fluoxuridine

Metabolism: This deoxyribonucleoside prodrug is bioconverted via 2'-deoxyuridine kinase-mediated phosphorylation to the same active 5-fluro-dUMP structure generated in the multistep biotransformation of fluorouracil.

Properties and uses: It is a white to off-white odourless powder, which is soluble in water, alcohol, or chloroform. Fluoxuridine is a prodrug of 5-fluorouracil. It is used for the palliation of gastrointestinal adenocarcinoma metastatic to the liver in patients who are considered incurable by surgery.

Cytarabine

1–β-D-Arabinofuranosyl cytosine

Synthesis

Properties and uses: Cytarabine is a white crystalline powder, soluble in water, very slightly soluble in alcohol and methylene chloride. It is used for acute leukaemia, chronic myclocytic leukaemia, meningeal leukaemia, acute lympholytic leukaemia, and chronic lympholytic leukaemia.

Assay: Dissolve the sample in anhydrous acetic acid, warm, if necessary, and titrate with 0.1 M perchloric acid. Determine the end point potentiometrically.

Dosage forms: Cytarabine injection I.P., B.P.

Capecitabine (Captabin, Capiibine, Xabine)

5'-Deoxy-5-fluoro-N^4-(pentyloxy carbonyl) cytidine

Synthesis

5'-Deoxy-5-fluorocytidine → (ClCOO(CH$_2$)$_4$CH$_3$, −HCl) → Capecitabine

Metabolism: The drug is actually another 5-fluoro-deoxy uridine monophosphate prodrug. When given orally, it is extensively metabolized to fluorouracil, which is then converted to the active fluorinated deoxyribonucleotide.

Uses: It is used in acute granulocytic leukaemia of adults and children.

Dose: The dose for colorectal cancer and breast cancer for adults is 1.25 g per m^2 two times a day for 2 weeks followed by a 1-week rest period. Therapy is to be given in 3-week cycles. Recommended treatment duration for colorectal cancer is 6 months. May be used in combination with docetaxel at 75 mg per m^2 given as a 1 h IV infusion, once in every 3 weeks for the treatment of breast cancer.

Gastric cancer: The dose for adults, used in combination with platinum-based compound, 1 g per m^2 two times a day for 14 days followed by a 7-day rest period. First dose is given on the evening of day 1 and the last dose on the morning of day 15.

II. b. Purine analogues

Mode of action: These drugs are converted into appropriate mono-ribonucleotides, which inhibit the conversion of inosine monophosphate to adenine and guanine nucleotides.

6-Mercaptopurine (Purinethol)

Purine-6-thiol

Properties and uses: Mercaptopurine is a yellow crystalline powder, practically insoluble in water, slightly soluble in alcohol, and dissolves in solutions of alkali hydroxides. It is used in the treatment of acute monocytic leukaemia.

Assay: Dissolve the sample in dimethylformamide and titrate with 0.1 M tetrabutylammonium hydroxide. Determine the end point potentiometrically.

Dose: The usual initial oral dose for children and adults is 2.5 mg per kg body weight daily, but the dose varies as per individual response and tolerance.

Synthesis

Route-I. From: 7H-Purin-6-ol

7H-Purin-6-ol $\xrightarrow{P_2S_5}$ 6-Mercaptopurine

Route-II. From: 6-Chloropyrimidine-4,5-diamine

6-Chloropyrimidine-4, 5-diamine $\xrightarrow{KSH}$ $\xrightarrow{\text{Conc. HCOOH}}$ 6-Mercaptopurine

Route III. From: Hypoxanthine

Hypoxanthine →[POCl$_3$ / Pyridine] 6-chloropurine →[NaSCN / −NaCl] 6-thiocyanatopurine →[H$_2$O] 6-Mercaptopurine

Dosage forms: Mercaptopurine tablets I.P., B.P, Mercaptopurine oral suspension B.P.

Thioguanine

2-Amino purine-6-thiol

Synthesis

2-Amino-9H-purin-6-ol →[POCl$_3$ / Pyridine] 2-amino-6-chloropurine →[NaSCN / −NaCl] 2-amino-6-thiocyanatopurine →[H$_2$O] Thioguanine

Properties and uses: It is used in treating acute leukaemia, especially in combination with cytarabine. The adverse effects are bone marrow depression, leucopenia, thrombocytopenia, and bleeding.

Fludarabine

Synthesis

Metabolism: This is a 3-halogenated adenosine based nucleoside, which undergoes conversion to active triphosphate nucleotides after active transport into the tumour cells.

Properties and uses: Fludarabine phosphate is a white crystalline hygroscopic powder, slightly soluble in water, soluble in dimethylformamide, and very slightly soluble in anhydrous ethanol. It shows activity against low-grade lymphoma and mycosis fungoides.

Assay: It is assayed by adopting liquid chromatography technique.

II. c Folic Acid Analogues

Mode of action: These drugs inhibit dihydrofolate reductase (DHFRase), which converts the dihydrofolic acid to tetrahydro folicacid, the co-enzyme required for one carbon transfer reaction in de novo purine synthesis and amino acid interconversion.

Methotrexate (Amethopterin)

4-Amino-N^{10}-methyl-pteroylglutamic acid

Synthesis

Route-I. From: Pyrimidine-2,4,5,6-tetraamine

Pyrimidine-2, 4, 5, 6-tetraamine   2, 3-Dibromo propanol

(i) $BaCl_2 \cdot H_2O$, NaOH
(ii) AcOH, I_2 / KI   pH 3.1

Methotrexate

Route-II. From: Pyrimidine-2,4,5,6-tetraamine

Pyrimidine-2, 4, 5, 6-tetraamine + 2, 3-Dibromopropanal → [intermediate] (−HBr)

→ (−H$_2$O, Cyclisation Dehydration) → 2-amino-4-amino-6-(bromomethyl)pteridine

+ RHN—C$_6$H$_4$—CONHCH(COOH)(CH$_2$)$_2$COOH

→ (−HBr) →

R = H   Aminopterin
R = CH$_3$ Methotrexate

Properties and uses: Methotrexate is a yellow or orange crystalline hygroscopic powder, practically insoluble in water, ethanol, and methylene chloride. It dissolves in dilute mineral acids and dilute solutions of alkali hydroxides and carbonates. It is used for the treatment of acute lymphocytic leukaemia, acute lymphoblastic leukaemia, breast cancer, and epidermoid cancer of the head, neck, and lung cancer.

Assay: It is assayed by adopting liquid chromatography technique.

Dose: For the maintenance therapy of acute lymphoblastic leukaemia, the dose is 15–30 mg per m^2 body surface once or twice weekly either orally or intramuscularly, with other agents, such as mercaptopurine.

Dosage forms: Methotrexate injection I.P., B.P., Methotrexate tablets I.P., B.P.

Azathioprine

6-[(1-Methyl-4-nitro-1H-imidazol-5-yl)thio]-1H-purine

Synthesis

9H-Purine-6-thiol + 5-Chloro-1-methyl-4-nitro-1H-imidazole $\xrightarrow{-HCl}$ Azathioprine

Properties and uses: Azathioprine is a pale-yellow powder, practically insoluble in water and alcohol. It is soluble in dilute solutions of alkali hydroxides and sparingly soluble in dilute mineral acids. It is used as an immuno-suppressant.

Assay: Dissolve the sample in dimethylformamide and titrate with 0.1 M tetrabutylammonium hydroxide. Determine the end point potentiometrically.

Dosage forms: Azathioprine tablets B.P.

Trimetrexate

5-Methyl-6-((3, 4, 5-trimethoxyphenylamino)methyl)quinazoline-2, 4-diamine

Synthesis

5-Methylquinazoline-2, 6-diamine

2, 3,-Trimethoxy bromobenzene

Trimetrexate

III. Antibiotics
III a. Anthracyclines

Anthracyclines occur as glycosides of the anthracyclinone. The glycosidic linkage usually involves the-7-hydroxyl group of anthraclinone and the β enentiomer of sugar with L-configuration. Anthracyclinone refers to an aglycone containing the anthraquinone chromophore within a linear hydrocarbon skeleton related to that of tetraycline.

Daunorubicin

Properties and uses: Daunorubicin is obtained from the fermentation of *Streptomyces peuletieues*. This drug bind to the DNA and inhibit nucleic acid synthesis, mitosis, and promote chromosomal aberration. These drugs are used for the treatment of acute myclocytic leukaemia, primary hepatocellular carcinomal, and ovarian endometrial carcinoma.

Doxorubicin

Properties and uses: Doxorubicin hydrochloride is an orange-red crystalline hygroscopic powder, soluble in water, and slightly soluble in methanol. Doxorubicin is 14-hydroxy daunoruibicin obtained from the cultures of *Streptomyces peuletiues*. It is one of the most effective antitumour agent. It is used in the treatment of acute lymphocytic leukaemia, breast, lung, ovarian, thyroid, gastric carcinoma, and Hodgkin's disease.

Assay: It is assayed by adopting liquid chromatography technique.

Dosage forms: Doxorubicin HCl injection I.P., Doxorubicin HCl tablets I.P., Doxorubicin injection B.P.

Idarubicin

Properties and uses: Idarubicin is demethoxy daunorubicin. It is a synthetic analogue of naturally occurring anthracyclines. It is used in acute myelogeneous leukaemia and acute lymphocytic leukaemia.

Valrubicin

Properties and uses: Valrubicin is a derivative of doxorubicin in which the amino group has a trifluoro-acetyl substituent and 14-hydroxy group is converted to valerate ester.

Bleomycin Sulphate

Bleomycinic acid R =	–OH
Bleomycin A$_2$ R =	–NH(CH$_2$)$_3$S$^{\oplus}$(CH$_3$)$_2$
Bleomycin B$_2$ R =	–NH(CH$_2$)$_4$NH–C(=NH)–NH$_2$

Properties and uses: Bleomycin sulphate is a mixture of cytotoxic glycopeptidase isolated from the strain of *Streptomyces verticillers*. It is mixture of closely related compounds with bleomycin A$_2$ and B$_2$, Bleomycins occurs naturally as blue copper chelates. Inside, the cell, bleomycin forms a complex with Fe (II), gives rise to hydroxyl radical and superoxide radicals. These radicals cleave the phosphodiesterase bond of DNA. This degradation of DNA strands is thought to be a lethal event in cells. It is effective in the treatment of testicular carcinomas. It is also useful in the treatment of squamous cell carcinomas of the head, neck, oesophagus, skin, and the genito-urinary tract, including the cervix, vulva, scrotum, and penis.

III. c. Mitomycin-C

Properties and uses: Mitomycin exists as blue-violet crystals or crystalline powder, slightly soluble in water, freely soluble in dimethylacetamide, sparingly soluble in methanol, and slightly soluble in acetone. It is obtained from *Streptomyces eqespitosus*; it contains three different carcinostatic functions, quinone, carbamate, and aziridine. The molecule is unreactive in its natural state. After intracellular enzymatic or spontaneous chemical reduction of the quinone and loss of the methoxy group, mitomycin becomes a bifunctional or trifunctional alkylating agent. The drug inhibits DNA synthesis at the O^6 and N^7 positions of guanine. In addition, single-strand breakage of DNA are caused by mitomycin. It is used in gastric and pancreatic carcinoma.

Assay: It is assayed by adopting liquid chromatography technique.

Dactinomycin or Actinomycin D

Properties and uses: It is obtained form the cultures of *Streptomyces antibioticus*. It consists of tricyclic phenoxazone ring in the quinone oxidation state and two identical polypeptide and intercalates into the double helical DNA. The main biochemical consequence of the intercalation of actinomycin into DNA is the inhibition of DNA and RNA synthesis, which in turn leads to depletion of protein and cell death.

Plicamycin (Mithramycin)

Properties and uses: It is an aureolic acid derivative obtained from *Stremyles plicatus* or *Streptomyces argillaceus*. It forms a complex with divalent metals, such as magnesium and calcium and such complex formation is required before binding with DNA. It inhibits DNA dependent RNA polymerase, which leads to cell death. It is used in the treatment of embryonal tumours of the testes and metastic cancers.

IV. Plant products

a. Vinca alkaloids

Vincristine R = CHO

Vinblastine R = CH_3

Mode of action: It binds to microtubular protein tubulin, prevents polymerization and assembly of microtubules, and causes mitotic spindle destruction. The chromosomes fail to move apart during mitosis and lead to metaphase arrest.

Properties and uses: Vinca alkaloids are isolated from *Catharanthus roseus*. They have complex structures composed of a dimeric indole-containing moiety named catharanthine and an indoline-containing moiety named vindoline. Four closely related compounds have antitumour activity, that is, vincristine, vinblastine, vinrosidine, and vinleurosine. Semisynthetic derivative vinorelbine is also used as an antitumour agent.

Vinorelbine

Properties and uses: They are used for the treatment of acute leukaemia, Hodgkin's disease, testicular cell tumour, lymphocytic lymphoma, histicytic lymphoma, and carcinoma of the breast.

b. Camptothecin derivatives

Name	R	R'
Camptothecin	–H	–H
Irinotican	–C$_2$H$_5$	–OCO–N(piperazine)N–N(piperidine)
Topotecan	–CH$_2$N(CH$_3$)$_2$	–OH

Properties and uses: Camptothecin is a pentacyclic alkaloid originally isolated from *Camptotheca acuminata*. These drugs are used for the treatment of colorectal and ovarian cancers.

c. Epipodophyllotoxins

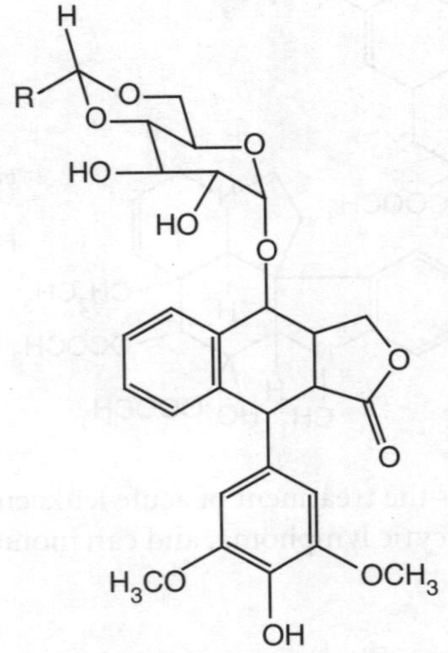

Etoposide R = CH$_3$

Teniposide R = (2-thienyl)

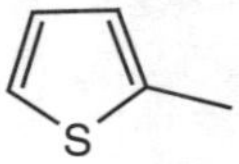

Mode of action: It arrests cells in G$_2$ phase and causes DNA breaks by affecting the DNA topoisomerase function and the resealing of DNA strand is prevented.

Properties and uses: Etoposide and teniposide are semi-synthetic derivatives of podophyllotoxin. It is obtained as extracts of May apple plant. It is effective in the treatment of lung cancer, testicular cancer, and Hodgkin's disease.

d. Taxol derivatives

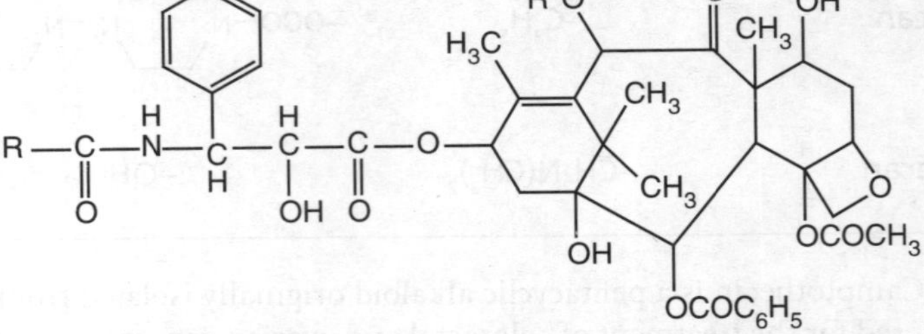

Name	R	R'
Paclitaxel	–C₆H₅ (phenyl)	–COCH$_3$
Docetaxel	$(CH_3)_3CO-$	–H

Mode of action: This stabilizes the polymerization of tubulin and the depolymerization is prevented.

Properties and uses: The taxol derivative, paclitaxel, is isolated from the Western row tree, *Taxus brevifolia*. It is the first member of the taxane family used in cancer therapy. It is used for metastatic ovarian and breast cancer, lung, mouth, oesophageal, and bladder carcinomas.

V. Enzymes

L-Asparaginase

It is an enzyme isolated from *Escherichia coli* and *Erwinia carotovora*. The enzyme has a molecular mass of 130,000. It consists of four equivalent subunits. It breaks down asparagin to aspartic acid and ammonia. It is active against tumour cells having lost the capacity to synthesize asparagines.

Properties and uses: It is used to treat childhood acute lymphocytic leukaemia in combination with vincristine and prednisone.

VI. Hormones

Mitotane

1,1-Dichloro-2-(*o*-chlorophenyl)-2-(*p*-chloro phenyl) ethane

Synthesis

2,2-Dichloro-1-(*o*-chlorophenyl) ethanol + Chlorobenzene $\xrightarrow[H_2SO_4]{-H_2O}$ Mitotane

Properties and uses: It is indicated only for treating adrenal cortex carcinoma.

Diethylstilbesterol

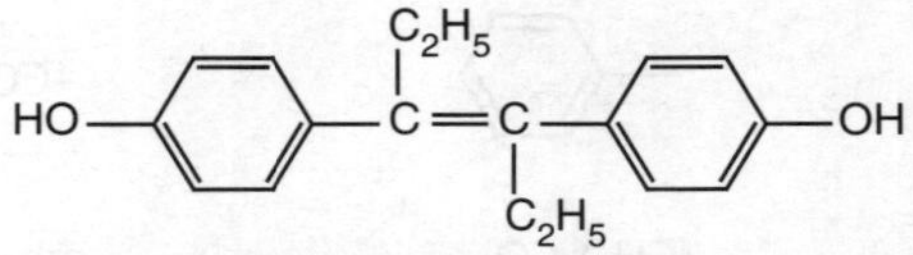

4,4'-(1,2-Diethyl-1,2-ethanediyl)bis-phenol

Synthesis

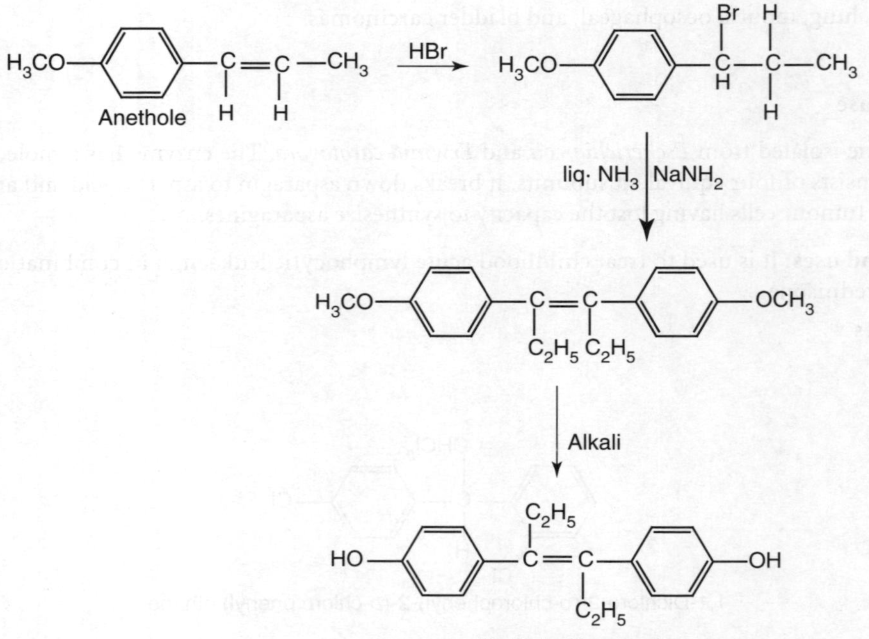

Anethole + HBr → brominated intermediate

liq. NH₃ | NaNH₂

Alkali →

Diethyl stilbesterol

Properties and uses: Diethylstilbesterol is a white crystalline powder, practically insoluble in water, and soluble in alcohol and alkali hydroxides solutions. It is used for pallative therapy and produces relief in primary as well as metastatic prostrate carcinoma.

Assay: Dissolve the sample in ethanol and dilute with the same solvent. To the resulting solution, add dipotassium hydrogen phosphate solution. Prepare in the same manner, a reference solution using diethylstilbestrol reference standard. Irradiate with mercury lamp and measure the absorbance of the irradiated solutions at the maximum of 418 nm, using water as a blank.

Dosage forms: Diethylstilbestrol pessaries B.P., Diethylstilbestrol tablets B.P.

Progesterone

17-Acetyl-10,13-dimethyl-1,7,8,10,11,12,13,15,16,17-decahydro-2H-cyclopenta[a]phenanthren-3(6H,9H,14H)-one

Synthesis

Properties and uses: Progesterone exists as white crystalline powder or colourless crystals, practically insoluble in water, soluble in ethanol, sparingly soluble in acetone and fatty oils. Progestins are pallative in 50% cases of advanced and metastatic endometrial carcinoma.

Assay: Dissolve the sample in alcohol, dilute with the same solvent, and measure the absorbance at 241 nm using ultraviolet spectrophotometer.

Dosage forms: Progesterone injection B.P.

Prednisone

(17R)-17-Hydroxy-17-(2-hydroxyacetyl)-10,13-dimethyl
-7,8,13,15,16,17-hexahydro-6H-cyclopenta[a]phenanthrene-3,11(9H,10H,12H,14H)-dione

Synthesis

Cortisone → *Corneybacterium simplex* → Prednisone

Properties and uses: Prednisone is a white crystalline powder, practically insoluble in water, slightly soluble in alcohol and methylene chloride. It is predominantly used in cancer chemotherapy, and in the treatment of acute exacerbations of multiple sclerosis. In paediatrics, it is widely used to treat nephrosis, rheumatic caslitis, leukaemia, and tuberculosis.

Assay: Dissolve the sample in alcohol, dilute with the same solvent, and measure the absorbance at 238 nm using ultraviolet spectrophotometer.

Tamoxifen

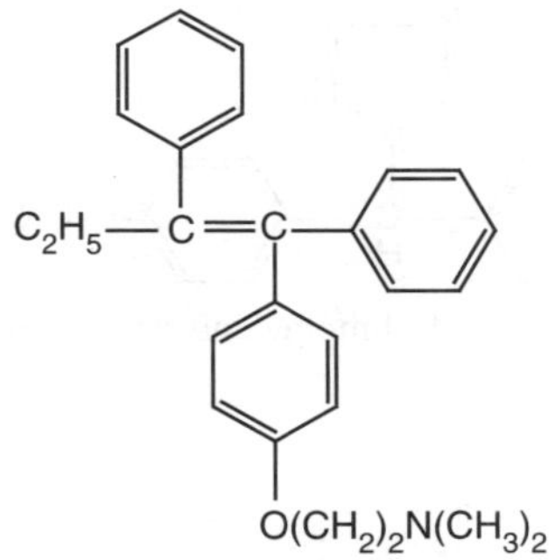
C_2H_5—C=C
$O(CH_2)_2N(CH_3)_2$

2-[4-(1,2-Diphenyl-1-butenyl)phenoxy]-*N*,*N*-dimethyl ethamine

Synthesis

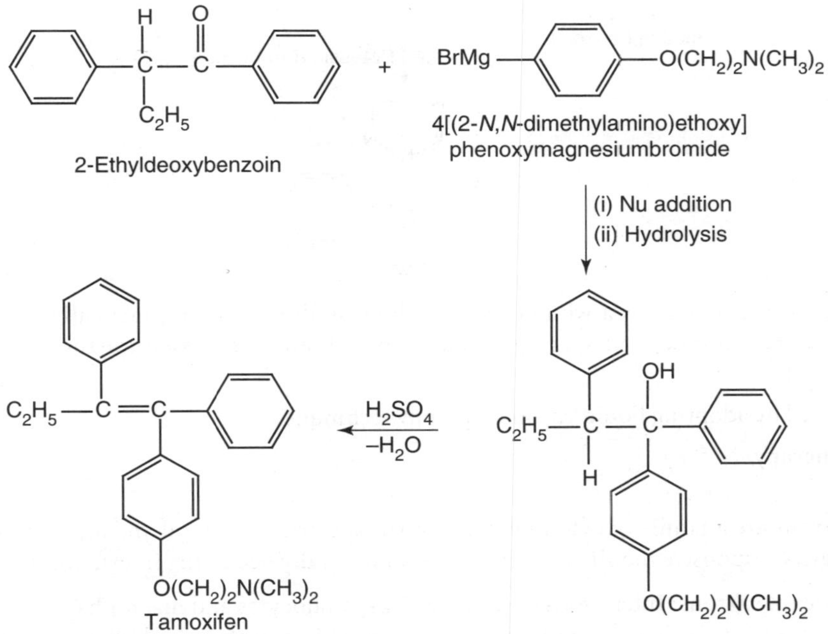
2-Ethyldeoxybenzoin
BrMg—
—$O(CH_2)_2N(CH_3)_2$
4[(2-*N*,*N*-dimethylamino)ethoxy] phenoxymagnesiumbromide
(i) Nu addition
(ii) Hydrolysis
H_2SO_4
$-H_2O$
Tamoxifen

Properties and uses: Tamoxifen citrate is a white crystalline powder, slightly soluble in water and acetone, but freely soluble in methanol. It is a nonsteroidal antiestrogen for palliative therapy of breast cancer in postmenopausal women. The drug competes with estrogens for cytosol estrogen receptors, and thus, blocks estrogens effects in the target tissue.

Assay: Dissolve the sample in anhydrous acetic acid and titrate with 0.1 M perchloric acid using naphthol-benzein as indicator.

Dosage forms: Tamoxifen citrate tablets I.P., Tamoxifen tablets B.P.

Letrozole

4,4'-(1H-1,2,4-triazol-1-yl-methylene)bis benzonitrile

Synthesis

4-((1H-1,2,4-Triazol-1-yl)methyl)benzonitrile + F—C6H4—CN

−HF | Potassium-t-butoxide

→ Letrozole

Properties and uses: Letrozole is a white or yellowish crystalline powder, practically insoluble in water, soluble in methylene chloride, and sparingly soluble in methanol. It is used for the treatment of breast carcinoma.

Assay: It is assayed by adopting liquid chromatography technique.

VII. Immunotherapy

Interferons

The interferons are a family of cytokines with broad-spectrum antiviral and anticancer activity making them biological responsive modifiers. Three types of naturally occurring interferons have been found:

1. Leukocytic interferons: Interferons α produced by lymphocytes and macrophages.
2. Fibroblast interferons: Interferons β produced by fibroblast epithelial cell and macrophages.
3. Immune interferons: Interferons γ synthesized by CD4[+], CD8[+], and natural killer lymphocytes.

IX. Micellaneous
Hydroxy Urea

$H_2N-\underset{\underset{O}{\|}}{C}-NHOH$

1-Hydroxy carbamide

Synthesis

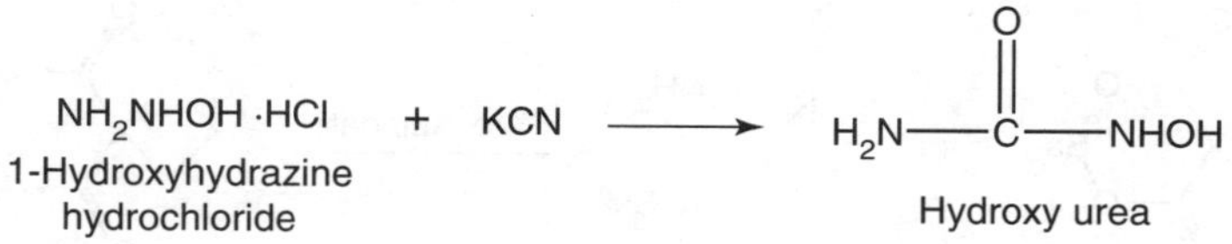

$$NH_2NHOH \cdot HCl + KCN \longrightarrow H_2N-\underset{\underset{O}{\|}}{C}-NHOH$$

1-Hydroxyhydrazine hydrochloride → Hydroxy urea

Uses: It is active against melanoma and chronic myelocytic leukaemia.

Gallium Nitrate

$Ga(NO_3)_3 \cdot 9H_2O$

Uses: It is used to treat cancer-related hypocalcaemia.

Cisplastin

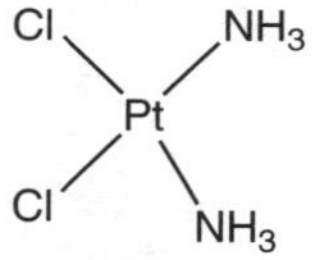

Cis-diamine dichloro platinum (CDDP)

Synthesis

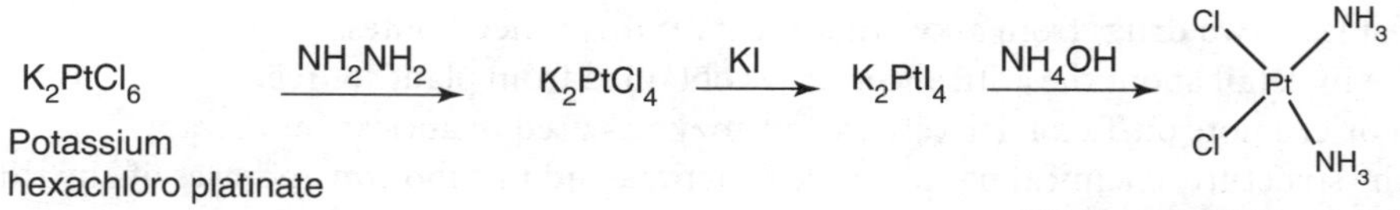

$$K_2PtCl_6 \xrightarrow{NH_2NH_2} K_2PtCl_4 \xrightarrow{KI} K_2PtI_4 \xrightarrow{NH_4OH} \text{Cis-diamine dichloro plati}$$

Potassium hexachloro platinate

Properties and uses: Cisplatin is a yellow powder or yellow or orange-yellow crystals, slightly soluble in water, sparingly soluble in dimethylformamide, and practically insoluble in alcohol, used in testicular tumour.

Assay: It is assayed by adopting liquid chromatography technique.

Dosage forms: Cisplatin injection B.P.

Carboplatin

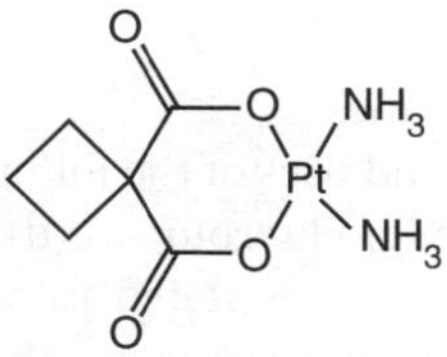

Cis-diamine(1,1-cyclobutane dicarboxylato) platinum

Synthesis

Barium cyclobutane-1,1-dicarboxylate + Pt(NH₃)₂I₂ →(Silver sulphate)→ Carboplatin

Properties and uses: Carboplatin is a colourless crystalline powder, sparingly soluble in water, very slightly soluble in acetone and alcohol. Food and Drug Administration (FDA) approved it for treatment of advanced ovarian cancer. It is cross-resistant with cisplatin in this tumour. Activity also has been reported in lung cancer, head and neck cancer, and testicular cancer. The usual dose-limiting toxicity is bone marrow suppression, especially, thrombocytopenia.

Assay: It is assayed by gravimetric method.

Dosage forms: Carboplatin injection B.P.

PROBABLE QUESTIONS

1. What is a neoplasm? What are the causations of neoplasm? Write the structure, name, synthesis, and uses of at least two drugs from alkylating agents and antimetabolites.
2. Describe in detail about the anticancer drugs obtained from plant source.
3. Write a brief a note on Taxol derivatives and enzymes used in anticancer therapy.
4. Write the structure, chemical name, mode of action, and metabolism and uses of any three anticancer drugs from different class.
5. How will you classify the antineoplastic agents? Write the structure, chemical name, and uses of two agents from each class.
6. Write an account on antibiotics used in anticancer therapy.
7. Mustards, methanesulphonates, ethylenimines, and nitrosoureas constitute four vital categories of the alkylating agents employed for the treatment of neoplasms. Outline the synthesis, metabolism, and uses of the following drugs:
   (a) Chlorambucil (b) Busulfan (c) Trithylene melamine (d) Carmustine
8. Recognition of antibiotics as an important class of antineolastic agents. Justify the statement with reference to the following drugs:
   (a) Dactinomycin (b) Daunorubicin.
   i. How would you classify 'antimetabolities'?
   ii. Give the structure, chemical name, and uses of the following:
   (a) Methotrexate (b) Meracaptopurine (c) Fluorouracil (d) Azaserine.
   iii. Discuss the synthesis of any one of the drug stated above.
9. Outline the synthesis of the following anticancer agents
   (a) Methotrexate (b) Lomustine (c) Cytarabine.

10. Give a comprehensive account of hormones that are potent as antineoplastic agents. Support your answer with suitable examples.
11. Give a brief account of the following:
    a. Immunotherapy in cancer
    b. Pharmacokinetics, pharmacodynamic, and mode of action of antineoplastic agents
12. What are alkylating agents. Explain with the chemical reaction about alkylating mechanism in anticancer therapy. Enumerate the agents used in this category and describe the synthesis and uses of any two of them.
13. Write the synthesis, mode of action, metabolism, and uses of the following agents: Cyclophosphamide, Thiotepa, and Azathiapurine
14. Write a note on cytoprotective agents.
15. Discuss the following with regard to antineoplastic agents:
    (a) Pteridines (b) Acyclic tertiary amines (c) Steroids

SUGGESTED READINGS

1. Abraham DJ (ed). *Burger's Medicinal Chemistry and Drug Discovery* (6th edn). New Jersey: John Wiley, 2007.
2. Bruntan LL, Lazo JS, and Parker KL. *Goodman and Gilman's: The Pharmacological Basis of Therapeutics* (11th edn). New York: McGraw Hill, 2006.
3. *British Pharmacopoeia*. Medicines and Healthcare Products Regulatory Agency. London, 2008.
4. Capizzi RL and Agrawal K. 'Drugs useful in the chemotherapy of the acute leukaemia'. In *Handbook of Experimental Pharmacology,* Fisher JW (ed), Vol. 101, pp. 523–64. Berlin: Springer-Verlog, 1992.
5. Dimmock JR and Kumar P. 'Anticancer and cytotoxic properties of Mannich bases'. *Curr Med Chem* 4: 1–22, 1997.
6. Dimmock JR, Murthi NK, Hetherington M, Quail JW, Pugazhenthi U, Sudom AM, Chamankhah M, Rose P, Pass, E, Allen TM, Halleran S, Szydlowski J, Mutus B, Tannous M, Manavathu EK, Myers, TG, Clercq E De, and Balzarini J. 'Cytotoxic activities of Mannich bases of chalcones and related compounds'. *J Med Chem* 41: 1014–1026, 1998.
7. Garnick MB, Griffin JD, Sack MJ, Blum RH, Israel M, and Frei E. 'Anthracycline'. In *Antibiotics in Cancer Chemotherapy*, Muggia FM, Young CW, and SK Carter (eds). The Hague: Martinus Nijhoff, 1982.
8. Gennaro AR. *Remington: The Science and Practice of Pharmacy* (21st edn). New York: Lippincot Williams and Wilkins, 2006.
9. Handchumacher RE. Cancer Chemotherapy-Examples of Current Progress and Future Perspective. In *IUPHAR, 9th International Congress of Pharmacology Proceedings* (Pt. 2.) W Paton, J Mitchell, and Turner P (eds). London: Macmillan, 1984.
10. *Indian Pharmacopoeia*. Ministry of Health and Family Welfare. New Delhi, 1996.
11. Klein E, Milgrom H, Stoll HL, Helm F, Walker HJ, and Holtermann OA. 'Topical 5-fluorouracil chemotherapy for pre-malignant and malignant epidermal neoplasma'. In *Cancer Chemotherapy* 11, Bradsky I and Kahn SB (eds). New York: Grune and Stratton, 1972.
12. Lednicer D and Mitscher LA. *The Organic Chemistry of Drug Synthesis*. New York: John Wiley, 1995.

13. Lemke TL and William DA. *Foye's Principle of Medicinal Chemistry* (6th edn). New York: Lippincott Williams and Wilkins, 2008.
14. Chabner BA and Collins JM (eds). *Cancer Chemotherapy: Principles and Practice*. Philadelphia: JB Lippincott, 1990
15. Sartorelli AC and Johns DG (eds). Antineoplastic and immunosupressive agents Pt II'. *Handbook der experimentellen Pharmakologie*, Vol. 38, pp. 348–72. Berlin: Springer-Verlog, 1975..
16. Pandeya SN. 'Chelation in anticancer activity'. In *Textbook of Inorganic Medicinal Chemistry*, pp. 79–83. SG Publisher, 1998.
17. Reynolds EF (ed). *Martindale the Extra Pharmacopoeia* (31st edn). London: The Pharmaceutical Press, 1997.
18. Skipper HT and Schabel FM (ed). 'Quantitative and cytokinetic studies in experimental tumour models'. In *Cancer Medicine* (3rd ed), Holland JF and Frei E (eds). Philadelphia: Lea and Febiger, 1973.
19. Skoda J. 'Azapyrimidine nucleoside'. In *Antineoplastic and Immunosuppressive Agents* (Pt II), Sarterelli AC and John GD (eds). Berlin: Handbuch de Experimentellen Pharmakology, 1975.
20. Umezava H. 'Cancer drugs of microbial origin'. In *Methods in Cancer Res*. *XVI*. *Cancer Drug Development* (Pt A), Deveta VT Jr (ed). New York: Academic Press, 1979.
21. Zubrod CG. 'Historical pespectice of curative chemotherapy'. In *Oncology,* Clark RL, Cumely RW, Mcloy JE, and Lopeland M (eds). Being the Proceedings of the Tenth International Cancer Congress Year Book. Chicago, 1970.

Chapter 12

Antileprotic Drugs

INTRODUCTION

Leprosy is a chronic disease caused due to acid-fast bacillus called *Mycobacterium leprae* and produces nodules on the skin and causes loss of sensation. Once the organism enters into the body, it multiplies and produces antigen–antibody reaction and causes cell-mediated immunity, and produces allergic reaction by the metabolite of the microorganism and finally produces lepra reaction.

Categories of Leprosy

1. Tuberculoid leprosy
2. Lepromatous leprosy
3. Intermediate leprosy
4. Borderline leprosy

Lepromatous leprosy: Large number of organisms that are present in the affected area and induce lepra reaction.

Tuberculoid leprosy: Is characterized by skin molecules with clear centre and well-defined margin.

Intermediate leprosy: Is localized hypo-pigmentation with some sensory loss.

Borderline leprosy: It is an intermediate stage between tuberculoid leprosy and lepromatous leprosy.

CLASSIFICATION

Antileprotic drugs are classified into the following:

  I. Sulphones
 II. Benzpyrazine derivatives: Clofazimine
III. Plant drugs

I. Sulphones

Dapsone (Diaminodiphenyl sulphone, DDS)

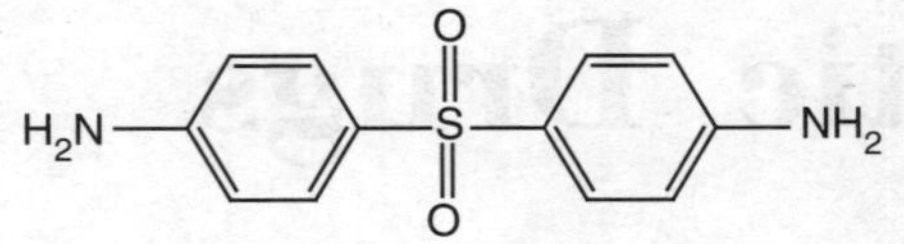

Acedapsone

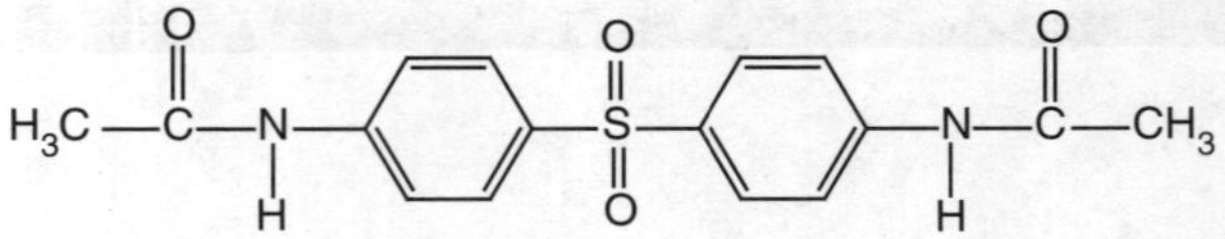

Solapsone sodium

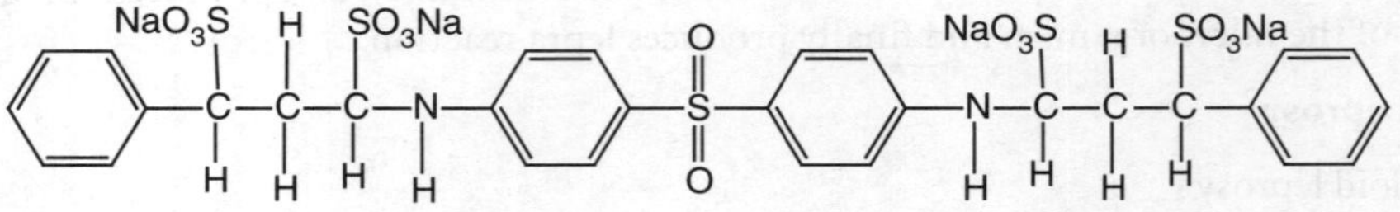

Sulfoxone sodium

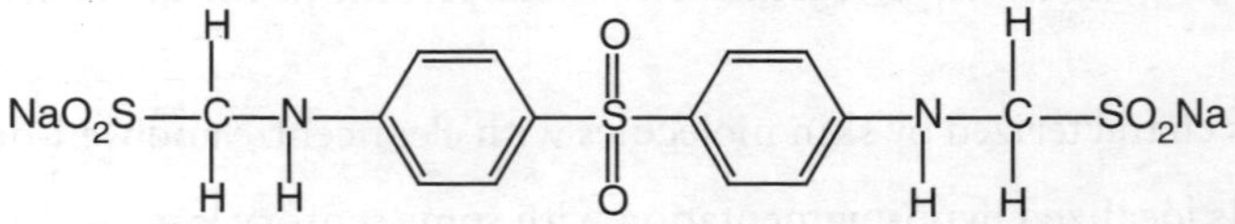

Gluco sulfone sodium

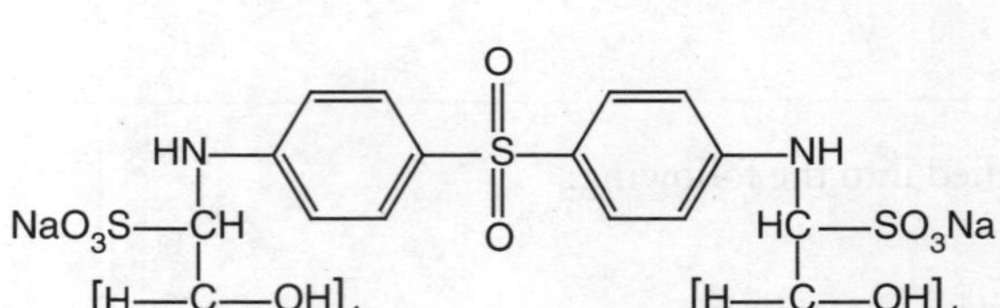

II. Dibenz pyrazine derivatives

Clofazimine (Lamprene)

III. Plant drug

i. Chaulmaogric acid

ii. Hydrocapric acid

SYNTHESIS AND DRUG PROFILE

I. Sulphones

i. Dapsone (DDS, Diaminodiphenyl sulphone)

4-(4-Aminophenylsulfonyl)benzenamine

Synthesis

Route I. From: 4-chloro nitrobenzene

$2\ O_2N\text{–}C_6H_4\text{–}Cl$ (p-Chloro nitrobenzene) + Na_2S $\xrightarrow{\text{(O) Chromic acid}}$ $O_2N\text{–}C_6H_4\text{–}SO_2\text{–}C_6H_4\text{–}NO_2$ $\xrightarrow[\text{Sn / HCl}]{\text{Reduction}}$ $H_2N\text{–}C_6H_4\text{–}SO_2\text{–}C_6H_4\text{–}NH_2$ (Dapsone)

Route II. From: 4-Chloro nitrobenzene

$2\ O_2N\text{–}C_6H_4\text{–}Cl$ (p-Chloronitrobenzene) + Na_2S $\longrightarrow$ $O_2N\text{–}C_6H_4\text{–}S\text{–}C_6H_4\text{–}NO_2$ $\xrightarrow[\text{Sn/HCl}]{\text{Reduction}}$ $H_2N\text{–}C_6H_4\text{–}S\text{–}C_6H_4\text{–}NH_2$ $\xrightarrow{\text{(O) Chromic acid}}$ $H_2N\text{–}C_6H_4\text{–}SO_2\text{–}C_6H_4\text{–}NH_2$ (Dapsone)

Metabolism: The major metabolic product of Dapsone results from *N*-acetylation in the liver by *N*-acetyl-transferase. It also undergoes *N*-hydroxylation to hydroxylamine derivative. These metabolic reactions are catalyzed by CYP3A4 isoforms. Neither of these compounds possesses significant leprostatic activity, although *N*-acetyldiamino-diphenyl sulphone may be deacetylated back to Dapsone. Products found in the urine consist of small amounts of Dapsone and the metabolites, that is, *N*-acetyldiamino-diphenyl sulphone and *N*-hydroxy-diamino-diphenyl sulfone, as well as glucuronide and sulphate of each of these substances.

N-Acetyldiaminodiphenyl sulphone   *N*-Hydroxydiaminodiphenyl sulphone

Glucuronide conjugation   Sulphate conjugation

Glucuronides and sulphats of the respective metabolites

Properties and uses: Dapsone is a white or slightly yellowish-white crystalline powder, very slightly soluble in water, soluble in acetone and dilute mineral acids, but sparingly soluble in alcohol. It is a folic acid synthesis inhibitor used in both lepromatous and tuberculoid leprosy.

Assay: Dissolve the sample in dilute hydrochloric acid and add potassium bromide. Cool in ice and titrate against 0.1 N sodium nitrate. Determine the end point electrometrically.

Dosage: The dose as tablets is 25 or 100 mg. For adults the dose consumed is 50 mg per day orally. For lepromatous leprosy, 100 mg Dapsone + 600 mg Rifampin and/or clofazimine 100 mg daily for at least 2 years followed by Dapsone monotherapy. For borderline tuberculoid disease, Dapsone 100 mg daily + Rifampin 600 mg once monthly for 6 months.

Dose : Dapsone tablets I.P., B.P.

ii. Solapsone Sodium

Chemotherapy

Synthesis

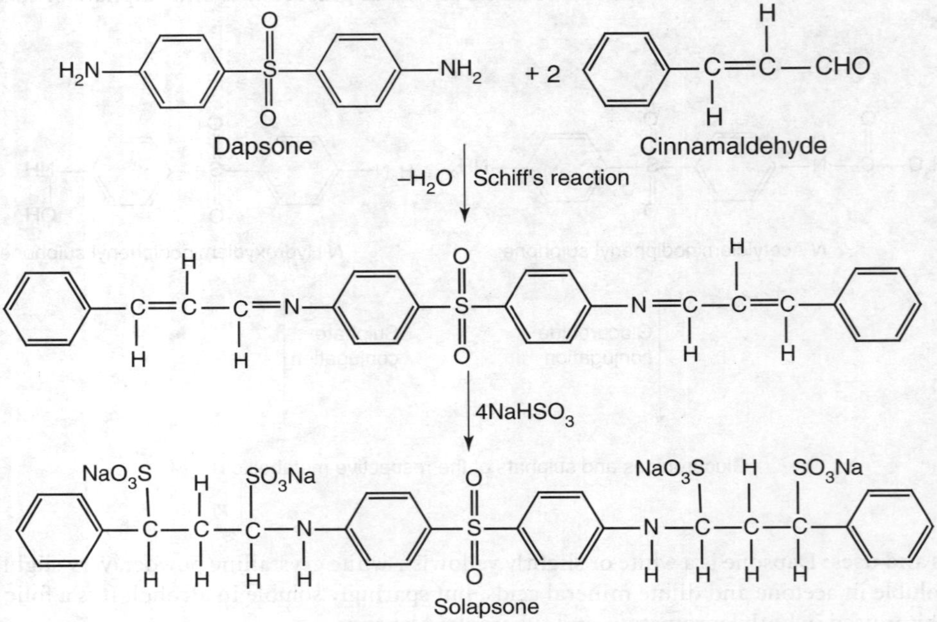

[Dapsone + 2 Cinnamaldehyde]

−H₂O | Schiff's reaction

[bis-Schiff base intermediate]

4NaHSO₃

Solapsone

Acedapsone

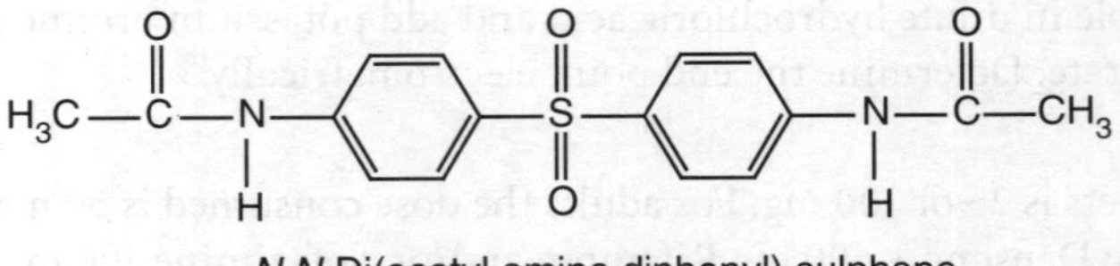

N,N-Di(acetyl amino diphenyl) sulphone

Synthesis

Route I: From Dapsone

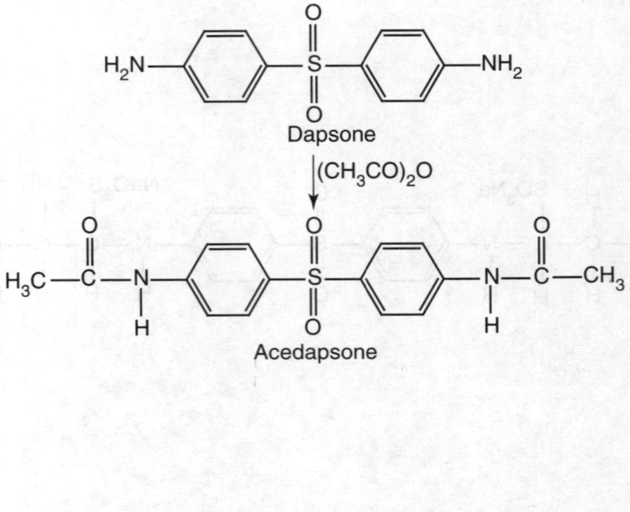

Dapsone

$(CH_3CO)_2O$

Acedapsone

Route II: From 4-Chloro nitrobenzene

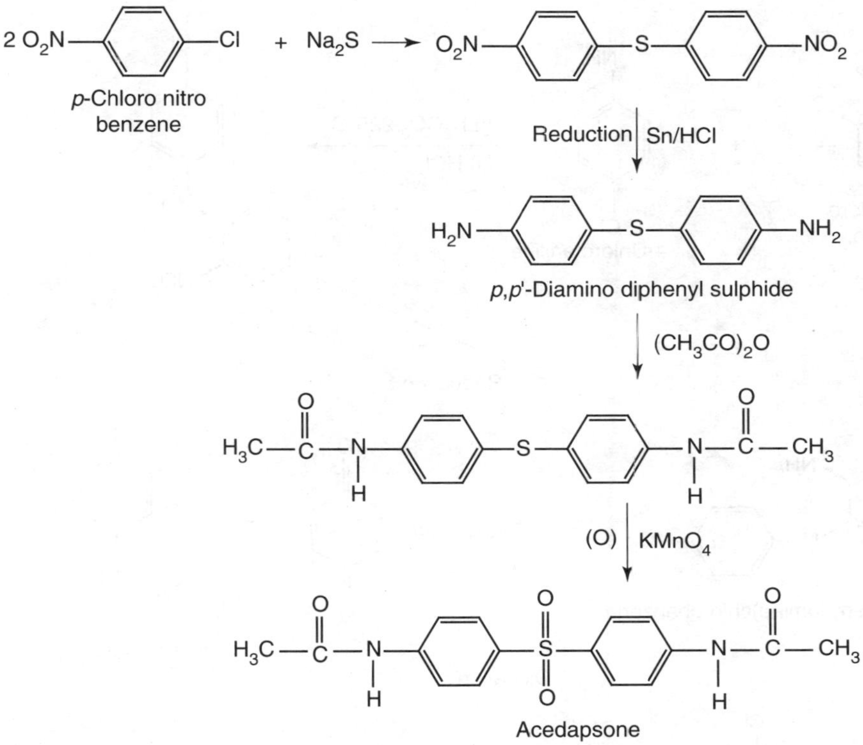

[Reaction scheme: 2 equivalents of p-Chloro nitrobenzene + Na₂S → 4,4'-dinitrodiphenyl sulphide → (Reduction Sn/HCl) → p,p'-Diamino diphenyl sulphide → ((CH₃CO)₂O) → bis-acetamido diphenyl sulphide → ((O) KMnO₄) → Acedapsone]

p-Chloro nitro benzene

p,p'-Diamino diphenyl sulphide

Acedapsone

Properties and uses: Acedapsone (prodrug of Dapsone) is used in the treatment of both lepromatous and tuberculoid type of leprosy.

II. Benzpyrazine derivatives

iii. Clofazimine (Lamprene)

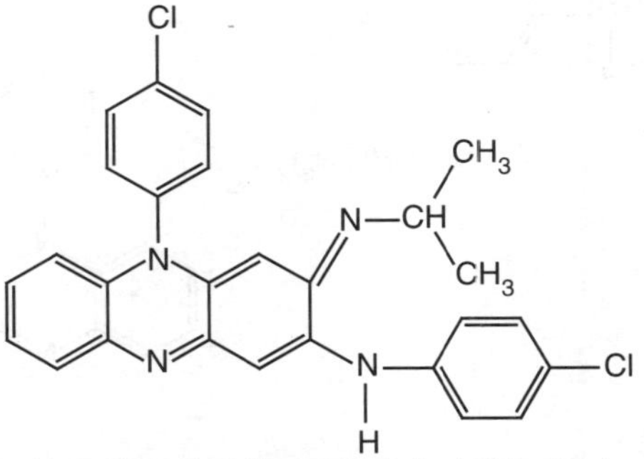

(*Z*)-*N*,5-Bis(4-chlorophenyl)-3-(isopropylimino)-3,5-dihydrophenazin-2-amine

Chemotherapy

Synthesis

2-Nitro chloro benzene + 4-Chloro aniline →(i) K₂CO₃/225°C (ii) HCl→ intermediate

$$\xrightarrow{\text{Reduction}}$$

2-(4-Chlorophenyllamine)chlorobenzene + FeCl₃ or benzoquinone

$$\xrightarrow{\text{Oxidation}}$$

$$\xrightarrow{NH_2CH(CH_3)_2}$$ **Clofazimine**

Metabolism: It is thought to undergo hydroxylic dehalogenation on the 4-chloroaniline, followed by sulphate conjugation. It also undergoes glucuronic acid conjugation.

Properties and uses: Clofazimine is a reddish-brown fine powder, practically insoluble in water, soluble in methylene chloride, and very slightly soluble in ethanol. It is used as antileprotic drug.

Assay: Dissolve the sample in methylene chloride, add acetone and anhydrous acetic acid and titrate with 0.1 M perchloric acid. Determine the end point potentiometrically.

Dose: The dose orally is 100 mg daily.

Dosage forms : Clofazimine capsules I.P., B.P.

iv Thalidomide (Thaloda, Thycad, Thalomid)

2-(2,6-Dioxopiperidin-3-yl)isoindoline-1,3-dione

Synthesis

Properties and uses: It is the drug of choice for *Erythema nodosum leprosum*. It must not be used in women during pregnancy because of its teratogenic activity.

Dose: Doses of 100–300 mg per day are effective.

PROBABLE QUESTIONS

1. Mention the different categories of leprosy, classify the drugs used, and outline the synthesis of any two of them.
2. Write a note on sulphones used in leprosy.
3. Outline the synthesis, metabolism, and uses of Clofazimine and Dapsone.

SUGGESTED READINGS

1. Abraham DJ (ed). *Burger's Medicinal Chemistry and Drug Discovery* (6th edn). New Jersey: Wiley, 2007.
2. Bruntan LL, Lazo JS, and Parker KL. *Goodman and Gilman's: The Pharmacological Basis of Therapeutics* (11th edn). New York: McGraw Hill, 2006.
3. Gennaro AR *Remington: The Science and practice of Pharmacy* (21st edn). New York: Lippincot Williams and Wilkins, 2006.
4. Lednicer D and Mitscher LA. *The Organic Chemistry of Drug Synthesis.* New York: Wiley, 1995.
5. Lemke TL and William DA. *Foye's Principle of Medicinal Chemistry* (6th edn). New York: Lippincott Williams and Wilkins, 2008.

Index

2. 19-Nor 2. Testosterone derivatives 200
3, 5-Pyrazolidinediones 67
4-Substituted quinolines 415
5-Fluorouracil 484
7-Chloro-4-amino quinolines 411
8-Amino quinolines 411
α-Anilinophenylacetamide 384
β-Lactam antibiotics 266

A

Acedapsone 516
Acetohexamide 166, 174
Acid degradation of erythromycin 324
Acridine derivatives 412, 424
Acrivastine 14
Acyclovir 372
Adamantane amines 368, 377
Albendazole 436, 441
Aldose reducatse inhibitors 169, 188
Alkylating agents 469
Alkyl sulphonate 457
Alkyl sulphones 477
Allopurinol 101
Altretamine 458, 480
Amantadine 368, 377
Amides 437, 449
Amidinopencillins 271
Amifloxacin 255
Amikacin 311, 341
Amino alkyl ether analogues 17
Aminocephalosporinic acid 292
Aminoglutethimide 468
Aminoglycoside antibiotics 308
Aminopenicillins 278
Amodiaquine 411
Amodiaquine HCl 418
Amopyroquine 411
Amoxicillin 269
Amphotericin B 346
Ampicillin 269, 278

Analgin 100
Androgens and anabolic agents 210
Aniline derivatives 216
Antazoline 37
Anthracyclines 460, 494
Anthranilic acid derivatives (Fenamates) 70
Antibiotics 346, 460, 494
Antifolates 412
Antimetabolites 459, 484
Antipseudomonal penicillins 270, 280
Antisecretory drugs 139
Apicycline 315
Artemether 431
Artesunate 415, 432
Arylalkanoic acids 72
Aryl and heteroaryl acetic/propionic acid derivatives 80
Asparaginase 501
Aspirin 59
Astemizole 13, 39
Atropine 140
Avermectins 450
Azatadine 35
Azathioprine 493
Azelastine 12, 40
Azidocillin 271
Aziocillin 270, 281
Aziridines 458, 479
Azithromycin 324
Azole antifungals 348

B

Bacampicillin 271
Bacitracin 322
Benzimidazoles 438
Benzonatate 111, 115
Benzotepa 480
Benzoxazinones 385
Benzpyrazine derivatives 517
Bifonazole 355

Biguanides 167, 179
Biosynthetic pathway of PGs 57
Bismuth subsalicylate 140
Bleomycin 462
Bleomycin sulphate 496
Both N-1 and N-4 substituted
    sulphonamides 234, 246
Bromopheniramine 10
Buclizine 10
Buformin 167
Busulfan 477
Butoconazole 354

C

Camptothecin 464
Camptothecin derivatives 463
Capecitabine 487
Caprofen 89
Caramiphen 111, 116
Carbenicillin 270, 280
Carbetapentane 111, 116
Carbimazole 218
Carbinoxamine 21
Carboplastin 468
Carbutamide 166
Carminomycin 461
Carmustine 477
Cefaclor 287
Cefadroxil 286, 294
Cefamandole 287, 301
Cefaparole 289, 307
Cefazolin 286
Cefepime 288
Cefmenoxime 288
Cefonicid 287, 302
Cefotaxime sodium 302
Cefotoxime 288
Cefoxitin 287, 300
Cefpirome 289, 305
Cefsulodin 295
Ceftazidime 288
Ceftizoxime 288
Ceftizoxime sodium 303
Ceftriaxone 288
Ceftriazone disodium 305
Cefuroxime 287, 298

Celecoxib 95
Centrally acting antitussive
    agents 112
Centrally active antitussive
    agents 110
Cephalexin 286, 293
Cephaloglycine 286
Cephaloridine 286
Cephalosporin C 284
Cephalosporin N 284
Cephalosporins 283
Cephalothin 286, 295
Cephapirin 286
Cephradine 286
Cetirizine 13, 40
Chaulmaogric acid 513
Chitin synthetase inhibitors 358
Chlophedianol hydrochloride 112
Chlorambucil 457, 470
Chloramphenicol or Chloromycetin 326
Chlorcyclizine 9, 25
Chloropropamide 166, 171
Chloroquine 416
Chlorpheniramine 10
Cholorquine 411
Ciclopirox 360
Ciglitazone 168, 185
Cimetidine 122, 125
Cinchona alkaloids 410
Ciprofloxacin 255, 258
Cis Pentacin 358
Cisplastin 468
Clemastine 9, 22
Clinafloxacin 256
Clomocycline 315
Clotrimazole 352
Cloxacillin 268
Codeine phosphate 111, 114
Cortisone 196
Cromolyn sodium 14, 43
Cyclic basic chain analogues orpiperazine
    derivatives 9
Cyclizine 9, 24
Cyclobendazole 436
Cyclophosphamide 472
Cyproheptadine 33
Cytarabine 486
Cytoprotective agents 468

Index

D

Dacarbazine 458
Dactinomycin C or Actinomycin D 462
Dactinomycin or Actinomycin D 497
Daunorubicin 460, 494
Decarbazine 483
Delavirdine 381
Dexamethazone 198
Dextromethorphan HBr 110, 112
Diamino pyrimidines 413, 426
Dibenzocycloheptenos 11
Dibenzocyclo heptene derivatives 33
Dibenzocyclo heptenes 11
Diclofenac 83
Dicloxacillin 268
Didanosine 386
Dienestrol 209
Diethyl cabamazine citrate 447
Diethyl carbmazine 437
Diethylstilbesterol 208, 502, 465
Diflunisal 62
Diloxanide furoate 402
Dimenhydrinate 18
Diphenhydramine 17
Diphenoxylate HCl 137
Diphenylpyraline 9, 22
Docetaxel 465, 501
Doxorubicin 460, 495
Doxycycline 315, 318
Doxylamine 20
Dribendazole 436
Dromostanolone 468
Drugs used in combination with sulphonamides 235, 250

E

Efavirenz 385
Emivirine 383
Enoxacin 255
Enzymes 465, 501
Epinastine 13, 43
Epipodophyllo toxins 464, 500
Epirubicin 461
Estorgenic derivatives 465
Estramustine 457, 475
Ethambutol HCl 335
Ethinyl oestradiol 206
Ethionamide 338
Ethylene diamine derivatives 7, 14
Etintidine 122, 128
Etodolac 91
Extra long-acting sulphonamides 234

F

Famotidine 122, 126
Fenbendazole 436
Fenoprofen 85
Fexofenadine 14
First-generation cephalosporins 293
Fleroxacin 256
Floxacillin 268
Flubendazole 436, 440
Fluconazole 353
Flucytosine 356
Fludarabine 490
Flufenamic acid 71
Fluorinated pyrimidines 356
Fluoroquinolones 257
Fluorouracil 484
Fluoxuridine 485
Fluoxymesterone 212
Flurbiprofen 87
Folic acid analogues 460, 491
Fourth-generation cephalosporin 305

G

Gallium nitrate 469
Ganciclovir 374
Gatifloxacin 256
Gentamycins 310
Glibenclamide 166, 174
Glibornuride 167
Gliclazide 167, 178
Glipizide 166, 177
Glucosidase inhibitors 169, 187
Griseofulvin 346
Guamecycline 315
Glucesufone sodium 512

H

H$_1$-antagonists with classical structure 14
H$_1$-antagonists with nonclassical structure 12, 39
Halofantrine 414, 429
Halofentamine 414
HIV protease inhibitors 370
Histamine induced gastric acid 5
Hormones 465, 501
Hydrocortisone 197
Hydroxychloroquine 411, 419
Hydroxyprogesterone caproate 203
Hydroxy urea 469, 506

I

Ibufenac 82
Ibuprofen 80
Idarubicin 461, 495
Idoxuridine 375
Ifosfamide 471
Imidazoles 215
Imidazothiazoles: Levamisole 437
Immunotherapy 468, 506
Indanyl carbenicillin 270
Indeneacetic acid derivatives 75
Indinavir 370, 394
Indole acetic acid derivatives 73
Indomethacin 73
Inhibition of histamine release (mast cells stabilizers) 14
Inhibition of histamine release 43
Interferons 506
Intermediate-acting sulphonamides 233
Intestinal antiseptics 139
Ionic inhibitors 216
Irinotecan 464
Isoaminile 112
Isoniazid 332
Isopentaquine 412

K

Kanamycin 311
Ketoconazole 350
Ketoprofen 86
Ketorolac 90
Ketotifen fumarate 37

L

Lamitidine 123
Lamitidine analogues 123
Lamivudine 390
Lansoprazole 124, 132
L-Asparaginase 501
Letrozole 468, 506
Levamisole 452
Levopropoxyphene napsylate 110, 113
Lincomycins 325
Linogliride 189
L Norvalyl—FMIP 358
Lomefloxacin 255
Lomustine and semustine 478
Long-acting sulphonamides 233
Loperamide 138
Loratadine 13, 42
Loviride 384
Loxtidine 123
Luminal amoebicides 402
Lupitidine 123
Lymecycline 315

M

Mafenide 235, 247
Mebendazole 436, 438
Mecillinam 283
Meclizine 10, 25
Meclocycline 315
Meclofenamate sodium 72
Medrylamine 9
Mefenamic acid 71
Mefloquine 414, 432
Meglitinide 167
Meglucycline 315

Meloxicam 94
Melphalan 474
Mestranol 206
Metabolism of salicylic acid derivatives 59
Metformin 167, 180
Methacycline 315, 317
Methapyrliene 8
Methdilazine 11, 32
Methicillin 268, 275
Methimazole 218
Methisazone 377
Methotrexate 491
Methylhydrazines 458, 487
Methyl testosterone 211
Metrifonate 451
Metronidazole 403
Miconazole 348
Midazothiazoles 452
Miglitol 188
Minocycline 315, 319
Miscellaneous 468
Mitomycin-C 462, 497
Mitomycins 462
Mitotane 501
Mitoxantrone 469
Mixed amoebicides 402, 403
Mode of action of antihistamines 6
Monoamino propylamine derivatives 26
Monoaminopropyl analogues 10, 29
Monoclonal antibodies 468
Moxalactam 287

N

N-1 Substituted sulphonamides 236
N-4 Substituted suphonamides 234
Nabumetone 98
Nafcillin 269
Naftifine 359
Nalidixic acid 255, 256
Naproxen 84
Nateglinide 168, 183
Natural products: Avermectins 437
Natural products 450
Natural tetracyclines 314
Nedocromil sodium 14, 44

Nelfinavir 370, 397
Neomycin 310
Netilmicin 312
Nevirapine 368
Niclosamide 437, 449
Nikomycin 358
Nimesulide 99
Nimorazole 406
Niridazole 437, 453
Nitazoxanide 406
Nitro derivatives 453
Nitrogen mustards 470
Nitrosourea 457, 477
Nizatidine 129
Non-nucleoside RT inhibitors 368, 380
Nonsedative H_1-antihistamines 13
Nonsedative H1-antihistamines
 (H1-antagonists) 40
Nonsteroidal anti-inflammatory drugs
 (NSAIDs) 56
Norethindrone 204
Norfloxacin 255
Norgestrel 205
Noscapine 111
NSAIDs 57
Nucleoside RT inhibitors 366
Nucleotide analogues 372
Nystatin 348

O

Octreotide 140
Oestradiol 206
Oestradiol benzoate 206
Oestradiol cypionate 206
Oestradiol derivatives 206, 207
Oestradiol dipropionate 206
Oestradiol valerate 206
Oestrogens 206
Ofloxacin 260
Omeprazole 124
Organo phosphorus: Metrifonate 437
Organophosphorus compounds 451
Ornidazole 405
Oxacillin 268, 275
Oxamniquine 436, 445

Oxantel 437
Oxibendazole 436
Oxicams 92
Oxmetidine 122, 129
Oxyphenbutazone 69

P

p-Amino phenol derivatives 63
Paclitaxel 465, 501
Pamaquine 412, 423
Pantoprazole 124, 133
Para-amino-salicylic acid 340
Paracetamol 66
Parbendazole 436
Pefloxacin 255, 261
Penam 266
Pencillanic acid derivatives 267
Penicillin-V 276
Penicillinase-resistant penicillins 269, 275
Penicillinase-susceptible penicillins 268, 276
Penicillin G 267
Penicillins 266
Penicillin V 267
Pentaquine phosphate 412
Peptides\proteins 358
Peripherally acting antitussives 111, 115
Phenacetin 65
Phenanthrine methanol 414
Phenethicillin 267
Phenformin 167, 179
Pheniramine 10
Pheniramine maleate 27
Phenylbutazone 68
Pholcodine 111, 114
Phthalylsulphathiazole 234, 246
Pifatidine 123
Pioglitazone 168, 184
Pipacycline 315
Pipemidic acid 255
Piperacillin 270, 282
Piperazine citrate 437, 446
Piperazine derivatives 24, 437, 446
Pipobroman 468
Piroxicam 92
Pivampicillin 279

Plant products 463, 498
Plant drug 513
Plicamycin 498
Plicamycin or Mithramycin 462
Polyhydric phenols 216
Polymyxin 323
Polypeptide antibiotics 322
Praziquantel 436, 443
Prednisolone 198
Prednisone 467, 504
Primaquine 412, 421
Pro-tetracyclines 315
Probenecid 102
Procarbazine 458, 481
Progesterone 201, 466, 503
Progesterone derivatives 200
Progestine derivatives 465
Progestogens 200
Proguanil HCl 425
Promethazine HCl 31
Promethazine hydrochloride 11
Prontosil 234
Propylthiouracil 217
Proton pump inhibitors 124
Purine analogues 488
Purine nucleosides and nucleotides 366, 372
Pyrantel 449
Pyrantel pamoate 437
Pyrazinamide 333
Pyridyl ethyl thiourea 384
Pyrilamine 8, 16
Pyrimdine analogues 459
Pyrimethamine 235, 251, 413, 426
Pyrimidine nucleoside and nucleotide inhibitors 375
Pyrimidine nucleosides and nucleotides 367
Pyrrobutamine 10
Pyrrole acetic acid derivative 78

Q

Quinacrine 424
Quinestrol 206
Quinicillin 271
Quinolide HCl 412
Quinoline and isoquinolines 436, 443

R

Rabeprazole 124, 134
Racecadotril 140
Radio-therapeutic agents 468
Ranitidine 122, 127
Release of histamine 4
Repaglinide 168, 182
Reserve drugs 338
Resorcinol 216
Ribavirin 379
Rifabutin 337
Rifampicin 328, 336
Rimantadine 368, 378
Ritonavir 370, 396
Rocastine 13, 43
Rofecoxib 96
Rolitetracycline 315, 320
Rosiglitazone 168, 185
Roxatidine 122, 130

S

Salicylates 58
Salsalate 60
Sancycline 315
Saquinavir 370, 392
SAR of *p*-amino phenol derivatives 65
Saturated analogues 10, 26
Semisynthetic tetracyclines 314, 317
Short-acting sulpha drugs 233, 248
Silver sulphadiazine 235, 248
Sitafloxacin 256
Sodium salicylate 60
Solapsone 235, 249
Somantadine 368
Sontoquine 411
Sorbinil 189
Sparfloxacin 255
Steroidal anti-inflammatory agents 467
Streptomycin and dihydrostreptomycin 309
Streptomycin sulphate 338
Structure activity relationship—H1 receptor antagonists 6
Succinyl sulphathiazole 234, 246
Sulindac 75

Sulphacetamide 232, 237
Sulphadiazine 232, 239
Sulpha dimethoxine 234, 242
Sulphadimidine 232, 240
Sulphadoxine 413
Sulphaisoxazole 233, 244
Sulphalene 234, 416
Sulphamerazine 241
Sulphamethizole 233
Sulphamethoxazole 233, 244, 414
Sulphamethoxy diazine 233
Sulpha methoxy pyridazine 243
Sulphanilamide 232, 236
Sulphaphenazole 234, 243
Sulphapyridine 232
Sulphasalazine 139, 237, 61
Sulphasomidine 233
Sulphasomizole 233
Sulphathiazole 232
Sulphinpyrazone 103
Sulphonamides and sulphones 413
Sulphones and sulphonamides 429
Sulphonylurea derivatives 170
Sulphonylureas 166
Sulphormethoxine 234
Systemic amoebicides 402

T

Talampicilin 269
Tamoxifen 505
Taxol derivatives 464, 500
Tazifylline 13, 40
Tefloxacin 256
Tenoxicam 93
Terbinafine 361
Terconazole 350
Testosterone 210, 466
Testosterone derivatives 466
Tetracycline antibiotics 313
Thalidomide 520
Thiabendazole 442
Thiacetazone 342
Thiazolidinediones 168, 184
Thioguanine 489

Thiosemicarbazones 367, 377
Thiotepa 458, 479
Thiouracil derivatives 215
Thioureylenes 215, 216
Third-generation cephalosporins 302
Thonzylamine 8, 17
Ticarcillin 270
Tinidazole 404
Tiotidine 123, 3
Tobramycin 312
Tolazamide 166, 172
Tolbutamide 166, 170
Tolmetin sodium 78
Tolnaftate 360
Tolrestat 189
Topically used sulphonamides 235, 247
Topotecan 464
Tricyclic ring system or phenothiazines 31
Tricyclic ring systems or phenothiazine derivatives 11
Triethylene melamine 458
Trimeprazine 11, 32
Trimethoprim 235, 250, 413, 428
Trimetrexate 493
Tripelennamine 8, 15
Triprolidine (Actidil) 29
Triprolidine 10
Tromantadine 368
Trovirdine 384

U

Unsaturated analogues 10, 29
Uracil Mustard 476
Ureido penicillins 270, 281

V

Valdeocoxib 97
Valrubicin 461, 496
Vinca alkaloids 463, 498
Vinorelbine 463
Vinyl pyrimidines 437, 449

Z

Zalcitabine 388
Zidovudine 389
Zinoconazole 355
Zomepirac 79